GW01424292

CASE RE

Gastrointestinal
Imaging

Series Editor

David M. Yousem, MD
Professor, Department of Radiology
Director of Neuroradiology
Johns Hopkins Hospital
Baltimore, Maryland

Other Volumes in the CASE REVIEW Series

Brain Imaging
Cardiac Imaging
General and Vascular Ultrasound
Genitourinary Imaging
Head and Neck Imaging
Breast Imaging
Musculoskeletal Imaging
Nuclear Medicine
OB/GYN Ultrasound
Pediatric Imaging
Spine Imaging
Thoracic Imaging
Vascular Interventional Imaging

Mosby

An Affiliate of Elsevier Science

St. Louis London Philadelphia Sydney Toronto

Peter J. Feczko, MD
Department of Diagnostic Radiology
Henry Ford Hospital and Medical Centers
Detroit, Michigan

Robert D. Halpert, MD
Professor of Radiology
Michigan State University
East Lansing, Michigan

WITH 275 ILLUSTRATIONS

CASE REVIEW

Gastrointestinal Imaging

CASE REVIEW SERIES

M Mosby

An Affiliate of Elsevier Science

Acquisitions Editor: Stephanie Smith Donley
Project Manager: Carol Sullivan Weis
Project Specialist: Christine Carroll Schwepker
Designer: Mark Oberkrom

Copyright © 2000 by Mosby, Inc.

All rights reserved. No part of this publication may be reproduced or transmitted in any form or by any means, electronic or mechanical, including photocopy, recording, or any information storage and retrieval system, without permission in writing from the publisher.

Permission to photocopy or reproduce solely for internal or personal use is permitted for libraries or other users registered with the Copyright Clearance Center, provided that the base fee of $4.00 per chapter plus $.10 per page is paid directly to the Copyright Clearance Center, 222 Rosewood Drive, Danvers, Massachusetts 01923. This consent does not extend to other kinds of copying, such as copying for general distribution, for advertising or promotional purposes, for creating new collected works, or for resale.

Mosby, Inc.
An Affiliate of Elsevier Science
11830 Westline Industrial Drive
St. Louis, Missouri 63146

Printed in the United States of America

Library of Congress Cataloging in Publication Data

Feczko, Peter J.
  Gastrointestinal imaging: case review / Peter J. Feczko, Robert D. Halpert.
     p. ; cm. — (Case review series)
  Includes bibliographical references and index.
  ISBN 0-323-00891-7
  1. Gastrointestinal system—Imaging—Case studies. I. Halpert, Robert D., M.D. II. Title. III. Series.
  [DNLM: 1. Gastrointestinal Diseases—diagnosis—Examination Questions. 2. Diagnostic Imaging—methods—Examination Questions. WI 18.2 F291g 2000]
  RC804.D52 F43 2000
  616.3'30754—dc21
                                                      00-028386

02 03 04 TG/MVY 9 8 7 6 5 4 3 2

To my wife, Claire, and Matthew, Julia,
and Andrea
PJF

To my mother,
with thanks
RDH

My experience in teaching medical students, residents, fellows, practicing radiologists, and clinicians has been that they love the case conference format more than any other approach. I hope that the reason for this is not a reflection on my lecturing ability, but rather that people stay awake, alert, and on their toes more when they are in the hot seat (or may be the next person to assume the hot seat). In the dozens of continuing medical education courses I have directed, the case review sessions are almost always the most popular parts of the courses.

The idea of this Case Review series grew out of a need for books designed as exam preparation tools for the resident, fellow, or practicing radiologist about to take the boards or the certificate of additional qualification (CAQ) exams. Anxiety runs extremely high concerning the content of these exams, administered as unknown cases. Residents, fellows, and practicing radiologists are very hungry for formats that mimic this exam setting and that cover the types of cases they will encounter and have to accurately describe. In addition, books of this ilk serve as excellent practical reviews of a field and can help a practicing board-certified radiologist keep his or her skills sharpened. Thus heads banged together, and Mosby and I arrived at the format of the volume herein, which is applied consistently to each volume in the series. We believe that these volumes will strengthen the ability of the reader to interpret studies. By formatting the individual cases so that they can "stand alone," these case review books can be read in a leisurely fashion, a case at a time, on the whim of the reader.

The content of each volume is organized into three sections based on difficulty of interpretation and/or the rarity of the lesion presented. There are the Opening Round cases, which graduating radiology residents should have relatively little difficulty mastering. The Fair Game section consists of cases that require more study, but most people should get into the ballpark with their differential diagnoses. Finally, there is the Challenge section. Most fellows or fellowship-trained practicing radiologists will be able to mention entities in the differential diagnoses of these challenging cases, but one shouldn't expect to consistently "hit home runs" a la Mark McGwire. The Challenge cases are really designed to whet one's appetite for further reading on these entities and to test one's wits. Within each of these sections, the selection of cases is entirely random, as one would expect at the boards (in your office or in Louisville).

For many cases in this series, a specific diagnosis may not be what is expected—the quality of the differential diagnosis and the inclusion of appropriate options are most important. Teaching how to distinguish between the diagnostic options (taught in the question and answer and comment sections) will be the goal of the authors of each Case Review volume.

The best way to go through these books is to look at the images, guess the diagnosis, answer the questions, and then turn the page for the answers. If there are two cases on a page, do them two at a time. No peeking!

Mosby (through the strong work of Liz Corra) and I have recruited most of the authors of THE REQUISITES series (editor, James Thrall, MD) to create Case Review books for their subspecialties. To meet the needs of certain subspecialties and to keep each of the volumes to a consistent, practical size, some specialties will have more than one volume (e.g., ultrasound, interventional and vascular radiology, and neuroradiology). Nonetheless, the pleasing tone of THE REQUISITES series and its emphasis on condensing the fields of radiology into its foundations will be inculcated into the Case Review volumes. In many situations, THE REQUISITES authors have enlisted new coauthors to breathe a novel approach and excitement into the cases submitted. I think the fact that so many of THE REQUISITES authors are "on board" for this new series is a testament to their dedication to teaching. I hope that the success of THE REQUISITES is duplicated with the new Case Review series. Just as THE REQUISITES series provides coverage of the essentials in each subspecialty and successfully meets that overwhelming need in the market, I hope that the Case Review series successfully meets the overwhelming need in the market for practical, focused case reviews.

David M. Yousem, MD

The goal of the Case Review series is to supplement and reinforce the concepts and teachings that are put in a more didactic form in THE REQUISITES series. It was recognized that whereas some students learn best in a noninteractive "study-book" mode, others need the anxiety or excitement of being quizzed, being put on the hot seat. The format that was selected for the Case Review series (i.e., showing a limited number of images needed to construct a differential diagnosis and asking a few clinical and imaging questions) was designed to simulate the boards experience. The only difference is that the Case Review books provide the correct answer and immediate feedback. Cases are scaled from relatively easy to very hard to test the limit of the reader's knowledge. In addition, a brief authors' commentary, a link back to THE REQUISITES volume, and an up-to-date reference to the literature are provided. Most importantly the images in the cases are of the highest pictorial quality and relevance.

Peter Feczko and Robert Halpert are well recognized as outstanding teachers of gastrointestinal radiology and have done an outstanding job of fulfilling the goals of the Case Review series. By integrating all modalities into this review, they cross the traditional boundaries of the barium slingers versus the sonar pingers versus the CT slip-ringers versus the MR gad flingers. Having recently published the second edition of *Gastrointestinal Radiology: THE REQUISITES*, they have produced timely, top-notch contributions to the imaging community. Trainees and practicing radiologists should certainly benefit from these recent works.

I am pleased to have the Gastrointestinal Imaging volume join the previously published Brain Imaging (by Laurie Loevner) and Head and Neck Imaging (by David Yousem) contributions to the Case Review series.

David M. Yousem, MD

I almost decided not to write this book. At the same time that Liz Corra from Mosby was asking me to write *Gastrointestinal Imaging: Case Review,* I was also involved in the American College of Radiology Continuing Physician Improvement program (ACR PCI). The ACR PCI enlists specialists to compile a series of questions for radiologists, who then take the examination and receive continuing medical education credit when they return the test. I delayed making my decision until I had completed my questions for the ACR PCI and had taken the ACR course on test making.

The ACR took the "test makers" to a hotel in Reston, Virginia, where we received instruction regarding question writing. We then broke into groups, and the experts attempted to compile the tests. Needless to say, it was a humbling experience. Our group was dominated by big-name East Coast radiologists who constantly berated the questions developed by radiologists from lesser-known institutions. I left the weekend feeling that this project was over my head, and I probably shouldn't write this book. However, the ACR submitted all the questions developed by the experts to other radiologists and to their own panel to determine which were "test worthy." Well, when the test was finally compiled, the majority of the questions included were those submitted by radiologists from nonuniversity institutions. Virtually all of my questions were included in the test, whereas the questions written by the "world-renowned" East Coast radiologists had been rejected. (Yes, there is a radiology God.) This experience renewed my interest in compiling this Case Review book and helped me see it as a task that would be fun and challenging.

Unlike other fields, gastrointestinal radiology has no certificate of additional qualification yet, and I hope never will. The field is too broad and general, and it encompasses almost all imaging modalities. This book was designed as a companion to THE REQUISITES series, which is published by Mosby. The Case Review series is developed so that residents, fellows, and practicing general radiologists can use the cases to review the material and sharpen their skills. I hope it will serve as a tool for board review as well.

The format I used dates back to my days as a resident at the University of Chicago. Our conferences were developed around viewing interesting cases, discussing the imaging findings, providing a working differential diagnosis for the findings, and then narrowing the diagnostic possibilities. In a sense, all radiologists follow these steps on a daily basis when confronted with an abnormality. Thus the format can be appropriate for the radiologist in training or the practicing radiologist.

The Case Review material is often presented so that the same findings are depicted on a conventional radiologic image and a cross-sectional image. The area of gastrointestinal radiology is increasingly dominated by CT, particularly since the proliferation of rapid helical scanning techniques. CT has become the primary imaging modality for most abdominal complaints, even in the emergency room setting. However, the role of ultrasound has diminished somewhat, and the future role of MRI in gastrointestinal imaging is yet to be determined. Because of these changes in the imaging approach to the abdomen, I attempted to include as much cross-sectional imaging as was warranted by the particular disease. A substantial number of barium studies are included. However, it was my intention to depict diseases using multiple modalities, reflecting current gastrointestinal imaging practice.

I would like to thank Liz Corra of Mosby and Stephanie Smith Donley of W.B. Saunders for their support in developing this book. The project initially was developed by Mosby, but Mosby was merged with W.B. Saunders during the writing of this book, and Stephanie completed the project without missing a beat. I would also like to thank Linda Galante of Henry Ford Hospital for her assistance in communicating information between myself and the publishers. Although many of the cases depicted came from my own teaching files, several other radiologists also made contributions. Dr. Ghiyath Habra from Henry Ford Hospital was a significant contributor to the book. Also, several studies were given to me by my former colleagues, Drs. Duane Mezwa and Michael Farah at William Beaumont Hospital in Royal Oak, Michigan.

Even though the book was written over a short period of time, it was during a major change in my life. During this time, two of my children started college. My son, Matthew, is a business major at Indiana University, and my daughter, Julia, who has just begun her studies at the University of Michigan, is going into the health profession. My youngest daughter, Andrea, still has a few more years before she begins college, but it is amazing how fast the time goes by. Even though I have written other books and chapters, this is the first time my children took notice of what I was doing (probably because I was using their computer so often). I hope it encourages them and provides an example. I also would like to thank my wife, Claire, who had to deal with having her dining room table covered with paper and images for almost a year. I keep telling her that the royalties from the book will help cover the cost of our ballroom dancing lessons.

Finally, I would like to thank all my former and future residents.

Peter J. Feczko, MD

CONTENTS

Opening Round Cases

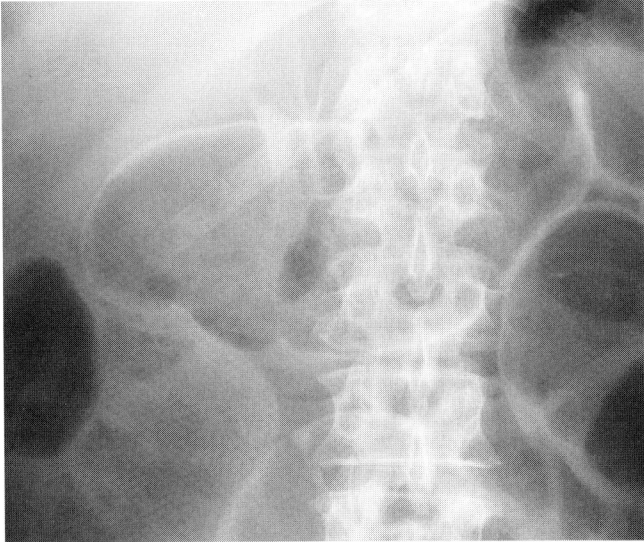

1. How much free intraperitoneal air is visible on an upright chest film?
2. What is meant by Rigler's sign?
3. What view or modality is best for demonstrating free intraperitoneal air?
4. What factors affect the absorption of air in the abdomen after surgery?

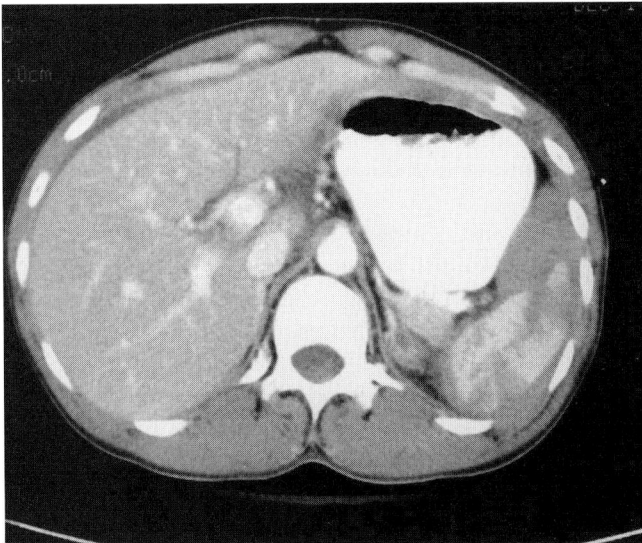

1. What is the most likely diagnosis?
2. What is the most important finding to identify on CT?
3. What is the diagnostic procedure of choice for patients who have suffered trauma but are stable?
4. What is the diagnostic procedure of choice for patients who have suffered trauma and are hemodynamically unstable?

Pneumoperitoneum

1. 1 to 2 ml of air.

2. Air is present on both sides of the bowel wall, creating a linear stripe.

3. CT.

4. Amount of air introduced, body fat, inflammation, and ileus.

Reference

Levine MS, Scheiner JC, Rubesin SE, et al: Diagnosis of pneumoperitoneum on supine abdominal radiographs, *Am J Roentgenol* 156:731-735, 1991.

Cross-Reference

Gastrointestinal Radiology: THE REQUISITES, ed 2, p 299.

Comment

Free intraperitoneal air is frequently encountered in the abdominal cavity. The most common cause of the free air is surgery. Air that is introduced into the abdomen during surgery usually takes 3 to 7 days to reabsorb and become inapparent. Under certain circumstances, this process may take several weeks. The more air that is introduced, the longer it takes to reabsorb. Thin patients take longer to reabsorb air, perhaps because overweight patients have a fatty omentum, which decreases the amount of air that can be introduced. If the patient has postoperative ileus or peritonitis, the ability of the peritoneum to absorb the air is reduced.

For many years, the upright chest film and the left lateral decubitus view of the abdomen were considered the best for demonstrating even minute amounts (1 to 2 ml) of air. However, CT has been shown to demonstrate free air even when these views cannot. CT is now considered the best modality for demonstrating even the tiniest amounts of free air.

Several signs have been described regarding the appearance of free intraperitoneal air on a supine abdominal radiograph. (Often the patient is too sick for horizontal views to be obtained, and the only view that can be obtained is a supine film.) The patient in this case shows several of these signs. Rigler's sign refers to the ability to see both sides of the bowel wall because there is gas on both sides. This sign is difficult to see unless there are large amounts of air and is often misinterpreted. Ability to see the patient's falciform ligament is another sign indicating free air, as in this case. Free air trapped between loops of bowel is often triangular or rhomboidal in configuration. This configuration does not occur with air within the bowel lumen, and it is another fairly reliable sign of free air. Also, free air over the liver produces a lucency that typically is not present on a supine film.

Notes

Splenic Laceration

1. Splenic laceration.

2. Evidence of active arterial extravasation.

3. CT.

4. Diagnostic peritoneal lavage.

Reference

Federle MP, Griffiths B, Miragi H, et al: Splenic trauma: evaluation with CT, *Radiology* 162:69-71, 1987.

Cross-Reference

Gastrointestinal Radiology: THE REQUISITES, ed 2, p 188.

Comment

The spleen is the organ most commonly injured after blunt abdominal trauma. It also can be injured during diagnostic procedures or surgery. Inadvertent surgical injury of the spleen is the second most common cause for splenectomy. The spleen can be injured directly by penetrating or blunt trauma or indirectly through stretching or a contrecoup mechanism. A scale has been developed to stage the extent of splenic injury and determine which patients require operative management and which may be followed conservatively. This scale is based on characteristics such as the depth of the capsular tear, the size of the hematoma, the number of tears, the presence of intraperitoneal hemorrhage, and any evidence of active bleeding. Some authorities suggest that the most serious finding is that of active arterial extravasation evident on CT, and immediate therapy, either surgical or embolic, must be considered to control it.

Diagnostic management of the patient who has sustained blunt abdominal trauma depends on his or her hemodynamic stability. Diagnostic peritoneal lavage (DPL) was once the mainstay for the diagnosis of serious abdominal injury. Its accuracy is said to be as high as 95%, although many feel that it is much lower than this, and a false positive is also possible. CT is considered to be much more accurate in determining the severity and site of bleeding and directing management. However, DPL is quicker and remains the primary diagnostic test for patients who are hemodynamically unstable and do not have time for CT. CT is the best modality when the patient is stable. Whenever possible, both oral and intravenous contrast should be used during CT. CT should also be considered if the DPL is equivocal.

Notes

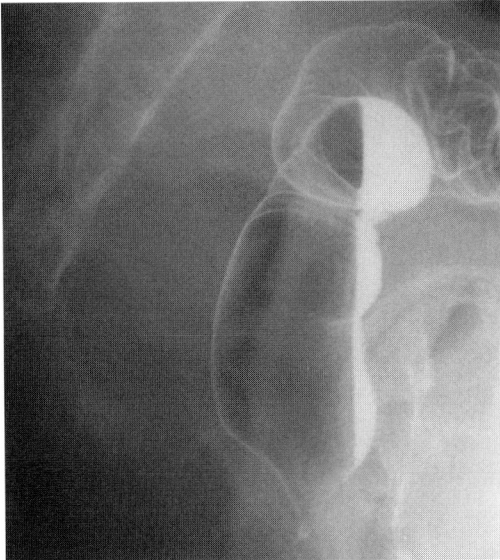

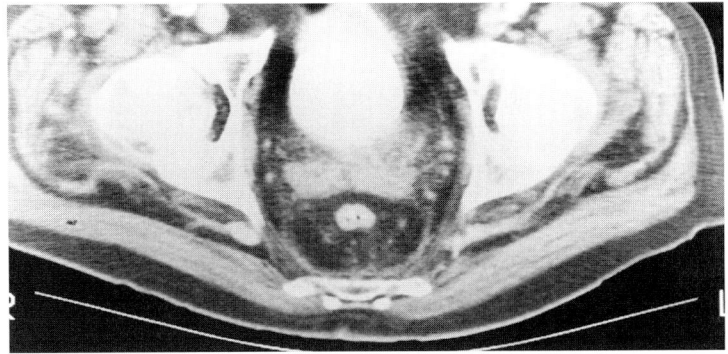

1. What measurement constitutes an enlarged retrorectal (presacral) space?
2. At what level is this measurement taken?
3. What occupies this space in patients with chronic ulcerative colitis?
4. What are common iatrogenic causes of this appearance?

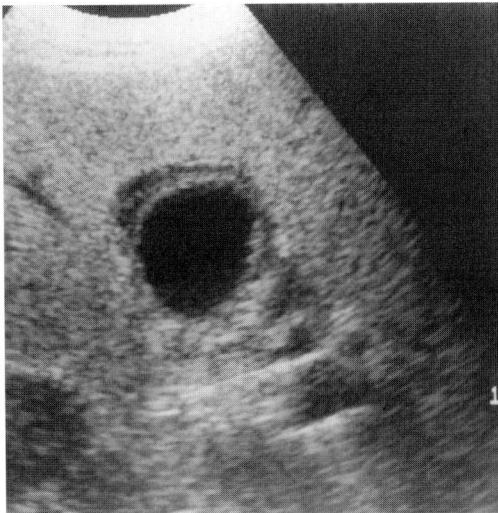

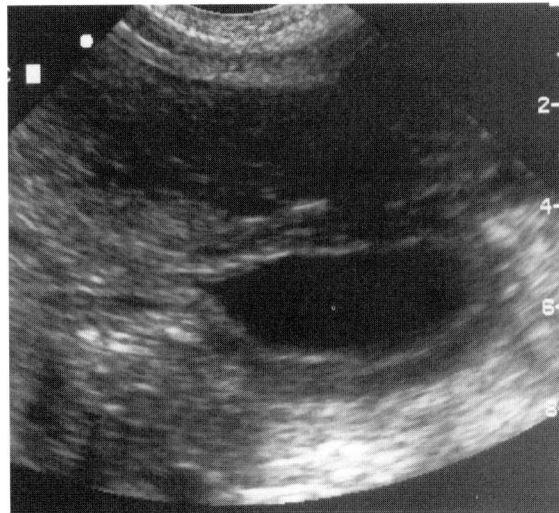

1. What condition may cause this appearance in a severely ill patient?
2. In the patient who has cirrhosis, what associated problems may produce this appearance?
3. What systemic conditions can produce this appearance?
4. What test may help improve the specificity of this finding?

CASE 3

Increased Presacral Space in Pelvic Lipomatosis

1. 1.5 or 2 cm.

2. Lower sacrum, preferably S4 or S5.

3. Normal connective tissue.

4. Radiation or pelvic surgery.

Reference

Kattan KR, King AY: Presacral space revisited, *Am J Roentgenol* 132:437-439, 1979.

Cross-Reference

Gastrointestinal Radiology: THE REQUISITES, ed 2, p 126.

Comment

The area between the rectum and the sacrum is one of the easiest areas to examine radiologically, but it still presents diagnostic dilemmas. The space behind the rectum is a potential space, with layers of fascia covering the anterior surface of the sacrum and the posterior wall of the rectum. The rectum becomes more mobile (in many patients it becomes much more mobile) as it approaches the peritoneal reflection, around the S2 level. Therefore the only correct measurement of the space is obtained along the lower sacrum, at either S4 or S5. Authors disagree on whether the space should be 1.5 or 2 cm wide at its maximum. The space can be measured only when the rectum is fully distended because a collapsed rectum does not fill this potential space.

Probably the best known causes of an increased presacral space are inflammatory processes of the rectum. Usually the increase is the result of a lack of distensibility of the rectum and not actual inflammation of the retrorectal soft tissues. The tissues may have some edema or may just be replaced by fatty or fibrous tissue. Once this space widens as a result of colitis or radiation, the space never fully returns to normal. However, if the patient develops an abscess or fistula in the region, the widening is due to this space-occupying process. Tumors can also cause widening of this region. They can be primary colonic tumors, which is quite obvious, or they can be tumors arising from the sacrum or the sacral neurogenic tissue.

Another large category that must be considered includes processes that produce infiltration of the retroperitoneum. The retroperitoneum can be infiltrated by fatty tissue (pelvic lipomatosis or Cushing's syndrome), edema (liver or renal failure), or hemorrhage. Infiltration by fatty tissue is probably one of the most common causes and is the cause for idiopathic presacral widening. Both CT and MRI can be helpful in distinguishing the various etiologies that produce this radiologic abnormality.

Notes

CASE 4

Gallbladder Wall Thickening

1. Acute cholecystitis.

2. Edema, gallbladder varices, and ascites.

3. Hypoproteinemia and anasarca.

4. Doppler imaging.

Reference

Weltman DI, Zeman RK: Acute diseases of the gallbladder and biliary ducts, *Radiol Clin North Am* 32:933-950, 1994.

Cross-Reference

Gastrointestinal Radiology: THE REQUISITES, ed 2, p 224.

Comment

The major finding in this patient is thickening of the wall of the gallbladder, as demonstrated by ultrasound. A similar finding also can be detected with CT. Either way the finding is somewhat nonspecific and can be caused by a variety of entities.

The most likely cause for this finding in a severely ill patient is acute cholecystitis. However, many physicians feel that other signs must be present before this diagnosis can be made. These signs include pain and rebound when the gallbladder is compressed and then released, the so-called sonographic Murphy's sign. The presence of gallstones is another indicator of possible cholecystitis. The gallbladder wall may appear thickened if it is contracted at the time of the examination. It also appears thickened in patients with chronic cholecystitis or hyperplastic cholecystosis. In patients with chronic cirrhosis, which is fairly common, the thickening may be the result of edema, gallbladder varices or collateral channels, or ascites, which is often present. Patients with ascites of any etiology have gallbladder wall thickening. Problems that affect areas other than the abdomen, such as hypoproteinemia, renal or heart failure, and other conditions producing fluid retention, also can result in thickening of the gallbladder wall.

Because of the variety of conditions causing this appearance, many authors are hesitant to place too much significance on the finding. Many do advocate the use of Doppler sonography during the examination. Increased arterial flow is believed to be present during inflammation, and it may help distinguish cholecystitis from other conditions.

Notes

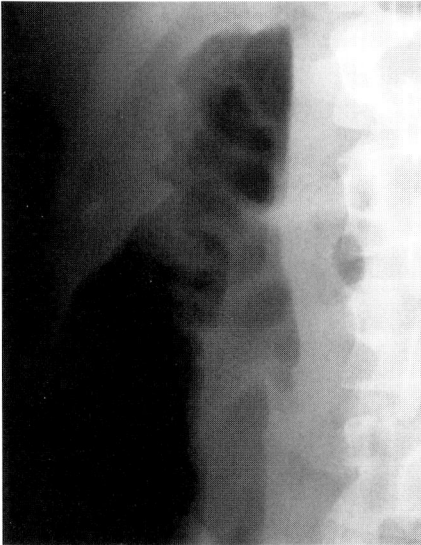

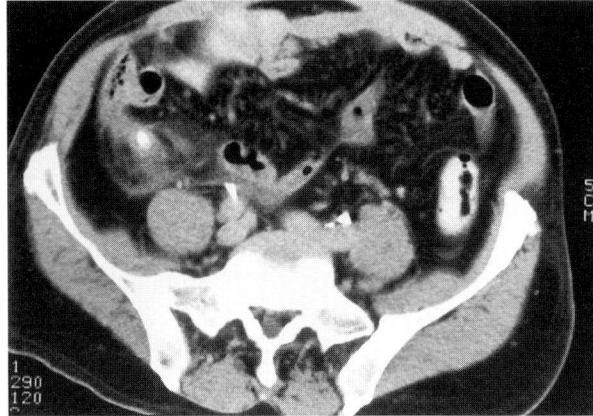

1. What is the most likely diagnosis?
2. What structures can develop laminated calcifications?
3. How often are appendicoliths identified in patients with appendicitis?
4. What is the significance of air in the appendix on abdominal radiographs or CT scans?

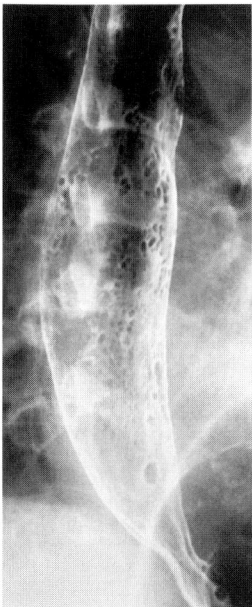

1. What is the most common cause of small nodules in the esophagus?
2. What condition produces plaquelike lesions in scleroderma?
3. What condition affecting the elderly may produce this appearance?
4. What skin condition may be associated with multiple tiny esophageal lesions?

Appendicitis with Appendicoliths

1. Appendicitis.

2. Gallbladder, appendix and bowel lumen in general, and urinary tract.

3. Less than 10% of the time.

4. It means nothing. It can be seen in healthy patients.

Reference

Brown SJ: Acute appendicitis: the radiologist's role, *Radiology* 180:13-14, 1991.

Cross-Reference

Gastrointestinal Radiology: THE REQUISITES, ed 2, p 285.

Comment

Appendicitis is one of the most common abdominal inflammatory processes encountered and is the cause of most surgical emergencies involving the abdomen, particularly in the younger population. CT has been advocated as the primary diagnostic tool in the evaluation of this process, and it probably will supplant all other diagnostic modalities for this purpose. However, conventional radiography remains the predominant method of evaluating the abdomen, and certain clues that may be visible on these studies indicate that the patient has appendicitis.

Possible diagnostic clues that are visible on plain abdominal radiographs include right lower quadrant fluid levels, either in the cecum and bowel loops or within a periappendiceal abscess. Mass effect with displacement of bowel loops also can be apparent. Loss of normal lines, such as the flank stripe or psoas margin, also may indicate an inflammatory process. Other possible abnormalities include small bowel obstruction, mottled air collections in an abscess, and scoliosis.

All of the aforementioned abnormalities are nonspecific. The one abnormality that is indicative of appendicitis is the appendicolith. These growths are small calcifications, which are often laminated, that develop in the lumen of the appendix. Not only are they strongly indicative of appendicitis, but appendicoliths are also associated with appendiceal perforation in up to 50% of patients who have appendicitis with appendicoliths. If the appendix is ectopically located, either in the middle or the right upper quadrant (as in this patient) of the abdomen, the presence of appendicoliths may be confusing. Perforation of the gallbladder with gallstone and abscess also is a consideration in this patient because of the position of the abnormality.

Notes

Candida Esophagitis in Scleroderma of the Esophagus

1. Artifact caused by the effervescent agent used in double-contrast esophagography.

2. Candida esophagitis.

3. Glycogen acanthosis.

4. Acanthosis nigricans with esophageal papillomatosis.

Reference

Levine MS, Macones AJ, Laufer I: Candida esophagitis: accuracy of radiographic diagnosis, *Radiology* 154:581-587, 1985.

Cross-Reference

Gastrointestinal Radiology: THE REQUISITES, ed 2, p 4.

Comment

Numerous small plaques or nodules of the esophageal mucosa are not an uncommon finding. A variety of conditions may produce these abnormalities. Often the correct diagnosis can be made based on the clinical information provided by the patient. These nodules are either diffuse or focal, and this determination has some bearing on the diagnostic possibilities.

Several infectious and inflammatory conditions may produce this abnormality. The most important is candidal infection. These small plaques, which are identified by the radiologist, correspond to the whitish plaques that are noted by the endoscopist. They are heaped-up areas of cellular debris that sometimes contain *Candida* organisms. They can be diffuse or quite focal. Typically the plaques are only a few millimeters in diameter, but they may be as large as 1 cm or more in diameter. In addition to immune-compromised patients, patients with scleroderma, achalasia, and other conditions associated with stasis of the esophageal contents may have *Candida* organisms visible on radiologic studies. Reflux esophagitis may produce plaquelike elevations in the distal esophagus, and these growths correspond to areas of edema and inflammation without ulceration. Rarely, herpetic esophagitis also may produce multiple small nodular lesions.

A common benign condition of the esophagus is glycogen acanthosis. This condition, which consists of swelling of the epithelium caused by increased cytoplasmic glycogen, predominantly affects the elderly. It is believed to be a degenerative phenomenon and of little or no clinical significance. Some malignant and premalignant conditions also may produce multiple plaques. Rarely, early esophageal cancer can present as a focal area of raised plaques, without a discrete mass. Superficial spreading carcinoma of the esophagus may have more diffuse nodules. Leukoplakia is a premalignant condition of the mouth that sometimes is found in the esophagus. Esophageal papillomatosis is a complication of acanthosis nigricans of the skin.

Notes

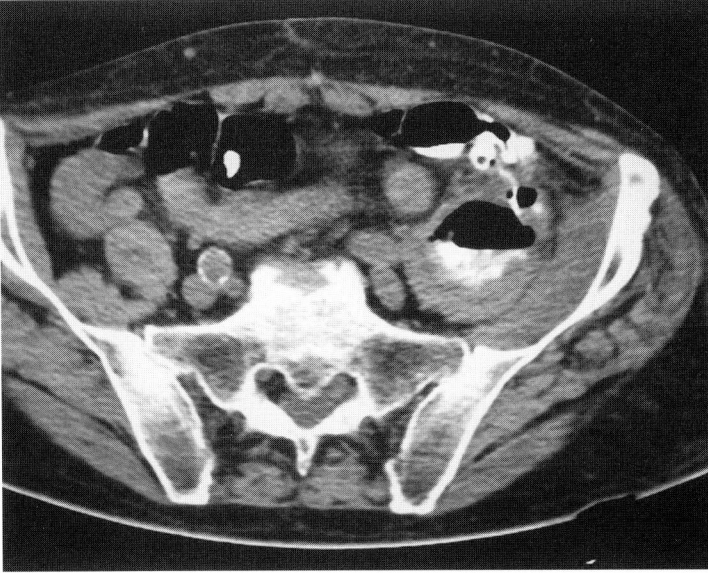

1. What modality is the most sensitive for evaluation of this condition?
2. What is the most common finding on CT?
3. What is the treatment of choice for this abnormality?
4. Is the performance of a barium enema contraindicated for patients with this condition?

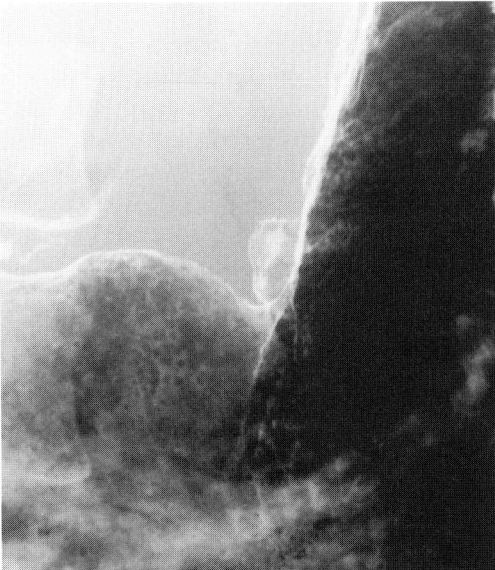

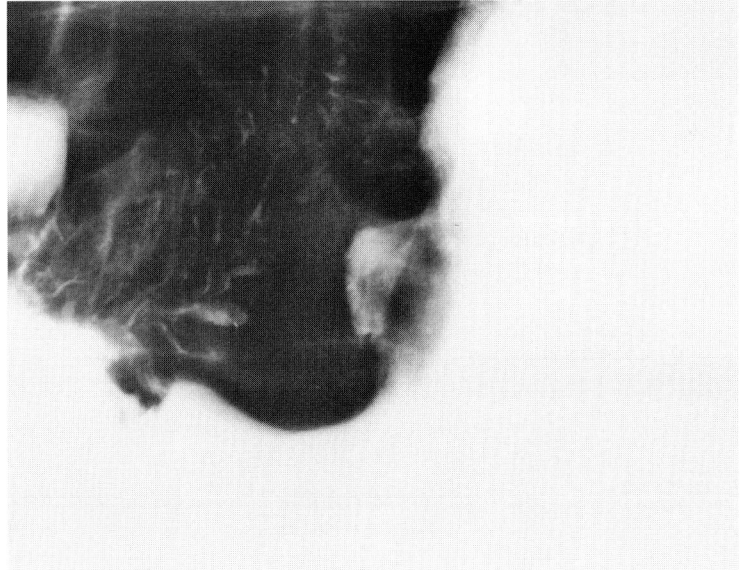

1. What is the most common location for a benign gastric ulcer?
2. What produces a so-called Hampton's line? What does it mean?
3. What do radiating folds that stop before the ulcer crater indicate?
4. Do all benign ulcers extend beyond the expected lumen of the stomach?

CASE 7

Pericolic Abscess Caused by Diverticulitis

1. CT.

2. Pericolic inflammatory changes.

3. Percutaneous abscess drainage and antibiotic therapy, followed by surgery.

4. No, the perforation is typically confined.

Reference

Birnbaum BA, Balthazar EJ: CT of appendicitis and diverticulitis, *Radiol Clin North Am* 32:885-898, 1994.

Cross-Reference

Gastrointestinal Radiology: THE REQUISITES, ed 2, p 271.

Comment

The presence of diverticula in the colon is common among those who live in industrialized societies, and it is believed that most people will develop colonic diverticula at some time during their life. It also is estimated that 10% to 25% of patients with diverticula will develop symptoms of diverticulitis at some point. Diverticulitis can occur at any age and has been reported even in patients in their twenties. Diverticulitis may occur when only a single diverticulum is present. The sigmoid is the most common site of diverticula formation, and it is also the most common site for the development of diverticulitis.

Computed tomography has become the definitive modality for the evaluation of this condition. A contrast enema is rarely necessary in the early phase and is typically employed only after therapy, usually to evaluate the colon with regard to the severity and extent of the diverticular changes. CT is extremely sensitive in detecting pericolic inflammatory changes, which often are not identified when other modalities are used. Many times such changes are the only abnormalities that are evident. Other abnormalities, such as fistulas, infected sinus tracts, and abscesses, are easily demonstrated by CT. It is believed that pericolic fluid collections occur in up to one third of patients, but communicating abscesses, such as that shown here, are much less common.

The treatment for this condition has also changed as a result of interventional radiology. In the past these patients often required three operations for definitive treatment. However, currently the typical treatment is percutaneous catheter drainage of the abscess along with antibiotic therapy. After several weeks, the surgery often can be performed in a single stage.

Notes

CASE 8

Benign Gastric Ulcer

1. The lesser curvature of the stomach.

2. Overhanging edematous mucosa at the margin of the ulcer. The ulcer is benign.

3. Nothing. Both malignant and benign ulcers may have folds that stop short of the crater.

4. No. Benign greater curve ulcers and those with a great deal of edema do not.

Reference

Levine MS: Erosive gastritis and gastric ulcers, *Radiol Clin North Am* 32:1203-1214, 1994.

Cross-Reference

Gastrointestinal Radiology: THE REQUISITES, ed 2, p 76.

Comment

Benign ulcers may occur anywhere in the stomach, although they do have a propensity to occur in the lesser curvature, particularly in the middle of the body. This type of ulcer is often seen in the older patient, but the cause for this is uncertain. As a corollary, the majority of ulcers found in the fundus are malignant. The size of an ulcer has no bearing on its malignancy, and giant gastric ulcers often represent a penetrating, walled-off, benign gastric ulcer. Also, the shape of the ulcer is not important, nor is the number of ulcers.

Much has been said about the gastric ulcer as seen in profile. Most benign gastric ulcers project outside the expected lumen of the stomach. However, if there is a great deal of edema, this may not be the case. Also, many benign ulcers along the greater curve do not extend beyond the lumen, probably as a result of muscle spasm. Another common sign of a benign gastric ulcer is Hampton's line, which is a thin lucent line at the neck of the ulcer as it passes through the mucosal layer. This line represents intact overhanging mucosa, which is more resistant to inflammation than the submucosal tissue. However, a very thick collar, particularly if it is asymmetric, at the neck of the ulcer is not a Hampton's line and may be noted in both benign and malignant ulcers.

Often, radiating folds are seen extending toward an ulcer. If these folds pass all the way to the edge of the crater, the process is most likely benign. Folds may stop short as a result of a large collar of edema (in benign ulcers) or as a result of neoplastic tissue (in malignant ulcers); therefore folds that stop short are not a differential feature. Also, the folds tend to be smooth and symmetric in benign ulcers and more irregular and "lumpy" in malignant ulcers. Finally, both benign and malignant ulcers may show signs of healing.

Notes

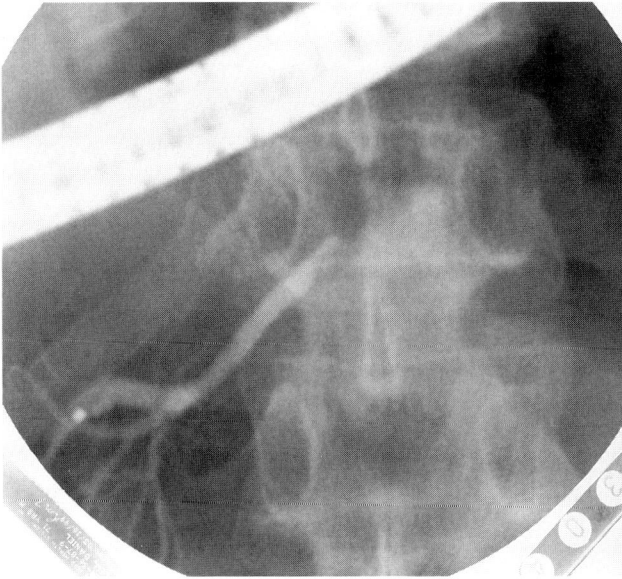

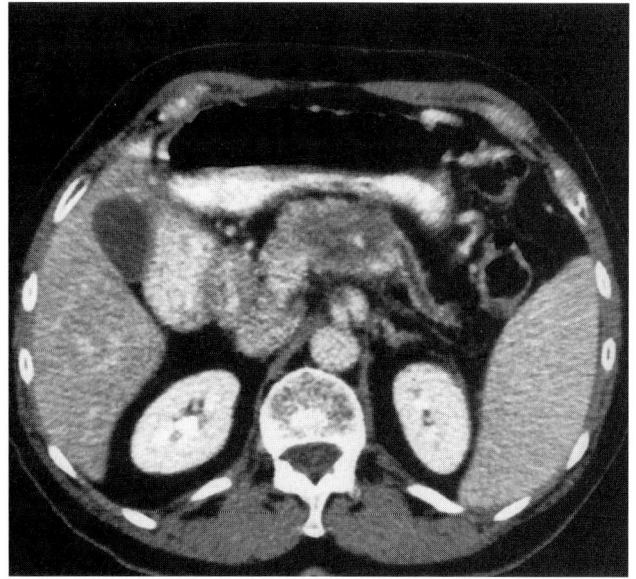

1. What is the most likely diagnosis?
2. From what cell does this tumor arise?
3. What indicates that the tumor is unresectable?
4. What is a paraneoplastic condition that is often associated with this tumor?

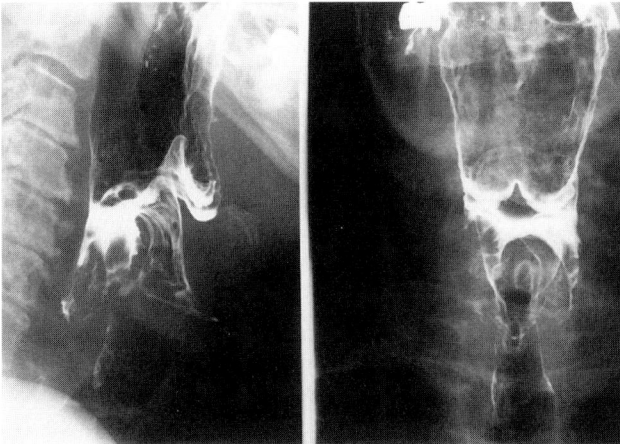

1. What is the most common tumor of the pharynx?
2. What is the second most common tumor of the pharynx?
3. Name some other tumors that may metastasize to the pharynx.
4. What is the significance of Plummer-Vinson syndrome?

Pancreatic Carcinoma

1. Pancreatic carcinoma.

2. Duct epithelium.

3. Vascular encasement, distant metastases, ascites, or invasion of adjacent structures.

4. Spontaneous venous thrombosis (Trousseau's sign).

Reference

Mergo PJ, Helmberger TK, Buetow PC, et al: Pancreatic neoplasms: MR imaging and pathologic correlation, *Radiographics* 17:281-301, 1997.

Cross-Reference

Gastrointestinal Radiology: THE REQUISITES, ed 2, p 144.

Comment

The most common primary tumor of the pancreas is ductal adenocarcinoma. As the name implies, the tumor arises from the ductal epithelium. With regard to abdominal tumors, this growth is one of the leading causes of death. It occurs twice as often in men as in women. Certain groups tend to have a higher incidence, and it tends to be more common in urban dwellers and in those who live in industrialized societies. Some possible risk factors include smoking, alcohol consumption, diabetes mellitus, prior pancreatitis, and a family history of ductal adenocarcinoma. A high-fat diet is believed to increase an individual's risk, and there is some controversy concerning a possible link between coffee consumption and this disease.

Pancreatic adenocarcinoma grows in a fibrous or scirrhous manner. It tends to grow along tissue planes and replaces the normal tissues in the region. It does not grow into a well-defined mass but rather has poor margins that are often difficult to delineate. Also, the tumor is poorly vascular and will rarely hemorrhage, calcify, or necrose. Affected patients have a poor prognosis because the tumor does not present clinically until very late in the course of disease. Also, the growth will invade adjacent vital structures in the region, making it virtually impossible to resect surgically. Most carcinomas arise in the head of the pancreas (60% to 70%), with the rest distributed throughout the gland. CT is currently the best modality for staging, although it still usually underestimates the extent of the disease. Major vascular encasement (SMA vessels), direct invasion of adjacent major organs, liver metastases, adenopathy, and ascites (which indicates peritoneal involvement) are all signs suggesting that the tumor is unresectable.

Patients with a ductal adenocarcinoma may have nonspecific abdominal pain, weight loss, jaundice, anemia, sudden onset of diabetes, or malabsorption. The occurrence of venous thrombosis in an otherwise healthy patient is an unusual condition often associated with the presence of pancreatic carcinoma.

Notes

Squamous Carcinoma of the Hypopharynx

1. Squamous carcinoma.

2. Lymphoma.

3. Although rare, pharyngeal metastases are seen with breast cancer, lung cancer, melanoma, and Kaposi's sarcoma.

4. Increased incidence of pharyngeal or esophageal carcinoma.

Reference

Low VHS, Rubesin SE: Contrast evaluation of the pharynx and esophagus, *Radiol Clin North Am* 31:1265-1291, 1993.

Cross-Reference

Gastrointestinal Radiology: THE REQUISITES, ed 2, p 3.

Comment

The majority of tumors involving the pharynx are squamous in origin. These tumors are seen radiologically as small nodules or masses or sometimes as a thickening or obliteration of the normal structures. Laryngoscopy is the method of choice for identification, but with the increase in swallowing studies being performed to diagnose conditions causing dysphagia, the radiologist may be the first to encounter these tumors.

The pharynx and hypopharynx are repositories of a substantial amount of lymph tissue. Thus it is to be expected that patients with lymphoma may develop neoplastic infiltration of these structures. In patients with lymphoma and dysphagia the hypopharynx must be studied closely. Squamous tumors of the hypopharynx typically arise in the vallecula, pyriform sinuses, or epiglottis. Lymphomas more frequently involve the posterior or lateral wall and may be submucosal in location, producing subtle changes. If a tumor is substantially posterior in location, lymphoma must be strongly considered. Potentially, all tumors may metastasize to this region. However, it is a rare event, given the number of patients with malignancies. Two common cancers—breast and lung—are known to metastasize to the pharynx on occasion. Also, cancers of the skin, such as melanoma and Kaposi's sarcoma, seem to metastasize to the hypopharynx relatively frequently. Patients with Plummer-Vinson syndrome have anemia associated with cervical esophageal webs. Although it is controversial, some authors believe that the syndrome is a premalignant condition and that affected patients have a higher incidence of pharyngeal and esophageal carcinoma.

Notes

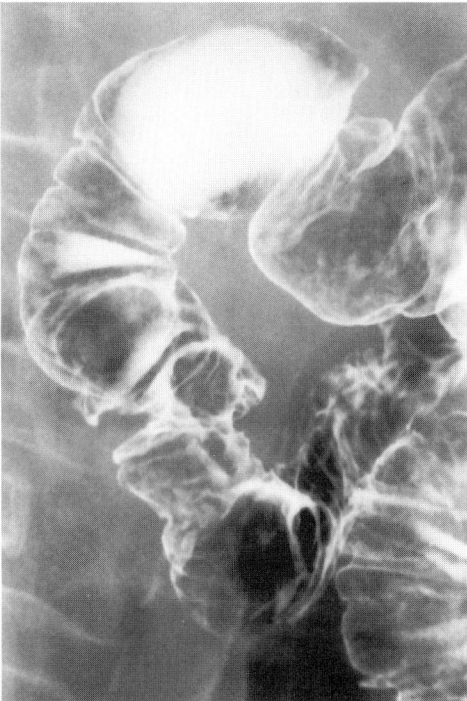

1. What is the size of a normal papilla?
2. What is the most common cause of benign enlargement of the papilla?
3. What biliary anomaly may produce an enlarged papilla?
4. Name the polyposis syndrome associated with tumors of the papilla.

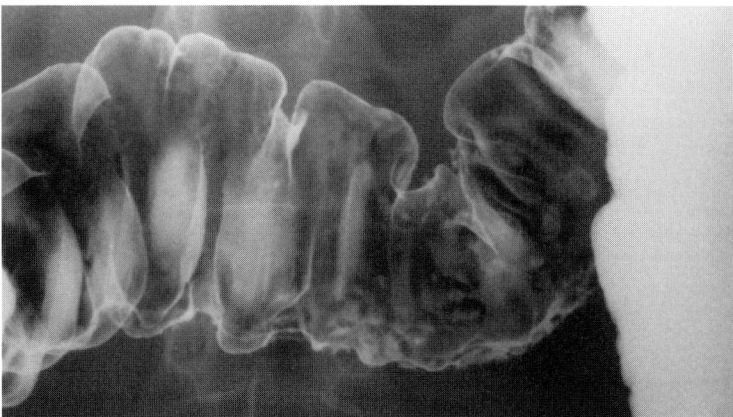

1. What inflammatory conditions produce collar-button ulcers?
2. What conditions produce aphthous ulcers?
3. What conditions produce long, fissuring ulcers?
4. What inflammatory bowel diseases result in fistula formation?

Enlarged Papilla Secondary to Neoplasm

1. 1.5 cm is considered the upper limit of normal.

2. Edema caused by stones in the distal bile duct.

3. Choledochocele.

4. Familial polyposis has an association with tumors developing near the papilla.

Reference

Buck JL, Elsayed AM: Ampullary tumors: radiologic-pathologic correlation, *Radiographics* 13:193-212, 1993.

Cross-Reference

Gastrointestinal Radiology: THE REQUISITES, ed 2, p 90.

Comment

On normal upper gastrointestinal tract examinations the papilla and associated structures may be identified along the medial wall of the second portion of the duodenum. The papilla is an elevated mound of tissue that is typically smaller than 1 cm. It is considered abnormal when larger than 1.5 cm, although healthy patients have been known to have papillae enlarged up to 3 cm. Inferior to the papilla, folds may be visible, extending up to 3 cm in length.

The papilla is usually enlarged as a result of benign disease. The most common cause of edema of the papilla is the presence of stones in the distal common bile duct. Other causes include pancreatitis (either short- or long-term), which may produce swelling (Poppel's sign). Typically the enlargement of the papilla with edema produces a smooth and symmetric enlargement. Rarely, acute duodenal ulcer disease produces papillary enlargement but is usually associated with duodenal fold thickening. A choledochocele, an abnormal enlargement of the most distal end of the common bile duct and ampullary region, also causes enlargement of the papilla.

Tumors arising in or about the papilla are called *perivaterian malignancies.* Carcinoma of the papilla is the most common tumor. Polyps or mesenchymal tumors, such as leiomyoma, may also arise in the region and produce enlargement. Certain polyposis syndromes—familial polyposis coli and the associated Gardner's syndrome—predispose patients to tumor development in the perivaterian region. Such a patient may require routine screening of the upper gastrointestinal tract throughout his or her life because of this association.

Notes

Crohn's Colitis

1. Almost all of them may produce collar-button ulcers.

2. Crohn's disease and some infectious colitides.

3. Crohn's disease.

4. Crohn's disease and tuberculosis.

Reference

Lichtenstein JE: Radiologic-pathologic correlation of inflammatory bowel disease, *Radiol Clin North Am* 25:3-24, 1987.

Cross-Reference

Gastrointestinal Radiology: THE REQUISITES, ed 2, p 261.

Comment

Several types of ulcers are encountered with inflammation of the colon, and these ulcers can also affect all portions of the gastrointestinal tract because the bowel has only a limited number of ways to respond to inflammation of the mucosa. When ulceration extends through the mucosa and muscularis propria, it reaches the submucosa. The epithelium is relatively resistant, but the submucosa has difficulty containing the inflammatory process. Thus ulcers tend to spread laterally when they reach the submucosa. With their thin necks and wide bases, the ulcers resemble collar buttons, hence the terminology. The collar-button shape can occur with virtually any type of ulceration from any cause.

Aphthous ulceration occurs in the colon as lymphoid follicles enlarge from inflammation and their overlying mucosa ulcerates. In other parts of the gastrointestinal tract, aphthous ulcers occur as focal ulcers, with surrounding edema. Either way, they produce a characteristic "bull's eye" appearance. These ulcers were initially described in association with Crohn's disease but can be found in a variety of infectious processes, particularly viral infections. Amebiasis, salmonellosis, and even ischemia have also been known to produce aphthous ulcers.

Long, fissuring ulcers are rare and much more specific to Crohn's disease. Rarely do other inflammatory conditions cause this type of ulceration, although tuberculosis is also a consideration. Fistulas between bowel loops are a sequela of inflammation of the bowel, occurring with Crohn's disease or tuberculosis. Fistulas are never seen in patients with ulcerative colitis. The possibility of malignancy and the sequelae of radiation or surgery are other considerations when fistulas are encountered. Diverticulitis also can produce fistulas.

Notes

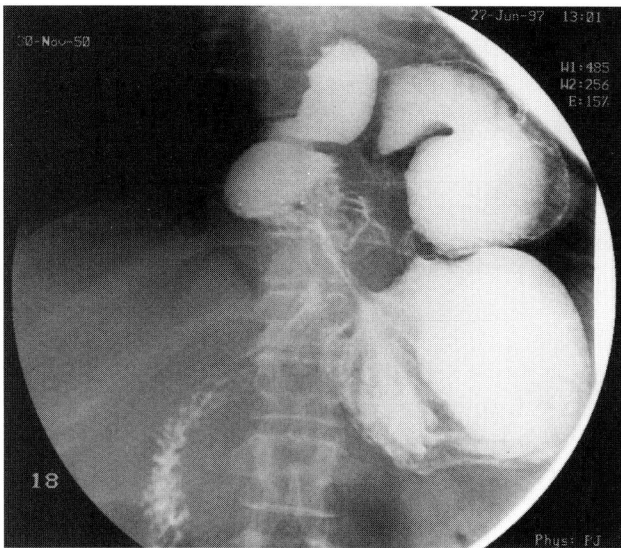

1. What abnormality is typically present, allowing this condition to occur?
2. What is the defect that is located anteriorly in the diaphragm and may contain a hernia?
3. Name the two types of this condition.
4. What other abnormalities may produce this condition?

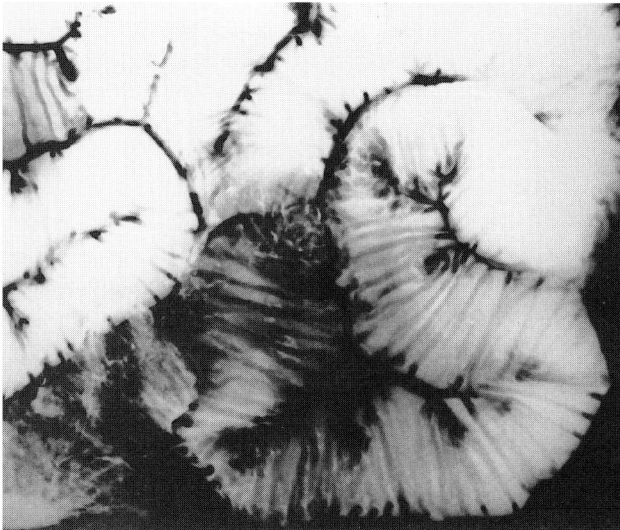

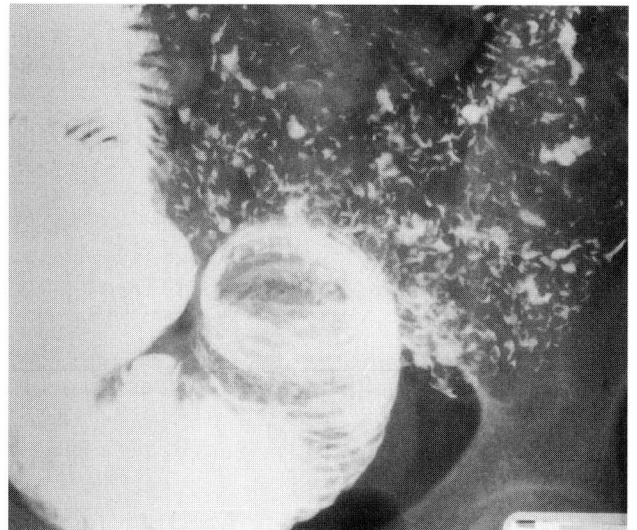

1. What happens to the number of folds per inch in patients with sprue? What happens to the number of folds per inch in patients with scleroderma?
2. What is meant by the term *jejunization?*
3. What are the malignant complications of sprue?
4. Do the lymph nodes enlarge in patients with sprue? What is the significance of this?

Gastric Volvulus

1. Most gastric volvulus occurs as a result of a large hiatal hernia or defect.

2. Foramen of Morgagni (Morgagni hernia).

3. Organoaxial and mesenteroaxial.

4. Paralysis or large eventration of the left hemidiaphragm.

Reference

Andiran F, Tanyel FC, Balkanci F, et al: Acute abdomen due to gastric volvulus: diagnostic value of a single plain radiograph, *Pediatr Radiol* 25:S240, 1995.

Cross-Reference

Gastrointestinal Radiology: THE REQUISITES, ed 2, p 54.

Comment

Volvulus of the stomach is an unusual entity but may be encountered more frequently in an elderly population. The stomach is relatively free to move within the upper abdomen, despite its multiple ligamentous attachments. The second portion of the duodenum fixes the duodenogastric region distally, and proximally there are gastrocolic and gastrolienal ligaments. The stomach is left to move freely between these points. Usually, patients with gastric volvulus have a large hiatal hernia or some other diaphragmatic defect permitting upward movement and rotation of the stomach. Left hemidiaphragm paralysis or large eventration may also lead to volvulus.

There are two types of volvulus. Organoaxial volvulus occurs when the rotation of the stomach is around its long axis (i.e., the axis from the cardia to the pylorus). The antrum and greater curvature rotate superiorly and occupy a position above the proximal stomach and fundal region. The other type of volvulus is mesenteroaxial volvulus. In this condition the stomach rotates from right to left about the axis of the gastrohepatic ligament. The antrum occupies a position to the left of the cardia and may even be above it. Clinically the volvulus may be long lasting and may produce no significant symptoms. This condition is often encountered in the elderly. The patient with acute volvulus may experience vomiting and severe pain. This condition is a surgical emergency because failure to decompress the volvulus may result in ischemia and necrosis. Radiologically the diagnosis often can be made on plain radiographs, particularly upright chest and abdomen films, where a double air-fluid level may be encountered. Barium study or even CT may also be of benefit.

Notes

Celiac Disease (Sprue) with Intussusception

1. In sprue, decreased number of folds per inch. In scleroderma, increased number of folds per inch.

2. Number of ileal folds increase, resembling the jejunum.

3. Lymphoma, carcinoma of the proximal small bowel, and esophageal carcinoma.

4. Yes. Often it indicates lymphoma, but benign enlargement may also occur.

Reference

Rubesin SE, Herlinger H, Saul SH, et al: Adult celiac disease and its complications, *Radiographics* 9:1045-1066, 1989.

Cross-Reference

Gastrointestinal Radiology: THE REQUISITES, ed 2, p 133.

Comment

Nontropical sprue (celiac disease) is a rare disorder caused by a sensitivity to gluten, a protein found in bread and other wheat products. There is believed to be a genetic predisposition to the condition. Sprue is more common in women and Europeans but is rare among those who live in Africa or the Orient. The protein gluten incites an immunologic response in the bowel wall, with an increased cellular infiltrate and inflammatory component. Clinically this sensitivity results in malabsorption and possibly steatorrhea and diarrhea. Symptoms are often vague and include neuropathies (vitamin B12 deficiency), anemia, glossitis, and changes in skin pigmentation. Diagnosis is made by small bowel biopsy, and villous atrophy is evident.

The radiologic changes in sprue can be fairly nonspecific and include bowel dilation, increased fluids or secretions, and sometimes fold thickening. Actual fold thickening occurs only in complicated sprue and is caused by edema (hypoalbuminemia) or lymphoma. A more specific radiologic finding is the overall decrease in folds per inch seen in the jejunum, with five or more folds per inch being considered normal. There is a paradoxical increase in ileal folds so that the ileum resembles the jejunum (the so-called jejunization of the ileum). With a gluten-free diet, these abnormalities are often corrected.

Numerous complications occur in patients with sprue. Transient small bowel intussusceptions occur and reduce spontaneously. A more sinister complication is the development of malignancy, although a gluten-free diet diminishes the likelihood of this complication. Lymphoma of the small bowel is the most common malignancy, but carcinomas of the small bowel, esophagus, and rectum have all been reported. Adenopathy detected by CT in sprue raises suspicions of lymphoma but can also be a benign condition and part of the cavitating lymph node syndrome. Hyposplenism, immunoglobulin deficiencies, and dermatitis herpetiformis are other complications.

Notes

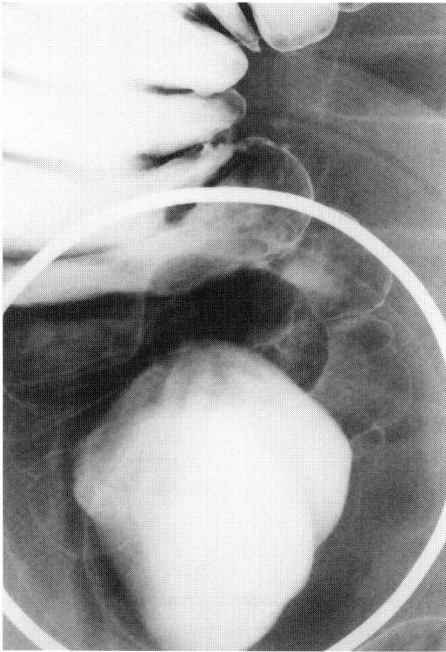

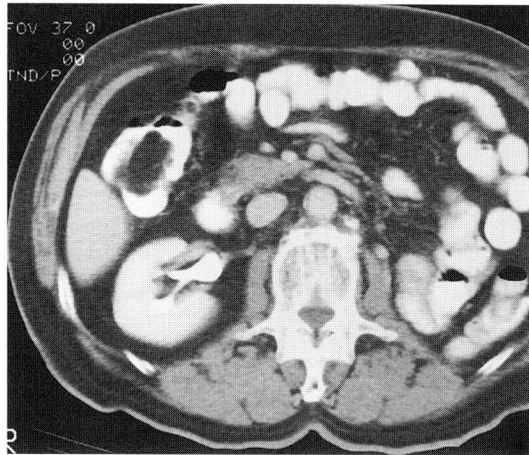

1. At what size should the ileocecal valve be considered enlarged?
2. What is the most common cause of an enlarged ileocecal valve?
3. What is the most common neoplasm of the ileocecal valve?
4. Name diseases of the ileum that can also enlarge the valve.

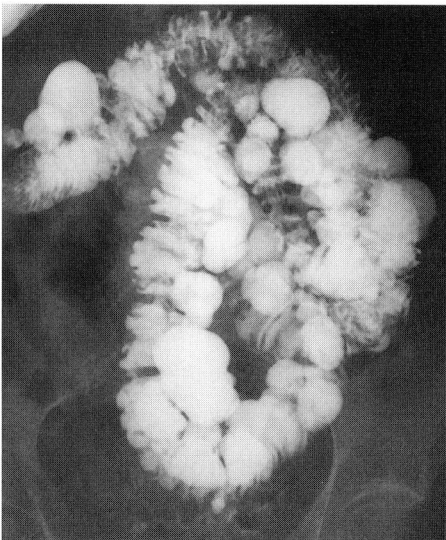

1. What conditions produce eccentric sacculations of the small bowel?
2. On which side of the bowel do "pseudosacculations" occur?
3. What layers of the bowel are in small bowel diverticula?
4. Name the major clinical problem associated with small bowel diverticula.
5. What vitamin deficiency may occur with small bowel diverticula?

Enlarged Ileocecal Valve Caused by Lipomatous Infiltration

1. 3 cm is the upper limit of normal; anything above 4 cm should be considered abnormal.

2. Lipomatous infiltration.

3. Lipoma.

4. Crohn's disease, lymphoma, and prolapsing ileal neoplasms.

Reference
Short WF, Smith BD, Hoy RJ: Roentgenologic evaluation of the prominent or unusual ileocecal valve, *Med Radiogr Photogr* 52:2-26, 1976.

Cross-Reference
Gastrointestinal Radiology: THE REQUISITES, ed 2, p 287.

Comment
The ileocecal valve must be thoroughly evaluated on every study (barium enema or CT) of the region. This structure is composed of two lips—upper and lower—that fuse at their corners. The lips have mucosal, submucosal, and muscular layers, with the mucosa being colonic in nature and the muscular layer resembling that of the ileum. The valve occurs at the first complete haustral segment of the cecal tip and defines the upper limit of the cecum. It is a true sphincter in that it functions to prevent retrograde flow of colonic contents back into the small bowel.

The normal ileocecal valve is usually 1.5 to 2 cm in height, with 3 cm being considered the upper limit of normal. Some authors consider the valve abnormal when it exceeds either 3 or 4 cm in height. By far the most common cause of enlargement is lipomatous infiltration, which occurs predominantly in women and is often related to generalized obesity. Lipomatous infiltration usually produces a symmetric enlargement of the structure, affecting both lips. A lipoma is a benign fatty tumor of the structure and is the most common neoplasm of the region. Its radiographic appearance is that of a smooth, well-demarcated polypoid lesion. However, malignant neoplasms of the ileocecal valve are also relatively common and account for a substantial proportion of overlooked lesions. Adenomas are frequently encountered, and adenocarcinomas also are found with some regularity. Lymphomas are another common neoplasm of the region and can produce enlargement of the valve. Also, virtually all diseases of the terminal ileum can produce valve enlargement as a result of edema.

Radiologically it may be quite difficult to determine the cause of the ileocecal valve enlargement. However, if the enlargement is eccentric or involves only one lip, the possibility of malignancy must be strongly considered. High-resolution CT of the region can be helpful in assessing the radiologic density of the tissue and determining whether it is fat containing. It can also assess possible disease in the terminal ileum.

Notes

Small Bowel Diverticulosis

1. Crohn's disease and scleroderma.

2. Antimesenteric side.

3. Mucosa, submucosa, and possibly some muscle layers.

4. Malabsorption caused by bacterial overgrowth.

5. Vitamin B12.

Reference
Ross CB, Richards WO, Skarp KW, et al: Diverticular disease of the jejunum and its complications, Am Surg 56:319-324, 1990.

Cross-Reference
Gastrointestinal Radiology: THE REQUISITES, ed 2, p 128.

Comment
Diverticula of the small bowel are frequently encountered during small bowel examinations, particularly in patients older than 40 years. There are actually two different types of diverticula—sacculations and pseudodiverticula (eccentric protrusions of the bowel along the antimesenteric side, containing all layers of the bowel). These protrusions are often caused by pathologic conditions of the bowel, which produce eccentric scarring or fibrosis that results in bulging of the opposite wall of the bowel. Crohn's disease and scleroderma are known to cause sacculation formation.

True small bowel diverticula occur predominantly in the jejunum. These diverticula occur on the mesenteric side of the bowel at the entrance of the blood vessels. They typically have a narrow neck compared with the wide-necked sacculations. Only portions of the bowel wall, typically mucosa, submucosa, and some longitudinal muscle, are found in diverticula. Most jejunal diverticula cause no symptoms. However, a major complication is that of malabsorption caused by stasis of the bowel contents and resultant bacterial overgrowth. As the number of bacteria increases in the small bowel, the amount of conjugated bile salts is reduced, diminishing fat absorption. Also, deconjugated bile salts irritate the mucosa and may induce electrolyte loss. All these factors result in malabsorption. There is also vitamin B12 deficiency as a result of its use by the bacteria. Management typically consists of antibiotic therapy, which reduces the bacterial load in the small bowel.

Rare complications include diverticulitis or perforation with abscess, which may be diagnosed by CT. Hemorrhage has also been reported. Patients develop obstructive symptoms on occasion, but typically this is a pseudoobstruction.

Notes

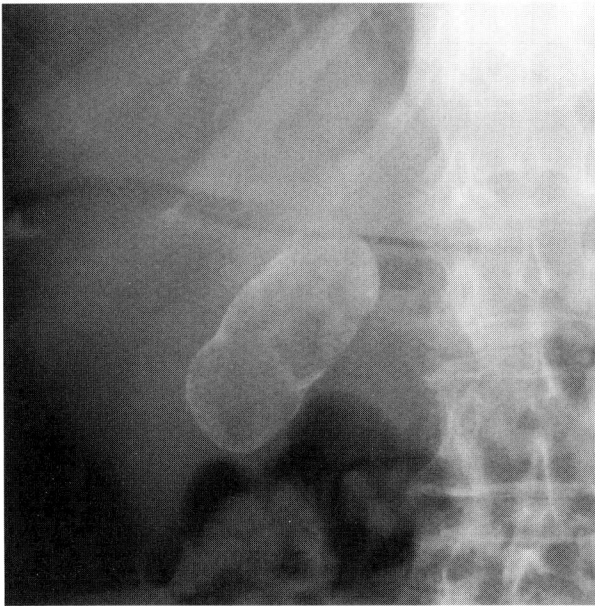

1. What is this condition called?
2. Does this condition affect men or women most commonly?
3. What problems often accompany this condition?
4. Name a major associated complication.

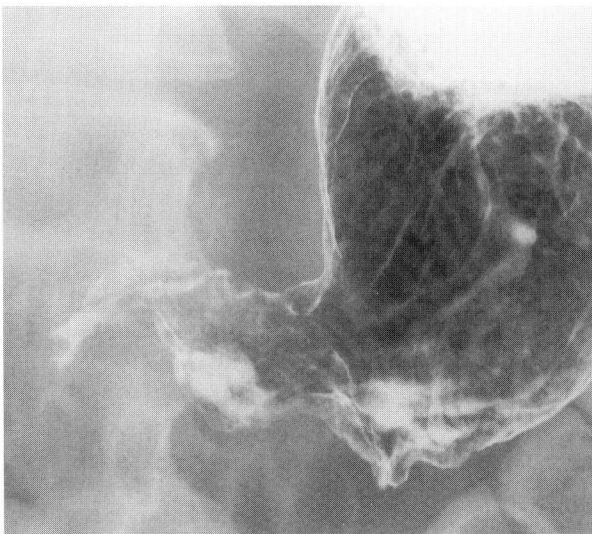

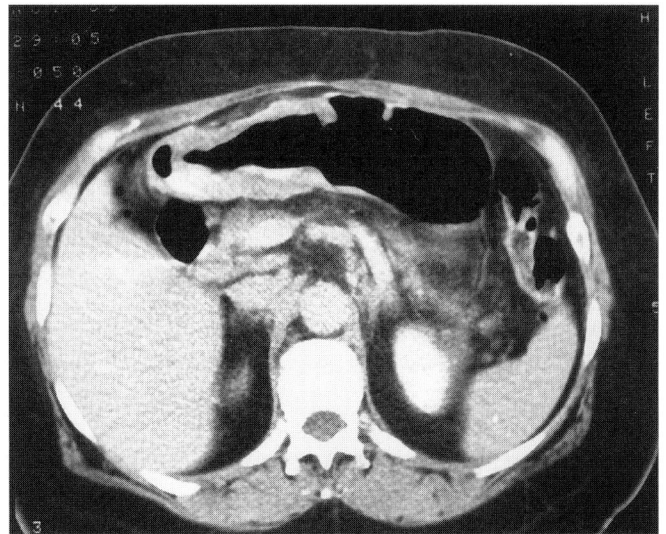

1. Does gastric adenocarcinoma cross the pylorus?
2. About how often is gastric lymphoma primary to just the stomach?
3. Where do intraperitoneal metastases invade the stomach?
4. What percentage of gastric lymphomas are of the Hodgkin's type?

Porcelain Gallbladder

1. Porcelain gallbladder.

2. Women.

3. Gallstones and cystic duct obstruction.

4. Gallbladder carcinoma.

Reference

Kane RA, Jacobs R, Katz J, et al: Porcelain gallbladder: ultrasound and CT appearance, *Radiology* 152:137-141, 1984.

Cross-Reference

Gastrointestinal Radiology: THE REQUISITES, ed 2, p 223.

Comment

A large, ovoid calcification in the right upper quadrant of the gallbladder can represent either a very large gallstone or calcification in the wall of the gallbladder. Calcification in the wall of the gallbladder is termed *porcelain gallbladder.* The name derives from the facts that the gallbladder can be quite brittle during surgery and may have a bluish discoloration. The calcification may develop within the muscular layer or in the glands of the gallbladder mucosa. If the calcification is continuous and smooth, it is usually in the muscular layer. This condition most frequently affects women, as does chronic cholecystitis. However, the reason this calcification develops is uncertain because it is a relatively rare finding compared with chronic cholecystitis, which is ubiquitous. There does not appear to be any underlying disorder of calcium metabolism.

Patients usually do not have many symptoms, and the finding is usually incidental on radiography or CT. Affected patients often have gallstones, and cystic duct obstruction is almost always present. The major complication associated with porcelain gallbladder is the development of gallbladder carcinoma, which occurs with such frequency (up to one half of all patients develop gallbladder cancer during their lifetime) that prophylactic cholecystectomy is advised. The tumor may be difficult to identify on ultrasound examination, but sometimes CT may demonstrate an intraluminal mass.

Notes

Gastric Lymphoma

1. Yes. Both carcinoma and lymphoma cross the pylorus and gastroesophageal junction.

2. In approximately one half of patients, lymphoma of the stomach involves only the stomach and the adjacent lymph nodes.

3. Greater curvature, usually because of the involvement of the omentum.

4. This is the rarest type; usually less than 10%.

Reference

Cho KC, Baker SR, Alterman DD, et al: Transpyloric spread of gastric tumors: comparison of adenocarcinoma and lymphoma, *Am J Roentgenol* 167:467-472, 1996.

Cross-Reference

Gastrointestinal Radiology: THE REQUISITES, ed 2, p 64.

Comment

The stomach is the area of the gastrointestinal tract most commonly affected by lymphoma. It may be part of generalized lymphoma involving other portions of the body and lymph system, or it may be primary, involving only the stomach and associated lymph nodes. Approximately half of all cases are primary lymphoma and half are associated with generalized disease. Lymphoma accounts for only 5% or less of primary gastric malignant neoplasms. Most lymphomas of the stomach are of the histiocytic or lymphocytic type, with Hodgkin's disease being the least common, typically accounting for less than 10% of cases. The disease predominantly affects men and is typically seen in an older age group (50 years and up).

Lymphoma has a variety of presentations in the stomach. It may appear as thickened gastric folds and be indistinguishable from gastritis and other causes of rugal fold thickening. It may also present as a solitary mass or as multiple masses and polyps. These masses are known to ulcerate. Rarely, it may infiltrate the entire stomach and produce more of a linitis plastica appearance, but this is more typically seen with Hodgkin's lymphoma. In these instances, mucosal biopsy may not detect the disease. Pliability of the gastric wall is usually still evident in lymphoma but not in adenocarcinoma. Lymphoma will readily cross the pylorus into the duodenum, somewhat more readily than does carcinoma. However, because both are known to cross the pylorus, it is not a distinguishing feature.

Surgical resection of the involved stomach is still the best treatment and may be supplemented by chemotherapy, depending on the situation. Patients with advanced primary disease or systemic lymphoma are best treated by chemotherapy first. Advanced lymphoma of the stomach has been known to perforate or ulcerate when the patient is undergoing this treatment.

Notes

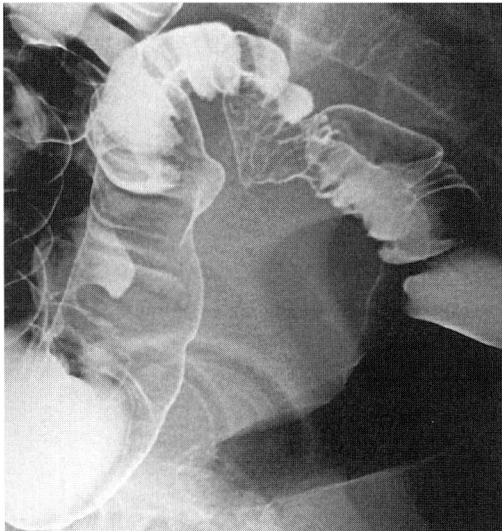

1. Name some malignancies that may affect this portion of the rectum.
2. What inflammatory conditions may occur in this area?
3. If this patient was a young woman, what would be a likely diagnosis?
4. What other imaging modalities may be helpful?

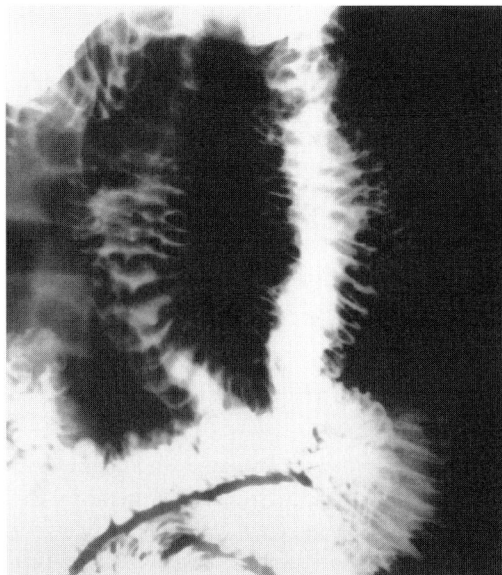

1. What medications may produce this appearance of the small bowel?
2. Name a malignancy that also may produce this appearance.
3. What types of vasculitis are known to cause this condition?
4. What inherited disorder can also produce this change?

CASE 19

Endometriosis Involving the Rectum

1. Serosal metastases to the cul-de-sac region from ovarian, gastric, and pancreatic malignancies.

2. Tuboovarian abscess, appendicitis, and diverticulitis.

3. Endometriosis.

4. Ultrasound and MRI.

Reference

Gordon RL, Evers K, Kressel HY, et al: Double-contrast enema in pelvic endometriosis, *Am J Roentgenol* 138:549-552, 1982.

Cross-Reference

Gastrointestinal Radiology: THE REQUISITES, ed 2, p 275.

Comment

The anterior wall of the rectum abuts some major structures and can be involved by disease processes arising from these organs. Most importantly, however, the lowermost portion of the peritoneal cavity, the cul-de-sac, overlies the anterior portion of the upper rectum. Typically this abuts the rectum above the first or second valve of Houston. In this location, any peritoneal process may reside and secondarily involve the rectum.

Malignancy is the most important factor, and any abdominal tumor may seed the peritoneal cavity with metastatic disease. The most important consideration in a female patient is ovarian carcinoma. Endometrial carcinoma is another possibility. In both sexes, gastric, pancreatic, or colon cancer can produce peritoneal metastases. The appearance of all these tumors is identical. Inflammatory processes include appendicitis, diverticulitis, and pelvic inflammatory disease. Because the region is the most dependent portion of the peritoneum, all pelvic inflammatory processes may spread to it, either before or after surgery.

Endometriosis is a condition produced when there are extrauterine deposits of endometrial tissue. The etiology is uncertain. When endometrial tissue becomes implanted on intraabdominal structures, it is typically on their serosal surface. The tissue is able to maintain viability, and it also responds to the monthly hormonal cycles. The tissue undergoes its normal cyclical changes, including proliferation and then desquamation, just as if it were in the uterine cavity. It is this recurrent shedding of tissue that can lead to complications, including fibrosis. The changes apparent on barium enema relate to fibrotic changes occurring in the wall of the bowel, with some mass effect produced by the tissue. In addition to the anterior rectum, the sigmoid colon, distal small bowel, cecum, appendix, and other pelvic structures may be involved. Rarely the condition may spread to the upper abdominal cavity.

Notes

CASE 20

Hemorrhage into the Bowel Wall in Henoch-Schönlein Purpura

1. Warfarin (Coumadin) or heparin.

2. Kaposi's sarcoma.

3. Henoch-Schönlein purpura, systemic lupus erythematosus, or any other type of vasculitis.

4. Hemophilia.

Reference

Lane MJ, Katz DS, Mindelzun RE, et al: Spontaneous intramural small bowel hemorrhage: importance of non-contrast CT, *Clin Radiol* 52:378-382, 1997.

Cross-Reference

Gastrointestinal Radiology: THE REQUISITES, ed 2, p 110.

Comment

Folds of the bowel are considered abnormally thickened when they exceed 3 mm in width. In this patient the folds are regularly thickened and somewhat symmetric in nature. The folds are not distorted or irregular and do not have any bizarre shapes. This symmetric thickening is seen in conditions such as edema and hemorrhage. Typically the changes that occur are most noticeable in the jejunum because the folds are somewhat closer together and better delineated in this portion of the bowel. With hemorrhage, there can sometimes be associated mass effect in the mesentery as a result of the development of hematomas.

A variety of conditions produce hemorrhage into the wall of the bowel. Anything that can produce bleeding has been associated with hemorrhage into the bowel. One of the most common conditions is that of hemorrhage associated with anticoagulant therapy, particularly with warfarin but sometimes with heparin. Ischemia of the bowel also has been reported to present as hemorrhage into the bowel, although the changes are often more bizarre. An unusual group of conditions is that of vasculitis. Inflammation of the small arterioles of the bowel can lead to hemorrhage, which can be a sequela of radiation therapy. It is also seen with Henoch-Schönlein purpura, which is an acute arteritis involving multiple organs of the body. Lupus, idiopathic thrombocytopenic purpura, thromboangiitis obliterans, and other types of vasculitis also produce small bowel bleeding. Hemophilia is a sex-linked recessive trait that occurs only in men. These patients have a congenital defect in their ability to form clots and thus suffer spontaneous hemorrhage into various parts of their body. Rarely, trauma can produce bleeding, which is often seen in patients who have been in a motor vehicle accident and suffered a seat-belt injury to their intestines. Kaposi's sarcoma may appear as distinct masses, often with central ulceration, or may be submucosal in location and produce hemorrhage, resulting in a radiologic appearance similar to that shown here.

Notes

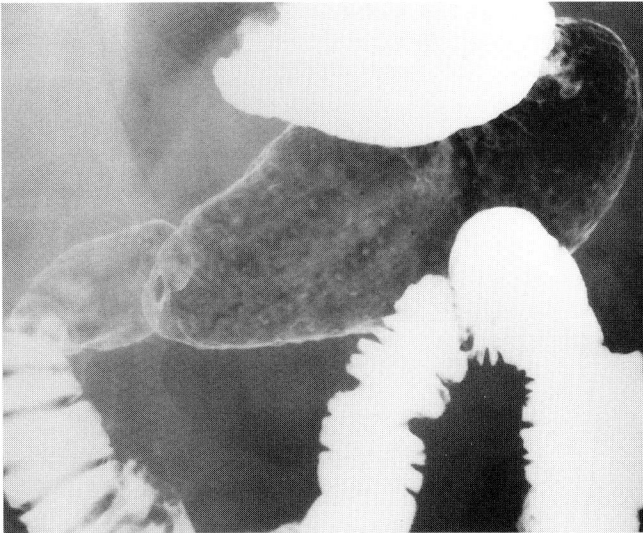

1. What medications may cause this appearance?
2. What group of patients often develops this condition?
3. What disease of the small bowel may have the same manifestation?
4. How often is there no underlying condition for the development of this pathologic condition?

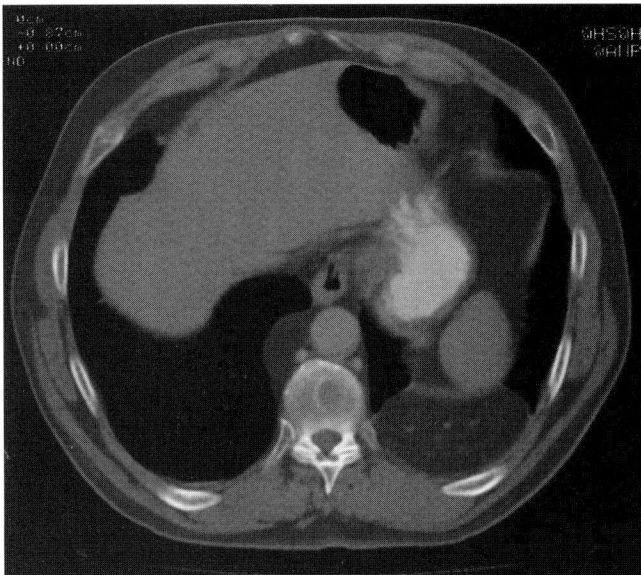

1. What are the major openings in which hernias occur in the diaphragm?
2. What is this type of hernia termed?
3. What is its prevalence?
4. On which side does this hernia most commonly occur?

CASE 21

Erosive Gastritis

1. Aspirin or nonsteroidal antiinflammatory drugs.

2. Alcoholics.

3. Crohn's disease.

4. More than half the time.

Reference

Levine MS: Erosive gastritis and gastric ulcers, *Radiol Clin North Am* 32:1203-1214, 1994.

Cross-Reference

Gastrointestinal Radiology: THE REQUISITES, ed 2, p 75.

Comment

This case is a good example of multiple erosions of the stomach. Erosions are shallow defects in the mucosal layer of the bowel (in this case the stomach) that do not penetrate beyond the muscularis mucosa. Barium collects in the shallow mucosal defects, and there is often a surrounding halo because of edema, which elevates the mucosa about the erosion. This type of mucosal lesion is nonspecific and can be produced by a variety of conditions and agents.

More than half of the patients with gastric erosions have no known predisposing condition. Erosions can be the result of aspirin ingestion or the use of nonsteroidal antiinflammatory drugs. These erosions are often found along the greater curvature of the distal stomach, where the aforementioned drugs come to rest on the stomach mucosa and produce a direct chemical effect. Crohn's disease of the stomach can also produce multiple erosions, or aphthous ulcers as they are called in that disease. The presence of numerous erosions throughout the body and antrum (as in this case) raises the possibility of severe erosive gastritis, which occurs in alcoholics. Alcoholics are prone to developing multiple erosions. If the ulcers are aligned along a fold, they are termed *varioliform erosions.* Patients who suffer from stress, burns, or trauma may also develop acute erosions and ulcers. Although *Helicobacter pylori* has been implicated in gastric and duodenal ulceration, there is not a strong association of *H. pylori* with this type of erosion.

Notes

CASE 22

Bochdalek Hernia

1. Esophageal hiatus, foramen of Bochdalek, and foramen of Morgagni.

2. Bochdalek hernia.

3. Some say it affects up to 3% of the population.

4. Left.

Reference

Miller PA, Mezwa DG, Feczko PJ, et al: Imaging of abdominal hernias, *Radiographics* 15:333-347, 1995.

Cross-Reference

Gastrointestinal Radiology: THE REQUISITES, ed 2, p 293.

Comment

Many types of hernias occur through the diaphragm. The most common is a hernia through the esophageal hiatus, which is probably the most frequent hernia encountered in industrialized societies. However, other defects in the diaphragm may contain hernias. Embryologically the bowel contents protrude into the lower chest, but eventually they enter the abdomen and are isolated from the chest by the diaphragm. The communication from the abdominal cavity and the lower chest may persist, however, due to the persistence of these pleuroperitoneal channels. Anteriorly, two pleuroperitoneal channels exist as the openings of Morgagni. Posteriorly there are another two channels, the foramina of Bochdalek. Morgagni hernias are rare, but Bochdalek hernias may affect between 3% and 5% of the population.

Bochdalek hernias occur more frequently on the left side of the diaphragm. The presence of the liver on the right side probably prevents many Bochdalek hernias from developing in that location. These hernias are located posteriorly and slightly medially. Often, only thin layers of peritoneum and pleura overlie the defects, and there is no diaphragmatic muscle. Most of these hernias are incidental findings on CT examination and contain only some retroperitoneal fat. Larger hernias may contain the kidney, adrenals, and rarely bowel. Most of these patients do not become symptomatic or require treatment in any way. Large Bochdalek hernias occurring in utero may result in pulmonary hypoplasia caused by large portions of bowel herniating into the lower chest.

Notes

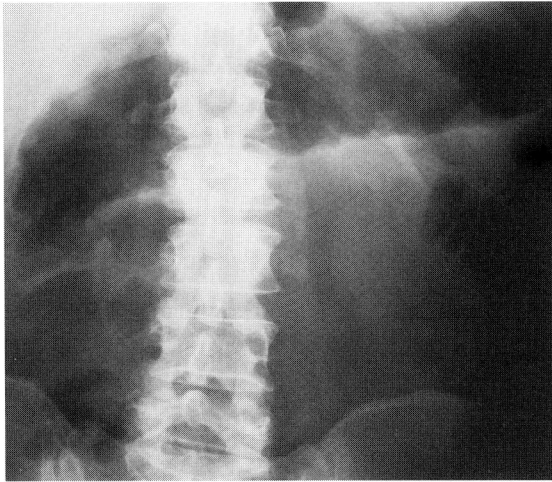

1. Name some diseases that produce this condition.
2. What measurements would indicate the seriousness of the disease?
3. What is the causal factor for the development of this condition?
4. What is the long-term outcome in this condition?

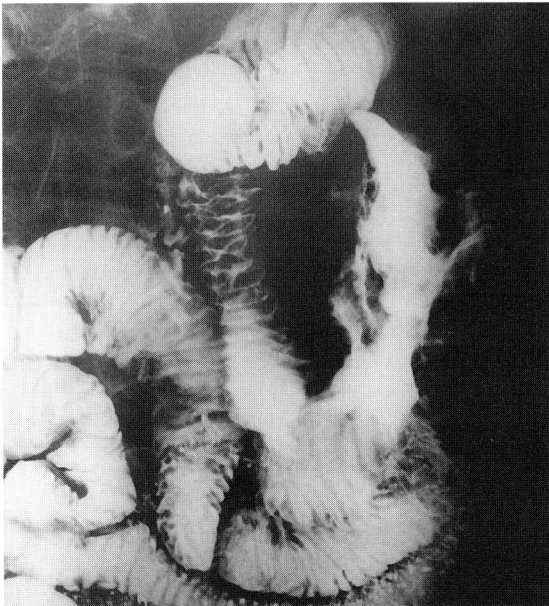

1. Among small bowel lymphomas, how many are caused by Hodgkin's disease?
2. What is the most common location for small bowel lymphoma?
3. Name some factors that predispose an individual to the development of small bowel lymphoma.
4. What virus is associated with lymphoma?

Toxic Megacolon in Ulcerative Colitis

1. Ulcerative colitis, Crohn's disease, infectious colitis, ischemia, and pseudomembranous colitis.

2. None. Measurements do not always indicate severity.

3. Transmural inflammation damaging the ganglion cells.

4. Usually poor. Surgery is often required even at a later date.

Reference

Halpert RD: Toxic dilatation of the colon, *Radiol Clin North Am* 25:147-155, 1987.

Cross-Reference

Gastrointestinal Radiology: THE REQUISITES, ed 2, p 280.

Comment

Toxic megacolon is a relatively uncommon complication of colitis but is one of the most life-threatening as well. Its incidence varies, but it probably affects fewer than 10% of ulcerative colitis patients. It has also been described in Crohn's disease, pseudomembranous colitis, ischemia, and infectious colitis (particularly in AIDS patients).

Toxic megacolon occurs when there is severe transmural inflammation extending into the muscularis propria. There is accompanying vasculitis of the arterioles and destruction of the ganglion cells in the myenteric plexuses. Inflammation can extend all the way to the serosa, producing peritoneal inflammation and clinical changes of peritonitis, even without perforation. The bowel wall becomes quite thin because the mucosa and submucosa are often sloughed as a result of the inflammation. There is an associated loss of muscle tone caused by the inflammation of the muscle layers and the ganglion cell destruction. Adding to this problem are the effects of the narcotic drugs and steroids that may be given to the patient for treatment, as well as possible electrolyte disturbances. These problems all lead to an atony of the bowel, with subsequent dilation. Some authors have stated that, if the transverse colon exceeds 8 cm, it is an indication of impending megacolon. The transverse colon usually dilates the most because it is in the least dependent portion of the colon and air accumulates in it. However, many authors try to disregard measurements because a large colon may be present without severe disease and perforation may occur without significant dilation.

Perforation is the most dreaded complication, with an associated high mortality rate. Often it is clinically occult because the high-dose steroids used to treat toxic megacolon mask the symptoms of peritonitis, which accompanies the perforation. The diagnosis can be made only on plain abdominal radiographs or CT scans. Patients who are successfully treated for toxic megacolon still do poorly in the future and are often at risk for recurrence or require colectomy at a later date.

Notes

Lymphoma of the Small Bowel

1. Few; it is considered relatively rare.

2. Distal small bowel and ileum.

3. Being a transplant recipient; having AIDS, sprue, or systemic lupus erythematosus; and receiving radiation therapy.

4. Epstein-Barr virus.

Reference

Rubesin SE, Gilchrist AM, Bronner M, et al: Non-Hodgkin lymphoma of the small intestine, *Radiographics* 10:985-998, 1990.

Cross-Reference

Gastrointestinal Radiology: THE REQUISITES, ed 2, p 117.

Comment

Lymphoma is one of the most common malignancies of the small bowel, occurring almost as often as adenocarcinoma. It may be either primary, involving only the small bowel and associated lymph nodes, or secondary, with lymphomatous involvement of extraintestinal sites. Lymphoma occurs most commonly in the distal small bowel (compared with adenocarcinoma, which is proximal), but it may occur anywhere within the bowel. A feature of lymphoma is that it may often be multicentric in location. The majority of small bowel lymphoma is the non-Hodgkin's type, with Hodgkin's disease of the small bowel being considered rare.

Lymphoma is difficult to characterize because of its variable morphologic appearance. Radiologic features include multiple nodules, solitary masses, endoexenteric masses, infiltrating tumors, and predominant mesenteric masses. Different studies have found different types to be the most common, but the infiltrating or the endoexenteric mass is believed to be the most common mass. The endoexenteric form, or aneurysmal dilation, is produced when lymphoma infiltrates and replaces the muscular layer and destroys the nerves in the area. This results in bulging of the abdominal wall, with resultant dilation. The bowel wall may become completely replaced by tumor. Perforation is a frequent complication, although the bowel can return to normal after therapy.

A variety of conditions may lead to the development of lymphoma. Any type of immunosuppression, such that associated with AIDS, can lead to lymphoma. Perhaps at highest risk are transplant recipients, who are 50 to 100 times more likely to develop lymphoma compared with the general population. Many of these patients have an associated infection with the Epstein-Barr virus. Other conditions that increase the incidence of small bowel lymphoma include celiac disease (sprue) and systemic lupus erythematosus.

Notes

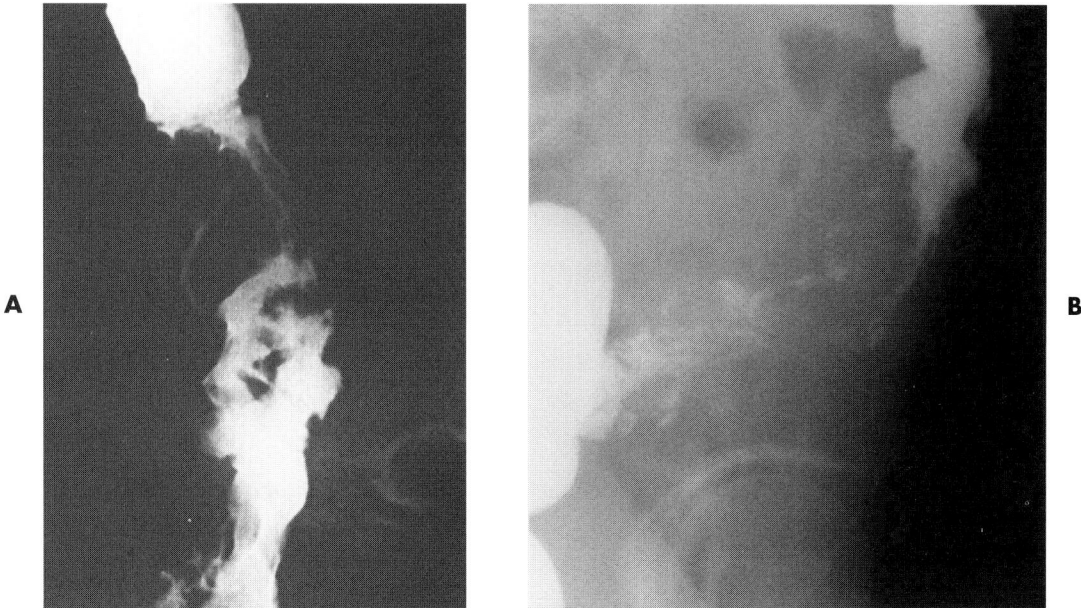

A

B

1. Name some conditions that produce intramural tracking of barium.
2. Does the intramural tracking disappear after treatment for benign disease?
3. What modality is best for evaluation of this abnormality?
4. What does parallel or intramural tracking indicate?

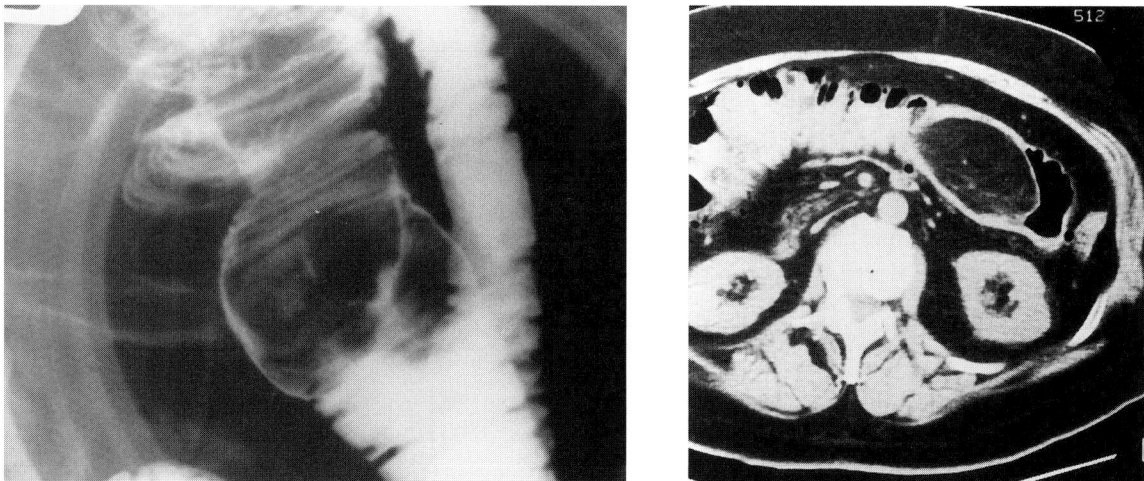

1. What is the most common benign tumor of the small bowel?
2. What are the most common symptoms of small bowel tumors?
3. What is the most common location for lipomas of the small bowel?
4. What polyposis syndromes involve primarily the small bowel?

CASE 25

Intramural Tracking in Colon Malignancy (A) and Diverticulitis (B)

1. Diverticulitis, Crohn's disease, and malignancy.

2. No. Sometimes the pericolic tracking remains even after the inflammation subsides.

3. High resolution CT.

4. An intramural fistula in the same segment of bowel.

Reference

Ferrucci JT, Ragsdale BD, Barrett PJ, et al: Double tracking in the colon, *Radiology* 84:307-312, 1976.

Cross-Reference

Gastrointestinal Radiology: THE REQUISITES, ed 2, p 285.

Comment

Barium tracking through the wall of colon in a parallel fashion is termed *parallel, double, longitudinal,* or *intramural tracking.* Three major conditions—diverticulitis, Crohn's disease, and malignancy of the colon—can produce this abnormality. Other conditions, such as tuberculosis, could produce this change, but this would be quite rare.

Intramural tracking is seen most commonly in patients with diverticulitis. It represents a focal perforation of a diverticulum in the portion that is still within the confines of the colon wall. The inflammation then dissects along the wall of the colon and recommunicates with the lumen through one diverticulum or even several other diverticula. At the time of the initial inflammation there is in essence an intramural, paracolic abscess that communicates with the colon through several tracts. It is likely that one tract initially occurs, and then others develop later. Once this tract develops, it may remain patent even after the inflammation has subsided.

Crohn's disease is known to produce fistulas and sinus tracts, arising from affected loops of bowel and extending for varying lengths. Sometimes these sinus tracts extend in a parallel fashion to the bowel and reenter the same segment in another area. Some suggest that the longer the tract (>10 cm) the more likely it is the result of Crohn's disease. Other signs of Crohn's disease in other portions of the gastrointestinal tract may help in differentiating this condition from diverticulitis.

One of the least common causes of parallel tracking is malignancy. Usually it is due to a primary colonic tumor that ulcerates and forms a paracolic abscess and inflammation. There may be a subsequent formation of a second sinus tract back into the bowel, forming a parallel channel. Usually, in malignancy this type of parallel tracking is more irregular and eccentric than it is in the other inflammatory conditions.

Notes

CASE 26

Lipoma with Intussusception

1. Leiomyoma.

2. Bleeding and abdominal pain.

3. Ileum.

4. Peutz-Jeghers syndrome.

Reference

Taylor AJ, Stewart ET, Dodds WJ: Gastrointestinal lipomas: a radiologic and pathologic review, *Am J Roentgenol* 155:1205-1210, 1990.

Cross-Reference

Gastrointestinal Radiology: THE REQUISITES, ed 2, p 118.

Comment

Benign tumors of the small bowel are infrequently encountered, in part because they cause no symptoms and in part because they are difficult to detect. Typically they occur in patients older than 50 years of age, with no particular gender predilection. Major symptoms include bleeding caused by ulceration of the overlying mucosa and pain caused by intussusception.

The most common benign small bowel tumor is the leiomyoma, which occurs slightly more commonly in the jejunum. These tumors are highly vascular and tend to bleed if injured. Their location is submucosal, and sometimes they may grow exoenteric, rarely intussuscepting because of this. Lipomas are the second most frequent small bowel tumor. They occur predominantly in the ileum. Because of their softness, lipomas grow intraluminally. Lipomas have a propensity to pedunculate and intussuscept. Because of their softness, they can radiologically change shape through peristalsis and conform to the lumen of the bowel. Adenomas occur predominantly in the proximal small bowel, duodenum, and jejunum. There is a high incidence of villous change in small bowel adenomas; thus they are considered premalignant. More rare benign small bowel tumors include hemangiomas, which occur proximally and have a strong propensity to bleed. Neurofibromas may occur as sporadic small bowel lesions, may be multiple, and may be associated with systemic neurofibromatosis.

Small bowel enteroclysis is considered the best modality for diagnosis. However, small bowel enteroscopy is increasingly being used to supplant this method. Many also advocate the use of CT for evaluating these lesions because leiomyomas and lipomas have characteristics that may be recognizable on CT examination.

Notes

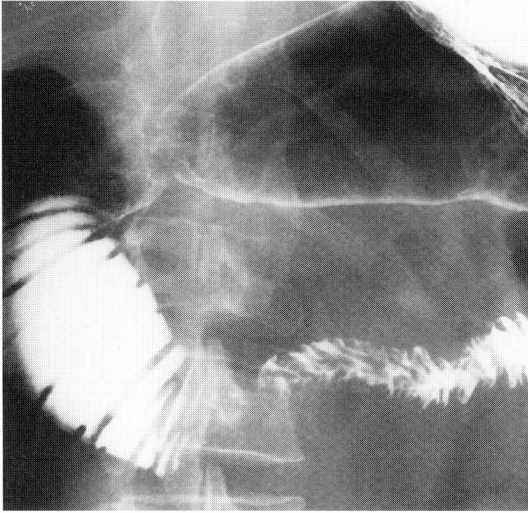
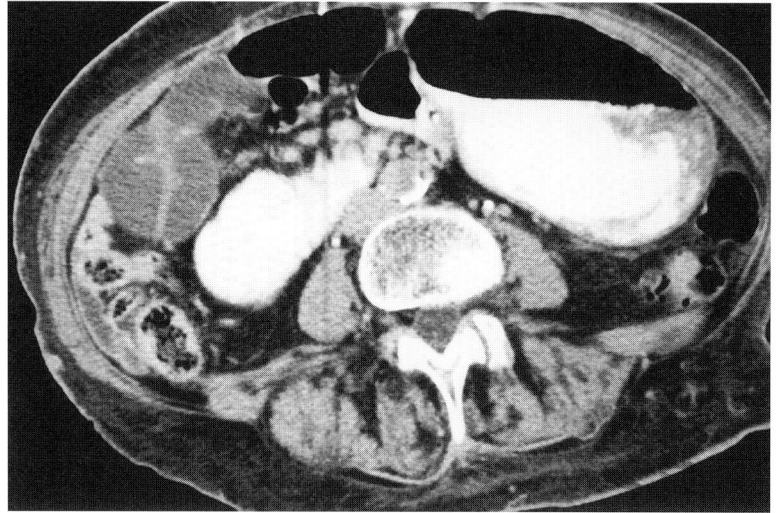

1. What is the mechanism for this abnormality?
2. Name possible etiologies for its development.
3. What motility disorder frequently results in development of this condition?
4. What neoplastic condition may produce this appearance?

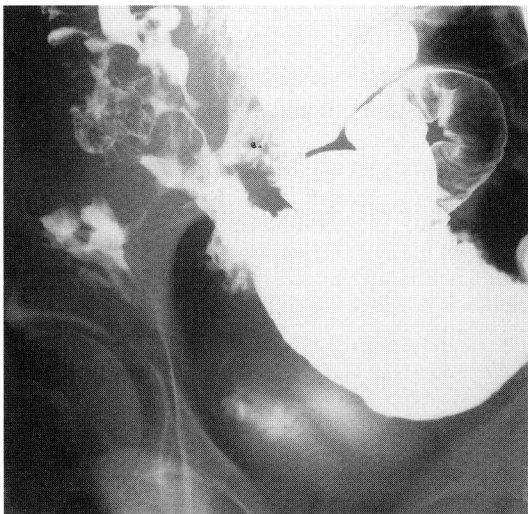

1. What is the most common cause of enterovesical fistulas?
2. What test is used to evaluate the urine in patients with a suspected fistula?
3. Name other conditions known to produce this finding.
4. What infectious process is known to produce intestinal fistula?

Duodenal Obstruction Caused by Superior Mesenteric Artery Syndrome

1. Duodenal compression caused by a narrow aortomesenteric window or angle.

2. Rapid weight loss, immobilization, wearing a body cast, decreased peristalsis, and consumption of certain drugs.

3. Scleroderma.

4. Adenopathy at the root of the mesentery.

Reference

Eisenberg RL: Miscellaneous abnormalities of the stomach and duodenum. In Gore RL, Laufer I, Levine MS: *Textbook of gastrointestinal radiology,* Philadelphia, 1994, Saunders.

Cross-Reference

Gastrointestinal Radiology: THE REQUISITES, ed 2, p 85.

Comment

The third portion of the duodenum—the aortomesenteric window or angle—traverses the midline and is located anterior to the aorta and posterior to the superior mesenteric vessels. Because of this anatomic positioning, this area of the duodenum is prone to physiologic compromise of the lumen caused by compression by the vessels, which have a much greater pressure than the intraluminal pressure of the duodenum. Even in healthy individuals, the transverse duodenum may show some narrowing or delay in transit. This finding may become more pronounced or pathologic in certain conditions.

Processes that cause narrowing of the aortomesenteric angle may lead to compression of the duodenum. These causes include sudden weight loss, which is usually the result of a debilitating condition, and fixed hyperextension, which is common among burn patients, patients wearing body casts, and those undergoing traction. Also, any condition that produces reduced peristalsis of the duodenum can lead to its dilation because pressure within the duodenal lumen is decreased. This is a classic finding of scleroderma and even other collagen vascular diseases. Other processes that can reduce duodenal peristalsis include consumption of certain medications, such as atropine and morphine, and vagotomy. Patients with neuropathies, such as diabetics, can occasionally develop this condition as well.

Another category that should be considered includes those processes that may infiltrate the root of the mesentery, producing its enlargement. This finding is seen in malignancies, such as lymphoma, where adenopathy could develop in the region. Inflammation of the root of the mesentery caused by pancreatitis is another possibility.

Notes

Enterovesical Fistula in Crohn's Disease

1. Diverticulitis.

2. Bourne test.

3. Malignancy, Crohn's disease, radiation therapy, and surgery.

4. Tuberculosis.

Reference

Kao PF, Tzen KY, Chang PL, et al: Diuretic renography findings in enterovesical fistula, *Br J Radiol* 70:421-425, 1997.

Cross-Reference

Gastrointestinal Radiology: THE REQUISITES, ed 2, p 127.

Comment

A fistula is defined as an abnormal tract extending from one mucosa-lined organ into the mucosal surface of another organ. The possible types include enteroenteric (between two loops of bowel), enterovesical (bowel to bladder), enterovaginal, and enterocutaneous, among others. A sinus tract is also a small communication with bowel, but it ends blindly or in a cavity that is not normally lined with mucosa.

Malignancy is one of the most common causes of fistula formation in the gastrointestinal tract. Usually the malignancy is fairly extensive or is already being treated (leading to necrosis) before the fistula occurs. Inflammatory conditions also lead to the formation of numerous fistulas. In the upper gastrointestinal tract, ulcer disease is the usual cause of fistulas. In the colon, diverticulitis is the most common cause of fistulas in industrialized society. Crohn's disease is a well-known cause of fistula formation between adjacent loops of bowel, as well as other structures. The most common infectious agent that may produce fistulization is tuberculosis. This chronic inflammatory process ulcerates and produces a variety of unusual fistulas. Fistulas may form as a complication of surgery, typically at an anastomotic site that dehisces. Radiation is a well-known cause of fistula development; this complication results from microvascular ischemic changes and fibrosis and "matting together" of organs.

Evaluation of fistulas can be quite difficult. Often, contrast will travel in only one direction through a fistula. Also, the fistula must be open at the time of the study or it cannot be demonstrated. CT is often considered the best modality for revealing the presence of a fistula, its complex communications, and the underlying cause of the complication. In the Bourne test a sample of urine is taken after the study, the material is centrifuged, and then the spun material is radiographed to detect barium. The presence of barium is believed to be indicative of an enterovesical fistula.

Notes

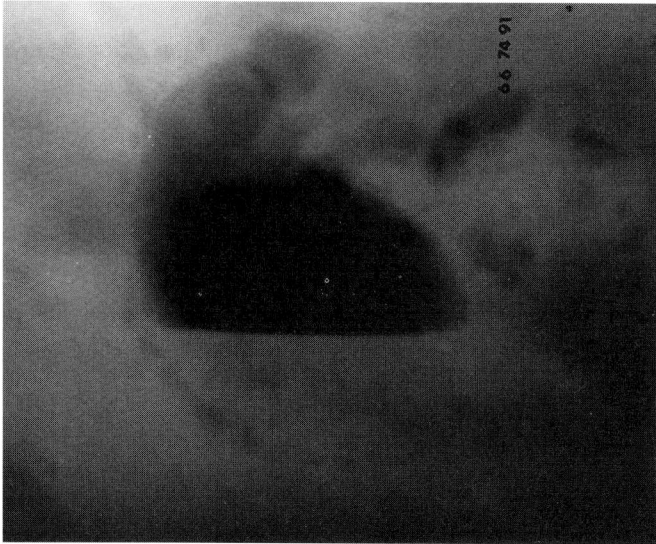

1. What organism typically produces the process shown in this image of the right upper quadrant?
2. What underlying condition does this patient probably have?
3. What is the major complication leading to a high mortality rate?
4. What other problem is often present when this condition occurs?

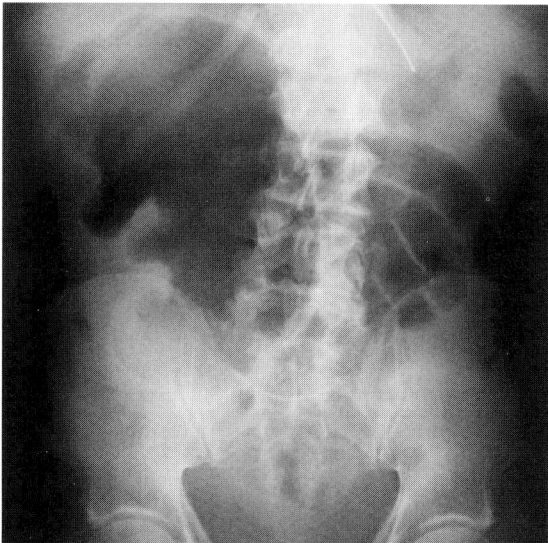

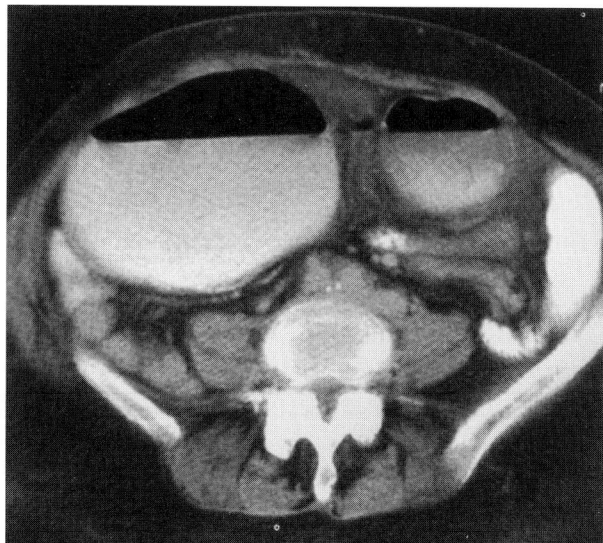

1. What is the most common type of volvulus?
2. What is the least common type?
3. What are the two categories of cecal volvulus?
4. What are the major complications associated with this condition?

Emphysematous Cholecystitis

1. *Clostridium* species (*Clostridium welchii* or *Clostridium perfringens*).

2. Diabetes mellitus.

3. Perforation.

4. Cystic duct obstruction.

Reference

Weltman DI, Zeman RK: Acute diseases of the gallbladder and biliary ducts, *Radiol Clin North Am* 32:933-950, 1994.

Cross-Reference

Gastrointestinal Radiology: THE REQUISITES, ed 2, p 227.

Comment

The appearance of air in the lumen or the wall of the gallbladder is diagnostic of a condition known as *emphysematous cholecystitis.* The air is the result of the gas-forming organism that is causing the cholecystitis. Most commonly, clostridial organisms are to blame. Patients who develop this condition are typically diabetic; rarely does emphysematous cholecystitis occur in individuals without diabetes as an underlying condition. Often the patient is older and has had diabetes for many years, resulting in vascular insufficiency to the gallbladder, which is probably a major underlying cause for the development of emphysematous cholecystitis. Usually, cystic duct obstruction is also present. Although air is present in the gallbladder lumen, air is rarely encountered in the rest of the biliary system. The risk of perforation in patients with emphysematous cholecystitis is five times higher than that in patients with ordinary acute cholecystitis.

Emphysematous cholecystitis is one of the few diagnoses that can be readily made based on conventional radiographs. When the patient is experiencing severe abdominal pain and there is air in the gallbladder lumen, particularly if the patient is diabetic, the diagnosis of emphysematous cholecystitis must be a primary consideration. Many conditions can result in the accumulation of air in the lumen of the gallbladder, but there is usually an abnormal connection of the biliary tract to the bowel lumen allowing this to occur. Also, in some instances air is visible in the wall of the gallbladder, which indicates necrosis of the gallbladder wall. On CT the abnormalities are shown quite well and pericholecystic complications of inflammation and abscess are demonstrated. This condition may not be readily diagnosed on ultrasound, however, because the air may mimic gallstones and produce acoustic shadowing.

Notes

Cecal Volvulus

1. Sigmoid.

2. Splenic flexure.

3. Axial torsion and bascule.

4. Obstruction and perforation.

Reference

Haskin PH, Teplick SK, Teplick G, Haskin ME: Volvulus of the cecum and right colon, *JAMA* 245:2433-2435, 1981.

Cross-Reference

Gastrointestinal Radiology: THE REQUISITES, ed 2, p 277.

Comment

The term *volvulus* describes a twisting or torsion of the bowel. It occurs where bowel is either on a mesentery or unattached. The most common complications are obstruction and perforation caused by necrosis of the bowel. In the colon the most common type of volvulus is that of the sigmoid (in 50% to 75% of cases). Volvulus of the cecum is the next most common type, accounting for 20% to 40% of cases of colonic volvulus. Other rare types of volvulus include the volvulus of the transverse colon and rarely of the splenic flexure.

The term *cecal volvulus* actually describes a volvulus of the cecum and a substantial portion of the right colon above the ileocecal valve. Typically the volvulated cecum occupies a position in the middle of the abdomen or left upper quadrant. The right side of the colon must be incompletely fused to the retroperitoneum for the volvulus to occur. On plain abdominal radiographs the cecum looks massively dilated, often with accompanying small bowel dilation because there is always associated small bowel obstruction. Typically there is little colonic gas beyond the cecum, but this finding is variable. Often there is not the typical coffee bean appearance that is seen with sigmoid volvulus. The definitive diagnosis can be made based on either barium enema, showing the "birds beak" appearance at the site of obstruction, or CT examination.

There are two types of cecal volvulus. The most common is the axial torsion or twisting type. The rare type of cecal volvulus is called a *bascule,* and it consists of a folding of the cecum and right side of the colon upon themselves without significant twisting. The case shown here illustrates this type of volvulus. Some believe that this is not a true entity, however. There is also a pseudocecal volvulus. In this condition the cecum massively dilates and moves into the middle of the abdomen during severe colonic mechanical obstruction or colonic ileus. This reaction occurs because the cecum is the portion of the colon that distends the most during colonic dilation for any reason and it is often mobile.

Notes

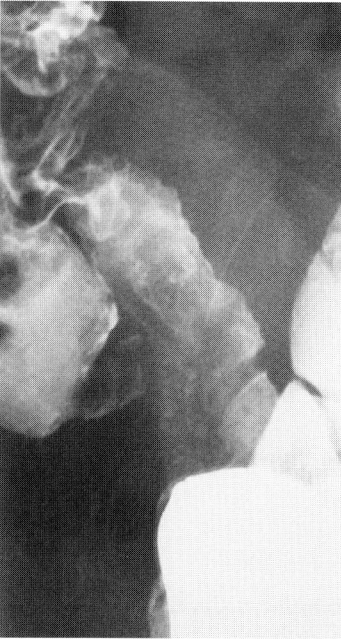

1. What is the most common type of tumor of the appendix?
2. What tumors of the appendix can produce pseudomyxoma peritonei?
3. Is Crohn's disease of the appendix ever isolated to that structure?
4. What is the major cause of appendiceal intussusception?

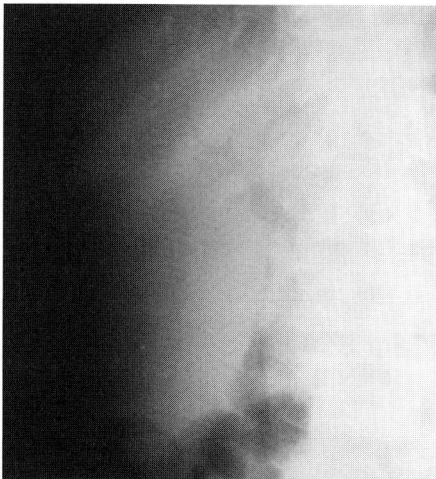

1. What is the most common cause of this appearance?
2. What other conditions may produce this appearance?
3. What is its relationship to emphysematous cholecystitis?
4. How is this finding distinguished from portal venous gas?

CASE 31

Intussusception of the Appendix

1. Carcinoid.

2. Mucocele, mucinous cystadenoma, and myxoglobulosis.

3. Yes.

4. Intraluminal mass, usually a tumor or fecalith.

Reference
Duran JC, Beidle TR, Perret R, et al: CT imaging of acute right lower quadrant disease, *Am J Roentgenol* 168:411-416, 1997.

Cross-Reference
Gastrointestinal Radiology: THE REQUISITES, ed 2, p 251.

Comment
Evaluation of the base of the cecum and appendix has changed dramatically in the past few years as sonography and CT have supplanted plain films and barium enemas in the evaluation of the right lower quadrant. However, all modalities have some shortcomings, and often numerous studies must be performed before a diagnosis can be made. Most studies are aimed at the evaluation of appendicitis, but other processes in the region occur and may produce symptoms similar to those of appendicitis.

Intussusception of the appendix occurs infrequently but can mimic appendicitis clinically, producing either acute or chronic recurrent pain in that region. Sometimes it is an asymptomatic finding on barium enema. Intussusception of this structure almost always occurs as a result of some mass within the lumen of the appendix. As the peristalsis of the appendix tries to expel the intraluminal mass, it can cause invagination and intussusception. Typically the mass is some type of tumor. Of the appendiceal tumors, carcinoid tumors are the most common, and they are typically benign when found in the appendix. Other benign mesenchymal tumors, as well as mucoceles and related lesions, also may occur. Rarely do endometriosis and metastases produce this intussusception because they are typically serosal in location.

The radiographic appearance is that of a filling defect at the base of the cecum or projecting into the lumen. Barium may outline a portion of the appendix and reveal a sausage-shaped filling defect in the lumen. The major differential diagnosis is an appendiceal stump resulting from previous appendectomy, but history would be helpful in this regard. Intussusception may reduce spontaneously during a barium enema. Appendiceal intussusception is rare but must be considered in the evaluation of the patient with right lower quadrant symptoms.

Notes

CASE 32

Air in the Biliary System

1. Previous surgery or endoscopic procedure.

2. Penetrating ulcers, erosion of gallstones into the bowel, traumatic fistula, neoplasms, and bowel obstruction.

3. None. Emphysematous cholecystitis rarely results in air in the biliary system.

4. Central in location in the liver.

Reference
Cho KC, Baker SR: Extraluminal air: diagnosis and significance, *Radiol Clin North Am* 32:829-844, 1994.

Cross-Reference
Gastrointestinal Radiology: THE REQUISITES, ed 2, p 209.

Comment
Air in the biliary system is fairly common and can be detected on both abdominal radiographs and CT. It typically indicates a connection between the biliary system and the bowel. It also can indicate an incompetent sphincter of Oddi, which would allow duodenal air in the biliary system. The cause is by far most commonly iatrogenic, usually the result of a surgical procedure in which the biliary tree has been anastomosed into a loop of bowel. Another common cause is sphincterotomy done with endoscopy. This procedure is becoming quite common and is performed either to remove bile duct stones or to aid in biliary drainage. Sometimes this procedure results in incompetence of the sphincter and allows air to gain access to the bile ducts.

Sometimes fistulas develop naturally between the bile ducts and the bowel. This finding is typically seen in penetrating ulcers in the duodenal bulb, which enter the common bile duct as it passes under the bulb. Sometimes, in patients with chronic cholecystitis and gallstones, the stones erode into the duodenum and less often into the colon or stomach. Rare causes of natural fistulas include carcinoma of the gallbladder or bowel and Crohn's disease. Patients who develop emphysematous cholecystitis, which is caused by a gas-producing organism, rarely have air in the bile ducts because emphysematous cholecystitis usually occurs with cystic duct obstruction, denying air the opportunity to enter the rest of the biliary system.

Air in the bile ducts is central in location. Portal venous gas is quite peripheral, although if it is severe enough it can be present in the main portal vein, which would be central and indistinguishable from the common bile duct. This difference in location helps distinguish these two entities, which have markedly different therapies and prognoses.

Notes

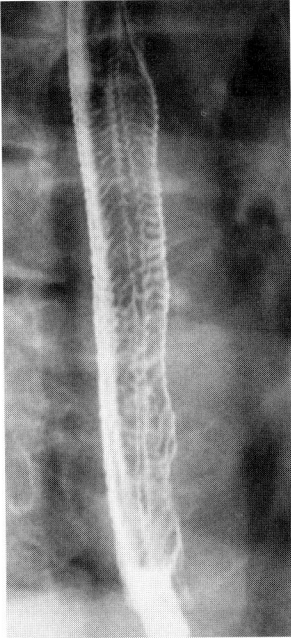

1. What muscle group contracts to produce a "feline" esophagus?
2. What is the significance of a "feline" esophagus?
3. What effect does glucagon have on esophageal motility and the lower esophageal sphincter?
4. What is the difference between presbyesophagus and diffuse esophageal spasm?

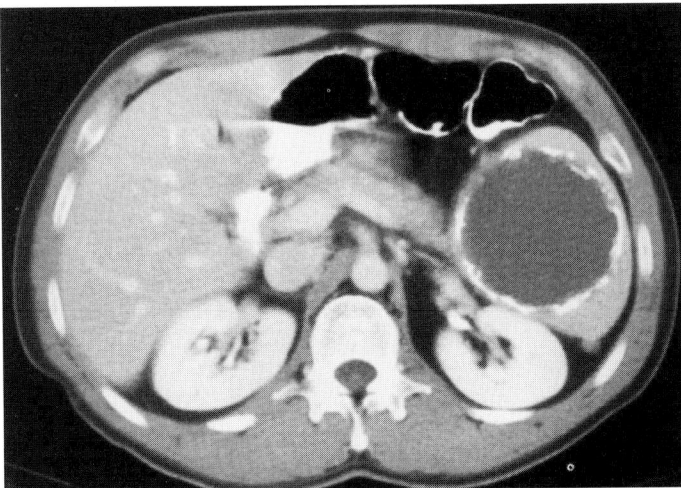

1. What are some diagnostic possibilities?
2. Do true splenic cysts calcify?
3. What is the difference between true splenic cysts and secondary (false) cysts?
4. What parasitic disease may have this appearance?

CASE 33

Transverse Esophageal Folds or "Feline" Esophagus

1. Longitudinal muscularis mucosa.

2. With rare exceptions, occurs in patients with gastro-esophageal reflux and other motor disorders.

3. Glucagon has no effect on esophageal motility but decreases lower esophageal sphincter pressure.

4. Diffuse esophageal spasm is symptomatic with chest pain.

Reference

Low VHS, Rubesin SE: Contrast evaluation of the pharynx and esophagus, *Radiol Clin North Am* 31:1265-1291, 1993.

Cross-Reference

Gastrointestinal Radiology: THE REQUISITES, ed 2, p 33.

Comment

One of the most unusual esophageal motor disorders that has been identified is fine transverse folds of the esophagus. This finding is termed a *feline esophagus* or *felinization of the esophagus* because barium studies in cats show that this is a normal phenomenon or appearance. This transverse folding of the mucosa is believed by some to be due to the contraction of the longitudinal muscularis mucosa of the esophagus, although this belief is somewhat controversial. When first described, the condition was associated with severe swallowing disorders, such as scleroderma. However, it is encountered with increasing frequency as it becomes better recognized. Several authors have indicated that the condition can be seen in healthy patients also. However, most of these "normals" actually have gastroesophageal reflux and often have subtle changes of esophagitis. Whenever a "feline" esophagus is encountered, other motility disorders or reflux should be considered.

Both presbyesophagus and diffuse esophageal spasm may cause large or coarse nonpropulsive contractions. Also, abnormal relaxation of the lower esophageal sphincter occurs in a substantial portion of patients with these conditions. The main differential feature is that chest pain is a clinical presenting feature in diffuse esophageal spasm, whereas presbyesophagus is a relatively asymptomatic condition. Both the age of the patient and the presenting clinical features help distinguish these entities from one another.

Notes

CASE 34

Splenic Cyst

1. Primary or secondary splenic cyst, echinococcal cyst, and pancreatic pseudocyst.

2. Less than 5% of true (primary) cysts calcify; secondary cysts calcify fairly commonly.

3. True cysts are epithelium lined.

4. Echinococcal disease.

Reference

Urrutia M, Mergo PJ, Ros LH, et al: Cystic masses of the spleen: radiologic-pathologic correlation, *Radiographics* 16: 107-129, 1996.

Cross-Reference

Gastrointestinal Radiology: THE REQUISITES, ed 2, p 191.

Comment

There are several diseases or processes that can produce cystic lesions of the spleen, including splenic cysts of various etiologies, echinococcal cysts, and possibly pancreatic pseudocysts. Several tumors may have cystic components, but they usually consist of multiple small cysts and not large solitary cysts.

Splenic cysts can be divided into primary, or true, and secondary cysts. True nonparasitic cysts of the spleen are epithelium lined. They are probably the result of an embryologic defect. Secondary cysts of the spleen occur as the sequela of prior infarction, hematoma, or even abscess. As these processes heal, they may leave behind a residual cyst. Secondary cysts are much more likely to calcify than are primary cysts. These cysts have the propensity to rupture, become infected, or even have hemorrhage within them, which is usually the only time they cause symptoms unless they become so big that they compress other abdominal structures. With both of these types of cysts, CT may demonstrate trabeculation of the wall or even septa.

It is not uncommon for intrasplenic fluid collections to develop after acute pancreatitis. These collections are generally believed to be extensions of pancreatic pseudocysts and have a similar appearance radiologically. Echinococcal cysts are always a consideration but actually occur in only a very small fraction (<5%) of patients with hydatid disease. However, echinococcal cysts frequently have peripheral calcification, as in this case.

Notes

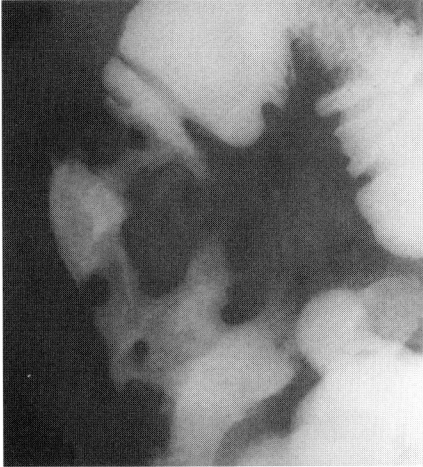

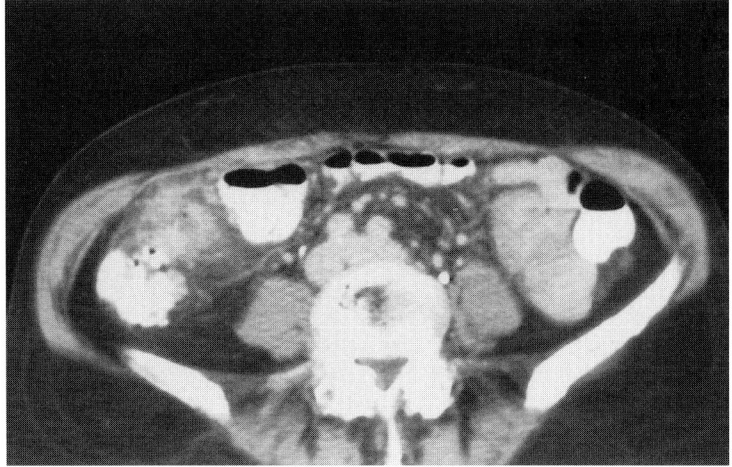

1. Name the possible diseases responsible for producing this appearance.
2. What is the cause of right-sided diverticula?
3. What are the demographic differences between left- and right-sided diverticulitis?
4. How numerous are right-sided diverticula in patients with this condition?

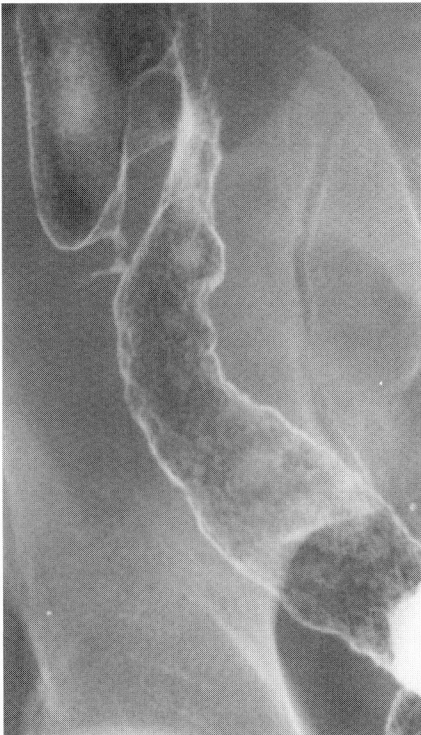

1. What inflammatory conditions produce dilation of the terminal ileum?
2. Does the terminal ileum become ulcerated in patients with ulcerative colitis?
3. What does *Yersinia* species infection of the ileum do to the bowel caliber?
4. How does amebiasis affect the terminal ileum?

Right-Sided Colonic Diverticulitis

1. Appendicitis, diverticulitis, infectious colitis, Crohn's disease, and perforated malignancy.

2. Congenital or acquired (same as left-sided diverticula).

3. Right-sided diverticulitis occurs in a younger age group and is common among those of Asian descent.

4. Most patients with right-sided diverticulitis have only a solitary diverticulum.

Reference

Katz DS, Lane MJ, Ross BA, et al: Diverticulitis of the right colon revisited, *Am J Roentgenol* 171:151-156, 1998.

Cross-Reference

Gastrointestinal Radiology: THE REQUISITES, ed 2, p 271.

Comment

Patients with inflammatory conditions of the right colon have flank and right lower quadrant pain. CT has become the primary modality for the evaluation of severe symptoms in that region, although some advocate the use of ultrasound, and rarely barium enema is employed. The entire spectrum of disease processes affecting this region must be considered when right lower quadrant symptoms are being investigated. The possibilities include appendicitis, diverticulitis, perforated neoplasm or bowel caused by a foreign body, and infectious and idiopathic inflammatory bowel disease.

Right-sided diverticulitis is rarely diagnosed preoperatively because the appearance on imaging studies, as well as clinically, may resemble that of appendicitis. However, location away from the cecum and identification of the appendix should help suggest the diagnosis. Right-sided diverticula were once believed to be congenital in nature, but most now agree that they are acquired in the same fashion as left-sided diverticula, by increased intraluminal pressures. However, right-sided diverticulitis tends to occur in a younger age group; often patients are in their forties or even younger. Also, in Asian populations the incidence of right-sided diverticulitis often exceeds that of left-sided diverticulitis. Interestingly the majority of patients with right-sided diverticulitis are found to have a solitary diverticulum, which is quite different from left-sided diverticulitis.

Computed tomography is the best modality for the evaluation of this region. The CT findings are similar to those of left-sided diverticulitis, including pericolonic inflammation, bowel wall thickening, and pericolic fluid or abscess. The presence of other diverticula or a normal-appearing appendix should strongly suggest the diagnosis. Although surgery is more commonly employed for the treatment of right-sided diverticulitis (often because of misdiagnosis), it is amenable to conservative antibiotic treatment.

Notes

Backwash Ileitis

1. Ileitis in ulcerative colitis and rarely infectious colitides.

2. Yes. It can develop granular mucosal–type ulcerations similar to those seen in the colon.

3. Usually, nothing; it remains the same.

4. Amebiasis does not affect the terminal ileum.

Reference

Caroline DF, Evers K: Colitis: radiographic features and differentiation of idiopathic inflammatory bowel disease, *Radiol Clin North Am* 25:47-66, 1987.

Cross-Reference

Gastrointestinal Radiology: THE REQUISITES, ed 2, p 115.

Comment

The appearance of the terminal ileum is a critical component in the evaluation of the different inflammatory conditions affecting the colon and the ileum. Often the appearance of this structure may help distinguish the idiopathic inflammatory bowel diseases and the infectious colitides from one another. Typically, Crohn's disease causes a progressive narrowing of the lumen of the terminal ileum. Early in the disease, the lumen may be of normal caliber and may demonstrate scattered (aphthous) ulceration. As the disease progresses and mural thickening develops, the lumen narrows. Infectious ileitis can cause variable changes in the diameter of the terminal ileum. Tuberculosis mimics Crohn's disease and causes narrowing. Patients with ileitis caused by *Yersinia* species typically have a normal-caliber terminal ileum. Rarely an infectious ileitis has been known to cause mild dilation. Some types of ileitis, such as amebiasis, spare the ileum, and this is an important differential point.

Ulcerative colitis typically affects only the colon, with no small bowel involvement. However, in patients with active pancolitis, particularly if it is severe, a condition known as *backwash ileitis* develops. This condition, which occurs in up to 40% of patients with pan-ulcerative colitis, is brought on by the loss of integrity of the ileocecal valve, causing reflux of bowel contents back into the terminal ileum (thus the term *backwash* or *reflux ileitis*). The lumen actually dilates, often considerably compared with other types of ileal inflammation. The ileum develops ulceration, usually with a fine, granular type of appearance on barium studies. Postinflammatory polyps can even develop in the ileum. Typically the backwash ileitis persists for several weeks during the most severe phases of the pancolitis and then subsides. The dilation may persist, however, particularly if there is a patulous ileocecal valve as a result of foreshortening of the colon.

Notes

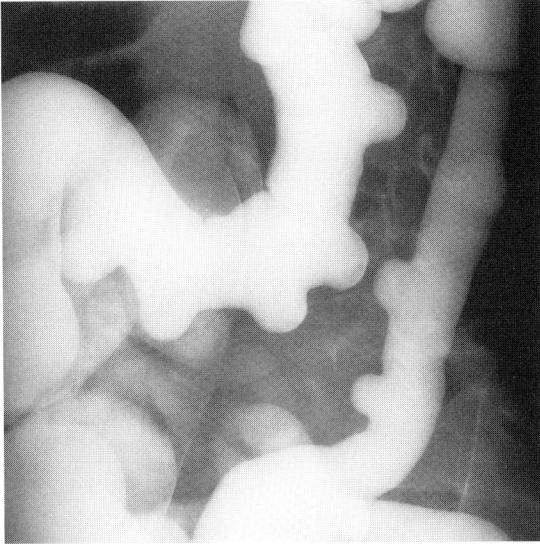

1. Name some disorders that may produce this appearance.
2. What is the difference between true diverticula and pseudodiverticula?
3. What disorders produce wide-mouth diverticula (pseudosacculations)?
4. What may develop within these diverticula?

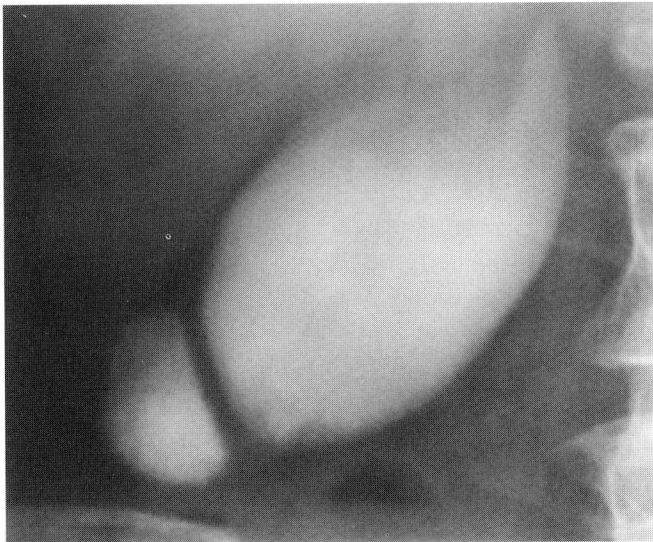

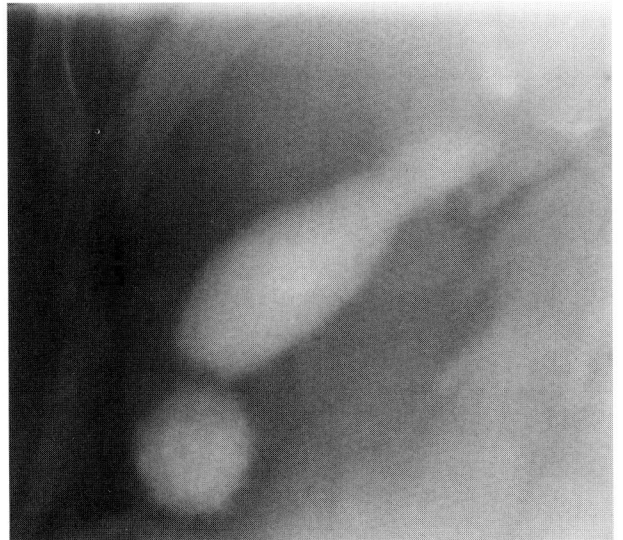

1. What is this condition called?
2. What is the underlying pathologic change?
3. Are there any long-term complications of this condition?
4. Name other conditions that may have a similar appearance on ultrasound.

Scleroderma of the Colon

1. Chronic colitis, laxative abuse, scleroderma, previous ischemia, and radiation.

2. True diverticula have all three layers of bowel wall. These large pseudosacculations are actually true diverticula.

3. Scleroderma, Crohn's disease, and ischemia.

4. Fecaliths, resembling tumors.

Reference

Plavsic BM, Raider L, Drnovesek VH, et al: Association of rectal diverticula and scleroderma, *Acta Radiol* 36:96-99, 1995.

Cross-Reference

Gastrointestinal Radiology: THE REQUISITES, ed 2, p 279.

Comment

The presence of large wide-mouth diverticula or sacculations in the colon can be an indication of several diseases. Many term these wide-mouth diverticula *pseudodiverticula* because they are not related to the typical diverticula seen in everyday practice. However, they contain all three layers of bowel and thus represent true diverticula. The small diverticula seen in everyday practice are not "true" diverticula. These large-mouth diverticula or sacculations occur when there is eccentric involvement of the bowel wall by some process, producing fibrosis on one side, with eccentric bulging of the opposite wall. A variety of processes can result in the loss of the haustral folds, but only some produce the eccentric diverticula. These processes include scleroderma, Crohn's disease, laxative abuse, and ischemia.

Scleroderma does not involve the colon as frequently as it does other portions of the gastrointestinal tract. Just as it does in other portions of the gastrointestinal tract, however, scleroderma of the colon produces patchy smooth muscle atrophy along with fibrotic replacement of the muscle. This effect leads to the formation of wide-mouth sacculations at weakened areas. There are also abnormalities of transit time, and patients often complain of constipation. The haustral fold pattern is often diminished. Fecal impaction is a complication, and patients often develop benign pneumatosis, which could be the result of a combination of steroid therapy and stasis in the colon. An interesting feature of these wide-mouth sacculations is their ability to retain material. They fail to contract and empty and are found outside the fecal stream in the colon. Thus these sacculations sometimes develop impacted fecal material or fecaliths within them. These fecaliths can become adherent and resemble polyps or tumors on barium enema studies. Colonoscopy is necessary to make the diagnosis.

Notes

Adenomyomatosis of the Gallbladder

1. Adenomyomatosis.

2. Proliferation of the smooth muscle and infolding of the mucosa.

3. No.

4. Chronic cholecystitis, cholesterolosis, and gallbladder carcinoma.

Reference

Berk RN, van der Vegt JH, Lichtenstein JE: The hyperplastic cholecystoses: cholesterolosis and adenomyomatosis, *Radiology* 146:593-602, 1983.

Cross-Reference

Gastrointestinal Radiology: THE REQUISITES, ed 2, p 224.

Comment

Two conditions—adenomyomatosis and cholesterolosis—are grouped together as the hyperplastic cholecystoses. These conditions are not pathologically or physiologically related in any way, but both produce an abnormal thickening of the gallbladder wall. In adenomyomatosis there is abnormal thickening of the smooth muscle layer of the gallbladder, which results in exaggerated infolding of the mucosal folds and epithelium. Sometimes the epithelium becomes surrounded by the muscle layers and forms cysts. The exact reason that this condition develops is uncertain. Adenomyomatosis is unusual in that frequently only portions of the gallbladder wall become involved; other gallbladder conditions usually involve the entire gallbladder.

On contrast examinations of the gallbladder, these infoldings of the mucosal surface trap contrast and appear as tiny diverticula-like projections in the wall. They become particularly pronounced when there is contraction of the gallbladder wall. If the proliferation is severe, there can be narrowing or deformity of the gallbladder lumen. A thickened gallbladder wall can be demonstrated on CT examination. If this thickening is focal, it may be impossible to distinguish the condition from gallbladder carcinoma. Thickening of the wall of the gallbladder also is apparent on ultrasound examination. Ring-down artifacts may be evident on the nondependent wall of the gallbladder. The wall of the gallbladder also may appear nodular or may appear to contain small polyps. Unlike other gallbladder conditions, there is little associated morbidity with adenomyomatosis, and there are no known long-term complications.

Notes

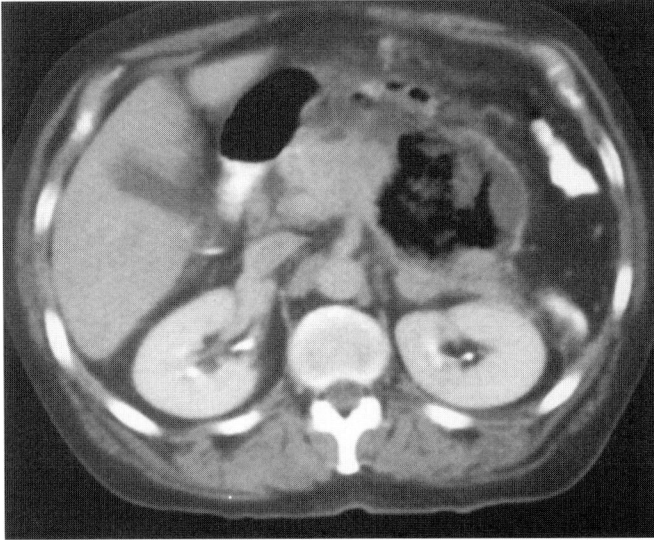

1. What pancreatic fluid collections may contain air?
2. How often is air present in pancreatic abscesses?
3. What is the density difference between an abscess and a pseudocyst?
4. When do pancreatic abscesses develop?

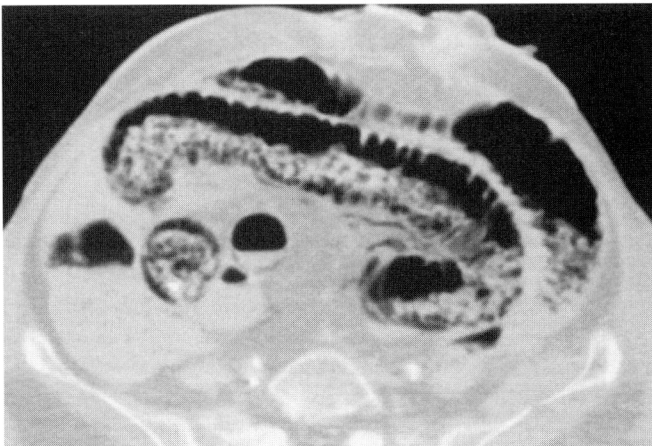

1. Where are these gas collections located in the bowel wall?
2. What collagen vascular disease may cause this condition?
3. List some pulmonary conditions associated with this condition.
4. What type of medication is believed to be strongly associated with this condition?

Pancreatic Abscess

1. Abscesses and communicating pseudocysts.

2. Around 20% of the time.

3. Abscess has higher density on CT (about 20 to 50 HU).

4. Usually within several days to weeks of an episode of acute pancreatitis.

Reference
Ros PR, Hamrick-Turner JE, Chiechi MV, et al: Cystic masses of the pancreas, *Radiographics* 12:673-686, 1992.

Cross-Reference
Gastrointestinal Radiology: THE REQUISITES, ed 2, p 151.

Comment
The presence of fluid collections and necrotic debris associated with acute pancreatitis represents an opportunity for infection to develop in the region. When bacteria gain access to the fluid collections, the potential for abscess development is significant. An abscess complicating acute pancreatitis is a very significant problem and was once a significant source of mortality in these patients. Abscesses probably occur in less than 10% of patients with acute pancreatitis. However, this complication must be rapidly diagnosed to prevent significant morbidity and mortality. Typically, abscesses develop within several days to weeks after an episode of acute pancreatitis. Those patients who develop this complication usually have a worsening of their symptoms. Of course, fever and abdominal pain often accompany the infection.

Computed tomography remains the primary modality for the evaluation of this complication. Abscesses appear as poorly defined fluid collections and may be difficult to distinguish from phlegmon. They are typically more dense than the fluid seen in pancreatic pseudocysts, which usually develop later anyway. The presence of air within a fluid collection has always been considered a pathonomonic sign of the development of an abscess or an infection. However, sometimes air is seen in fluid collections or pseudocysts that develop communication to the intestinal tract. Yet, whenever air is seen in peripancreatic fluid collections, the possibility of abscess must be strongly considered. Air is visible within abscesses approximately 20% of the time. Another indication of abscess complication is a poorly defined, thick-walled fluid collection persisting several weeks after the initial episode. Sometimes there is enhancement of the periphery of the fluid collection.

Notes

Pneumatosis of the Bowel

1. Usually subserosa, then submucosa.

2. Scleroderma, systemic lupus erythematosus, and dermatomyositis.

3. Asthma, chronic obstructive pulmonary disease, and cystic fibrosis.

4. Steroids.

Reference
Feczko PJ, Mezwa DG, Farah MC, White BD: Clinical significance of pneumatosis of the bowel wall, *Radiographics* 12:1069-1078, 1992.

Cross-Reference
Gastrointestinal Radiology: THE REQUISITES, ed 2, p 302.

Comment
Pneumatosis of the bowel describes a condition in which air collects in the layers of the wall of the bowel. Histologically the collections usually are found in the subserosa, with the submucosal layer being less commonly involved. There are many causes for this condition, and there are also several theories regarding its development. The most plausible theory is that the condition is bacterial in origin, based on the facts that the air cysts contain hydrogen gas, which is a byproduct of anaerobic bacteria, and hyperbaric oxygen often resolves the condition. However, for the bacteria to gain access to the bowel wall, there must be some disruption of the mucosal integrity, and the conditions in the bowel wall must be such that the anaerobes will grow.

Numerous conditions have been associated with the development of pneumatosis, despite the fact that there may be no known (idiopathic) etiology. Ischemia is a very common cause. Inflammatory conditions, such as necrotizing enterocolitis; pseudomembranous colitis; Crohn's disease; and even infectious agents also are known to produce pneumatosis. It often affects individuals who take steroids. Patients with collagen vascular diseases, such as scleroderma, may develop pneumatosis. Also, obstruction, trauma, prior endoscopy, malignancies, chemotherapy, and organ transplantation are associated with the development of pneumatosis.

The radiologic appearance may be one of multiple bullae or air cysts or may be linear in nature. The appearance does not have any particular significance. Overall, location and distribution are not helpful in prognosis. Pneumoperitoneum sometimes develops in association with the pneumatosis, but this may be a benign finding, a so-called balanced pneumoperitoneum. Portal venous gas in a patient with pneumatosis often indicates the presence of bowel necrosis, and this is probably the most significant associated finding.

Notes

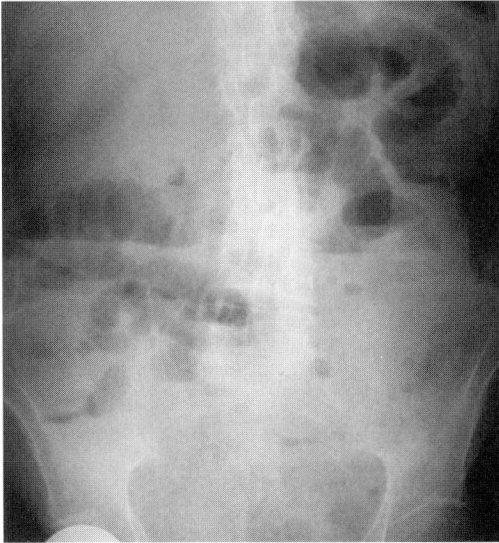

1. What is this condition called?
2. What are the three radiographic features associated with this condition?
3. Where does the stone most often have an impact?
4. What is necessary for the condition to develop?

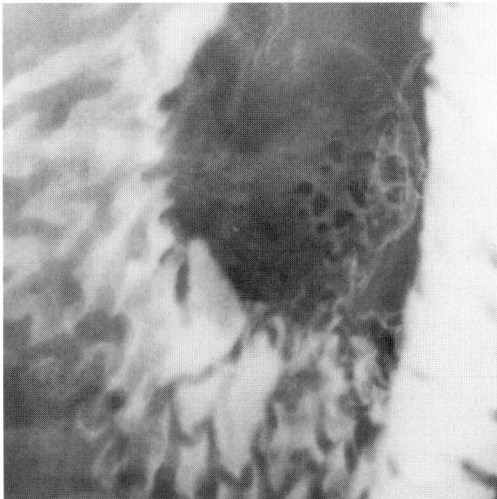

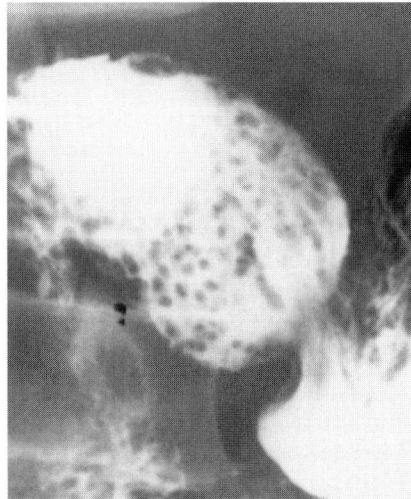

1. What causes benign lymphoid hyperplasia of the duodenum?
2. Approximately what percentage of people have heterotopic gastric mucosa in the duodenal bulbs?
3. What may occur as a response to increased acidity in the duodenal bulb?
4. Where do most benign duodenal tumors occur?

Gallstone Ileus

1. Gallstone ileus.

2. Gallstone in the bowel, small bowel dilation, and air in the biliary system.

3. Terminal ileum.

4. Cholecystenteric fistula must develop.

Reference

Weltman DI, Zeman RK: Acute diseases of the gallbladder and biliary ducts, *Radiol Clin North Am* 32:933-950, 1994.

Cross-Reference

Gastrointestinal Radiology: THE REQUISITES, ed 2, p 229.

Comment

The term *gallstone ileus* refers to an unusual set of circumstances that develop in conjunction with chronic gallbladder disease and stone formation. In this condition a large gallstone or gallstones develop. There must also be associated chronic cholecystitis. During this inflammation, a portion of the bowel becomes adherent to the gallbladder, which is actually a common occurrence in patients with chronic gallbladder inflammation. With time, the gallstone erodes through the gallbladder wall and into the lumen of the bowel, resulting in a cholecystenteric fistula. The fistula most commonly extends into the duodenum, but extension into the colon and even the stomach also has been reported. As the large gallstone travels through the bowel lumen, it becomes impacted at a site where the lumen narrows, resulting in bowel dilation or obstruction.

The classic triad in this condition consists of air in the biliary system, bowel obstruction, and a radiopaque stone evident in the abdomen. The biliary air is secondary to the fistula that is now present between the gallbladder and bowel. Often, the amount of air is quite small. The stone is the most difficult finding to establish because of the bowel dilation. If it is not obscured by the contrast material, the stone often can be demonstrated on CT. Finally, the bowel obstruction usually occurs in the terminal ileum at the ileocecal valve. Less commonly the stone obstructs the third portion of the duodenum, or the sigmoid colon. Only rarely (probably less than a third of the time) is the entire triad of radiologic findings present. Any time two of the entities are visible, the diagnosis of gallstone ileus should be considered.

Notes

Heterotopic Gastric Mucosa and Brunner's Gland Hyperplasia

1. Unknown. Although sometimes it may occur in conditions such as hypogammaglobulinemia.

2. Some authors claim as many as 20%.

3. Brunner's gland hyperplasia.

4. Proximal half of the duodenum.

Reference

Valls C, Lopez-Calonge E, Guma A: Polypoid heterotopic gastric mucosa of the duodenum, *Eur Radiol* 5:553, 1995.

Cross-Reference

Gastrointestinal Radiology: THE REQUISITES, ed 2, p 89.

Comment

It is not uncommon to encounter nodular filling defects within the duodenal bulb. These may be solitary or multiple and of variable size. Certain distinguishing features may help differentiate the conditions that are known to produce this radiologic appearance.

Heterotopic gastric mucosa in the duodenal bulb occurs more frequently than most radiologists recognize, occurring in up to 20% of patients in pathologic series but encountered in less than 1% of patients in radiologic series. The radiologic appearance is that of slightly elevated lesions measuring only a few millimeters in diameter and often clustered in only a segment of the duodenal bulb. A distinguishing feature is their sometimes angulated or plaquelike margins. These lesions are believed to have no clinical significance. Benign lymphoid hyperplasia of the bulb and proximal duodenum is characterized by multiple tiny (1- to 2-mm) smooth filling defects, which are usually diffuse throughout the region. Often there is no known reason for their appearance, but they occur more frequently in patients with decreased immune competence, such as those with hypogammaglobulinemia or agammaglobulinemia. Brunner's gland hyperplasia has a different radiologic appearance than the two aforementioned entities. The filling defects in this condition are larger, often ranging up to 1 cm. These lesions are smooth and diffuse, often producing a cobblestone appearance. They may be associated with hyperacidity, although this belief is controversial.

Benign tumors of the duodenum, such as leiomyomas, adenomas, and neurofibromas, occur more frequently in the proximal duodenum, particularly the duodenal bulb. Also, polyposis syndromes, such as Peutz-Jeghers, Cronkhite-Canada, and familial polyposis, are known to cause multiple polyps in the duodenum.

Notes

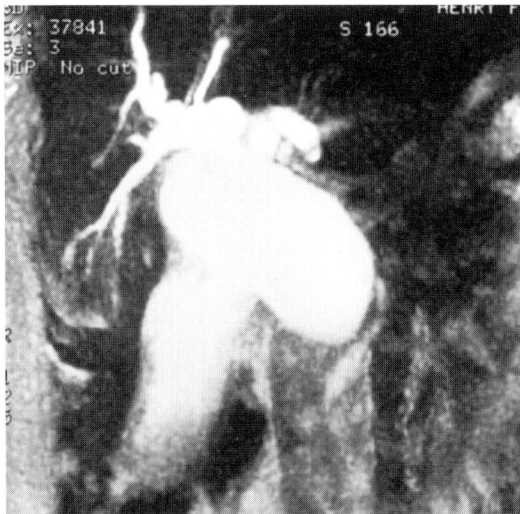

1. What is the most likely diagnosis?
2. What is the supposed etiology for this condition?
3. What is a long-term complication?
4. Which gender is affected more commonly?

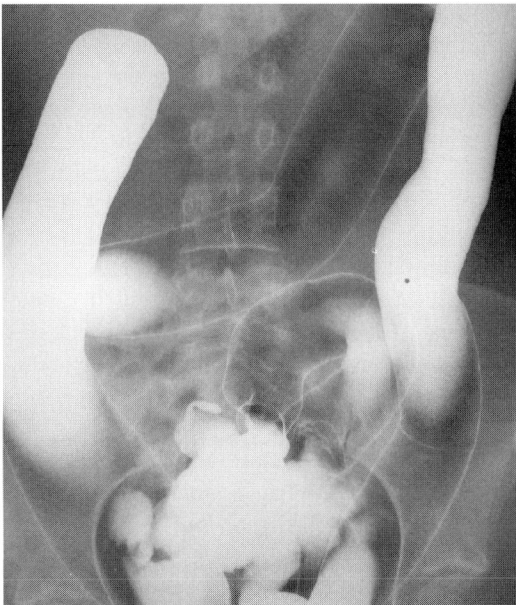

1. What conditions may result in loss of the haustral folds of the colon?
2. Do the haustral folds return to normal as ulcerative colitis heals?
3. What is the incidence of rectal sparing in ulcerative colitis?
4. What type of ulceration is present in Crohn's disease but not in ulcerative colitis?

CASE 43

Choledochal Cyst

1. Choledochal cyst.

2. Anomalous junction between the bile and pancreatic ducts.

3. Cholangiocarcinoma.

4. Female.

Reference
Kim OH, Chung HJ, Choi BG: Imaging of the choledochal cyst, *Radiographics* 15:69-88, 1995.

Cross-Reference
Gastrointestinal Radiology: THE REQUISITES, ed 2, p 208.

Comment
Cystic dilation of the bile ducts is a congenital abnormality with serious consequences. There are several types, and categories have been developed for these biliary cysts or ectasia, commonly termed *choledochal cysts.* The most common type is cystic dilation of the extrahepatic bile ducts (type I). This cystic dilation may be small and focal or may extend for some length, involving both common and hepatic ducts. The condition is proposed to begin development in a long common segment of duct where the bile and pancreatic ducts join together in the head of the pancreas. This joint allows reflux of pancreatic enzymes into the bile ducts, producing weakness of the wall and eventual dilation. Unfortunately, few of the patients with choledochal cyst have this anomaly. Choledochal cysts occur three to four times more often in women.

Clinically, patients develop jaundice of varying degrees, pain in the right upper quadrant, and a palpable right upper quadrant mass. Most patients develop some of these symptoms in childhood, and the majority are diagnosed as infants and children. However, many patients may live to adulthood before this condition is diagnosed. Ultrasound, CT, hepatobiliary scans, or direct injection of the ducts can all demonstrate this anomaly.

There is often an association with other bile duct anomalies. Also, patients are prone to development of infection and calculus formation. Some who have associated hepatic fibrosis may progress to cirrhosis and portal hypertension. The best known complication is that of cholangiocarcinoma, which develops after many years. Surgery is the only known therapeutic approach, but the decision to operate is dependent on the size and number of complications.

Notes

CASE 44

Chronic Ulcerative Colitis

1. Most types of colitis, laxative abuse, and scleroderma.

2. Yes.

3. Generally less than 5%.

4. Aphthous ulceration.

Reference
Caroline DF, Evers K: Colitis: radiographic features and differentiation of idiopathic inflammatory bowel disease, *Radiol Clin North Am* 25:47-66, 1987.

Cross-Reference
Gastrointestinal Radiology: THE REQUISITES, ed 2, p 279.

Comment
The colon has only a limited number of ways to manifest inflammation, and ulceration and foreshortening of the bowel are the results of several of the inflammatory conditions of the colon. Ulcerative colitis typically results in a granular type of appearance of the mucosa, which is caused by hyperemia and edema of the mucosa in the early phases of inflammation. Also, the decrease in the amount of mucus produced by the mucosa, which commonly occurs in many inflammatory conditions, affects mucosal coating with barium, producing this granular appearance. Any type of inflammation may produce this change.

Loss of the normal haustral fold pattern is a hallmark of many colitides. Early in the inflammation, the folds become edematous and thickened. Later, there is complete loss of the haustra. Haustral folds are the result of the discrepancy between the circular muscle and taenia coli or longitudinal muscle bands. In ulcerative colitis these haustra are lost because of alterations in the taenia coli (longitudinal fibers), which for some reason become relaxed. At the same time, there is hypertrophy of the muscularis mucosa, which also becomes contracted and fixed, producing foreshortening. Interestingly, as the inflammation subsides, these muscular changes revert, and the haustra reappear. In contrast, in Crohn's disease, strictures and loss of haustra are the result of inflammation and fibrosis. The fibrosis maintains the stricturing even after the active inflammation subsides.

Chronic laxative abuse may produce similar changes in the colon and is considered predominantly a muscular phenomenon, not unlike ulcerative colitis. Scleroderma of the colon also causes loss of the haustral pattern, but it is related to fibrotic changes in the wall of the bowel and is not a muscular change.

Notes

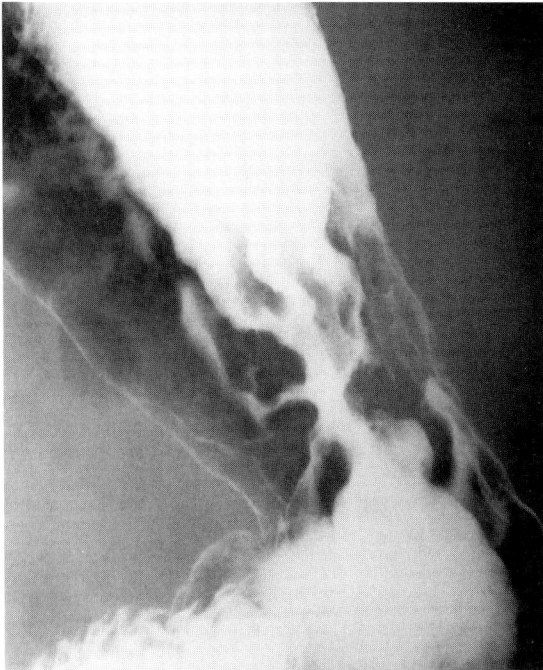

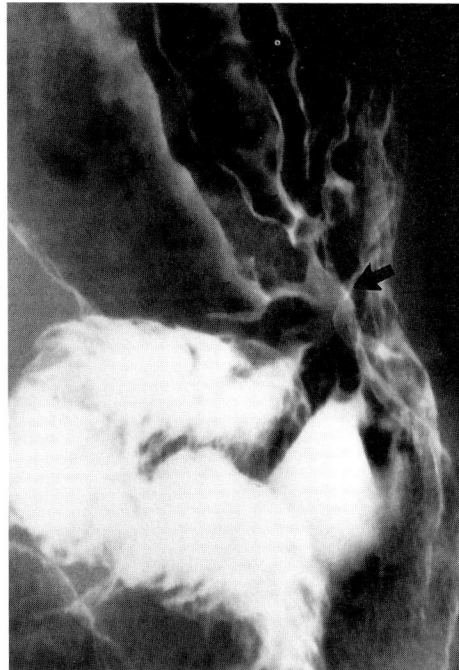

1. In what part of the stomach are gastric ulcers predominantly malignant?
2. What is the significance of a linear configuration of a gastric ulcer?
3. What are the features of a Kirklin complex, and what does it signify?
4. Where do most malignant ulcers occur?

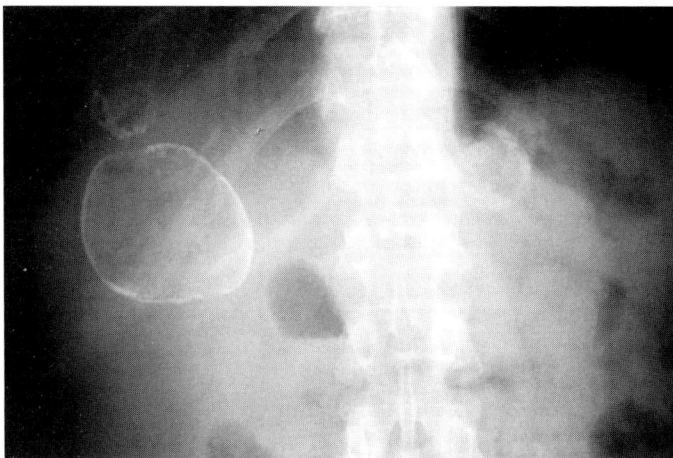

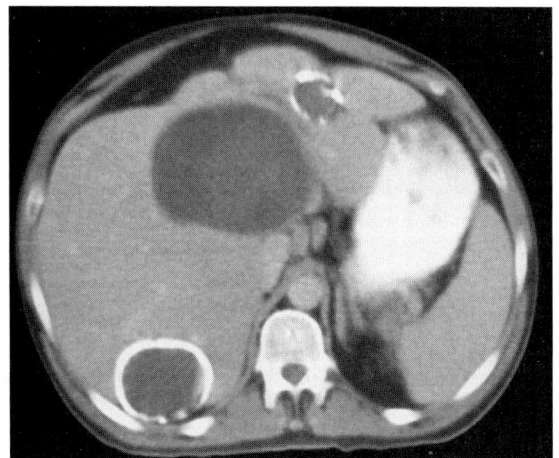

1. Which cystic structures of the liver calcify?
2. What organisms produce this disease?
3. Where do these cysts spontaneously drain?
4. Can these cysts be drained percutaneously?

Malignant Gastric Ulcer

1. Fundus.

2. Linear ulcers are typically benign and often develop this configuration during healing.

3. Barium fills the ulcer crater, and there is a mound of soft tissue surrounding the ulcer. This complex typically is seen with malignant ulcers.

4. Antrum.

Reference

Levine MS: Erosive gastritis and gastric ulcers, *Radiol Clin North Am* 32:1203-1214, 1994.

Cross-Reference

Gastrointestinal Radiology: THE REQUISITES, ed 2, p 77.

Comment

With the advent of double-contrast radiography, there has been an increased emphasis on the detection of early neoplasm of the stomach based on subtle radiologic signs. Double-contrast radiography can demonstrate subtle changes in the folds about the ulcer and reveal mucosal irregularities.

The antrum is a very common location for ulcerous disease of the stomach. The majority of these ulcers are benign, often the sequela of ingestion of antiinflammatory drugs. However, the antrum is still the most common area for malignant ulcers of the stomach. Interestingly, ulcers in the fundus are exceedingly uncommon, and the majority of these are malignant. A number of features indicate that an ulcer may be malignant rather than benign. Evaluation of the fold pattern is of extreme importance. Folds about a benign ulcer are typically smooth and of decreasing size. Malignant folds may be irregular in outline and may be clubbed (become larger or bulbous as they approach the ulcer crater). The folds of both benign and malignant ulcers may stop short of the crater. Benign ulcers are typically round or linear, whereas malignant ulcers may be irregular in outline.

Some of the classic signs of malignant ulceration are Carman's sign and Kirklin complex. This description applies to ulcers in the distal stomach, which can be compressed radiologically during fluoroscopy. Upon compression, the heaped-up margins of the ulcer encircle a collection of contrast within the ulcer crater. The entrapped barium has a crescentic shape. If the inner margin is convex toward the lumen, the ulcer is malignant. Benign ulcers have their margin toward the lumen concave, the "crescent" sign. The Kirklin complex consists of the barium-entrapped ulcer crater along with a heaped-up mound of tissue about the ulcer margin, creating an irregular lucent halo about the ulcer.

Notes

Echinococcal Cyst (Hydatid Disease)

1. Echinococcal cysts and sometimes simple liver cysts.

2. *Echinococcus granulosis* and *Echinococcus multilocularis.*

3. Biliary system and rarely the peritoneal, pleural, or pericardial region.

4. Yes.

Reference

Murphy BJ, Casillas J, Ros PR, et al: The CT appearance of cystic masses of the liver, *Radiographics* 9:307-322, 1989.

Cross-Reference

Gastrointestinal Radiology: THE REQUISITES, ed 2, p 201.

Comment

Echinococcal cysts are produced by two types of tapeworms—*E. granulosus* and *E. multilocularis. E. granulosus* is the species most commonly seen in North America. These tapeworms live in the intestinal tract in dogs. Humans and more commonly sheep are intermediate hosts, harboring the parasite in its larval stage. Humans contract the parasite by eating contaminated food, such as unwashed vegetables, or through contact with an infected dog or sheep. When the eggs of the parasite are ingested, they penetrate the mucosa of the intestine and then are carried via the portal vein to the liver. Sometimes the lungs, spleen, and kidneys are involved as well. The embryos then develop in a hydatid stage in which they form cysts in the liver. The life cycle is completed when the intermediate host dies and is consumed by the final host.

Hydatid cysts consist of three layers. The outer pericyst is a rigid fibrous structure that is vascular and may enhance on CT. There is an intermediate layer, and finally the inner layer or endocyst is the living parasite. These cysts represent the larval stage, and there are often multiple small cysts seen within the larger cyst. Debris produced by brood capsules may be visible on the dependent portion of the cysts. Most cysts cause no symptoms until they are large enough to produce pressure on adjacent structures. Approximately 20% to 30% of the cysts calcify, which is much higher than the percentage of simple hepatic cysts that calcify. Sometimes the cysts spontaneously rupture into the biliary system or the peritoneal, pleural, or pericardial surfaces. Symptoms vary, but this complication can produce cholangitis or inflammation of the structures it comes in contact with. A fatal anaphylactic reaction is also possible.

Hydatid cysts must be drained for treatment. Surgery was once considered necessary for treatment of this condition because of the possibility of anaphylactic reaction if the cyst drained into the peritoneum. However, it is now recognized that these cysts can be managed by percutaneous catheter drainage and instillation of scolecoidal agents.

Notes

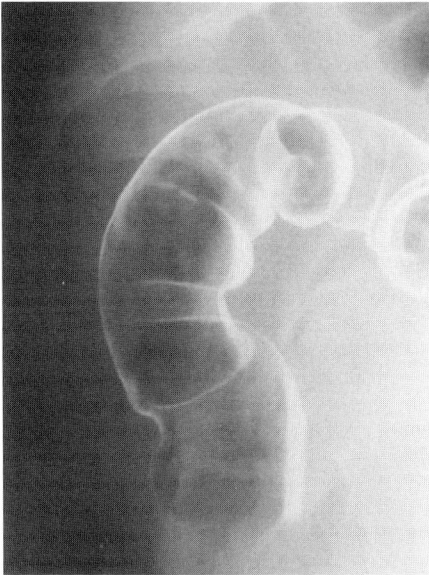

1. What is the normal width of the rectal valves (valves of Houston)?
2. What is the significance of their absence?
3. How often is the rectum spared in ulcerative colitis?
4. What is the distance of a normal presacral space?

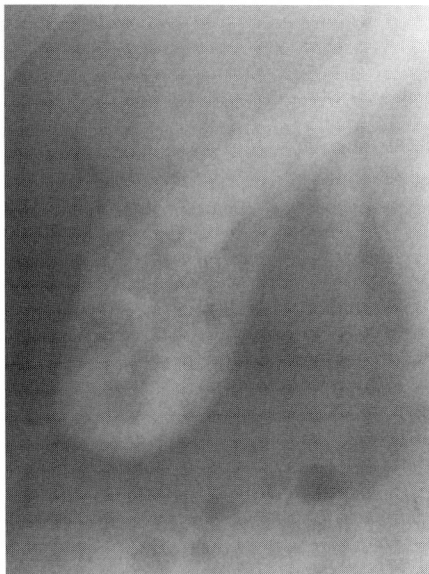

1. What may produce multiple mural lesions of the gallbladder?
2. What is the most common type of gallbladder polyp?
3. What tumors may produce mural nodules?
4. What benign condition can produce nodularity of the wall of the gallbladder?

C A S E 4 7

Nonspecific Proctitis

1. 5 mm or less. Width in excess of 7 mm is usually abnormal.

2. Nothing. They may be absent in healthy people.

3. Approximately 5% of the time.

4. Less than 2 cm, measured at S4.

Reference
Russell JGB, Donoghue V: Rectal fold thickness as an indicator of disease, *Clin Radiol* 34:427-431, 1983.

Cross-Reference
Gastrointestinal Radiology: THE REQUISITES, ed 2, p 260.

Comment
Inflammation of the rectum can be caused by a variety of conditions. The most common cause is idiopathic ulcerative colitis. Almost all patients with ulcerative colitis have rectal inflammation, with rectal sparing occurring in a small minority (5%) of cases. Sometimes the inflammation is confined to the rectum, a so-called nonspecific proctitis. Crohn's disease frequently involves the rectum as well, although its appearance is different from that of nonspecific proctitis. Other diseases that may mimic this condition include infectious proctitis, particularly as seen in patients with acquired immunodeficiency syndrome, and radiation proctitis.

The radiologic findings in patients with proctitis can be quite subtle. In this patient the valves of Houston (rectal valves) are slightly thickened and indistinct. The rectal valves usually measure 5 mm or less on the cross-table lateral view. Anything in excess of 7 mm is typically considered abnormal, and a careful evaluation to determine the possible cause should be considered. Also, rectal valves are typically sharply defined, and the barium should not have a hazy or indistinct margin. This type of margin is usually indicative of edema and mucosal inflammation. Another area that should be considered in the evaluation of possible proctitis is the presacral space. This space is measured at the S4-S5 level and measures 2 cm or less in healthy individuals. Numerous conditions can produce widening of this space, but rectal inflammation of some type is one of the most common causes. Usually the presacral widening occurs with more severe inflammatory changes. Other features, such as granularity of the mucosa caused by ulceration, are more specific to proctitis but may not always be present.

Notes

C A S E 4 8

Gallbladder Polyps

1. Polyps, adherent stones, metastases, adenomyomatosis, and blood clots.

2. Cholesterol.

3. Metastases.

4. Adenomyomatosis.

Reference
Rosenthal SJ, Cox GG, Wetzel LH, et al: Pitfalls and differential diagnosis in biliary sonography, *Radiographics* 10:285-311, 1990.

Cross-Reference
Gastrointestinal Radiology: THE REQUISITES, ed 2, p 221.

Comment
Although calculi are by far the most common cause of filling defects within the gallbladder, several noncalculous lesions can produce filling defects within the gallbladder lumen. One of the more common noncalculous causes is a gallbladder polyp. Polyps in the gallbladder produce echogenic filling defects within the lumen but are fixed, often along the nondependent surface of the gallbladder. They do not move with changes in position. Polyps of the gallbladder, particularly when they are multiple, are most often cholesterol polyps. The patient with multiple cholesterol polyps is considered to have a type of cholesterolosis. If the polyp is solitary, it could be cholesterol, an adenoma, or a papilloma.

Rarely, other conditions produce multiple mural nodules or protrusions that simulate gallbladder polyps. Adenomyomatosis with prominence of the Rokitansky-Aschoff sinuses sometimes results in some mural nodularity. Adherent stones may also produce polyplike lesions that can be difficult to differentiate from true polyps. Metastases are quite uncommon in the gallbladder, but when they occur, they can produce mural polyps. Melanoma, breast cancer, or lymphoma infiltrating the gallbladder can cause gallbladder metastases. Primary gallbladder carcinoma can result in the formation of a solitary polypoid lesion but rarely results in multiple mural polyps. Potentially, blood clots, hemorrhage, or even varices could produce mural polyps or nodularity, but this is quite uncommon.

Notes

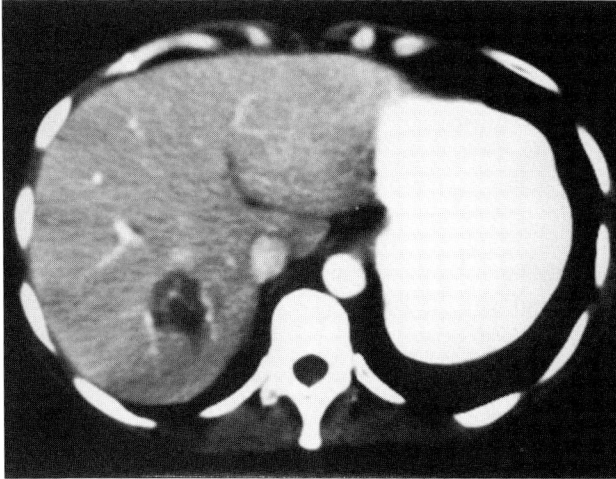

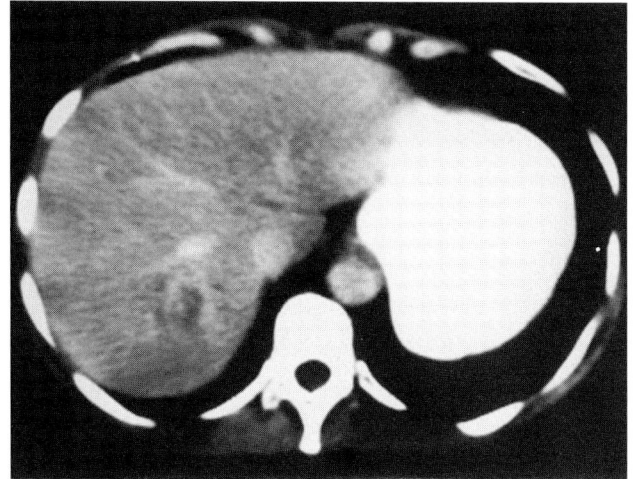

1. What is the most likely diagnosis?
2. What percentage of these lesions calcify?
3. What type of activity does this lesion have on a nuclear sulfur-colloid scan?
4. What type of activity is seen on a tagged red blood cell scan?

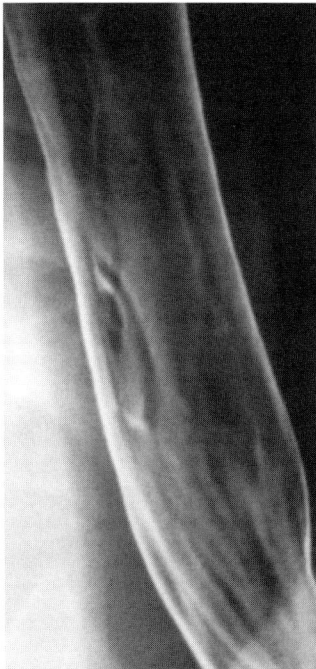

1. In an immune-compromised patient, what is the most likely diagnosis?
2. What disease entities produce this type of esophageal ulceration?
3. What small bowel disease can be associated with this type of esophageal ulceration?
4. Name several groups of medications that produce esophageal ulcerations.

Liver Hemangioma

1. Hemangioma of the liver.

2. Less than 10%.

3. None. Produces a cold defect.

4. Defect in the early phase, with increasing and prolonged activity over time.

Reference
Freeny PC, Marks WM: Hepatic hemangioma: dynamic bolus CT, *Am J Roentgenol* 147:711-719, 1986.

Cross-Reference
Gastrointestinal Radiology: THE REQUISITES, ed 2, p 169.

Comment
Hemangiomas of the liver are the most common benign neoplastic tumors of the liver. There are two types of hemangiomas—capillary and cavernous. It is thought that these tumors affect 2% to 5% of the population. They are more common in women and occur most frequently in the right lobe of the liver. Multiple hemangiomas occur in 10% to 15% of patients. By themselves, hemangiomas are rarely symptomatic and are of no consequence to the patient. Their importance lies more in the fact that their appearance can mimic that of more sinister conditions of the liver, such as metastases or malignant tumors.

Most discussions regarding hemangiomas concern the diagnostic tests that may help distinguish them from other lesions. Dynamic scanning of the liver by CT is quite helpful. In this case, initial CT scans show the hemangioma to be a low density lesion in the liver. Delayed images of the lesion over the next several minutes demonstrate increasing opacification of the hemangioma from the periphery toward the center, the so-called centripetal opacification. However, not all cavernous hemangiomas show the classic findings, and often other studies are required. Ultrasound often shows a well-defined echogenic lesion, although the findings are not always pathognomonic. MRI is often useful because hemangiomas have a high signal intensity on T2W images, but cysts and even some metastatic lesions may have a similar appearance. Radionuclide scanning is quite helpful for evaluating the liver hemangioma. On tagged red blood cell studies the hemangioma typically appears as a cold defect during the early scans, but in later images the lesion fills in and actually has increased activity on delayed images. With all these imaging studies, the most difficulty is encountered when the hemangioma has a central area of necrosis or fibrosis, which can mimic other lesions.

Notes

Herpetic Esophagitis

1. Viral esophagitis, usually caused by herpesvirus or cytomegalovirus.

2. Viral esophagitis, Crohn's disease, and medication-induced ulcers.

3. Crohn's disease.

4. Antibiotics (tetracycline), nonsteroidal antiinflammatory drugs (aspirin), potassium chloride tablets (when taken by patients with cardiac disease), and ascorbic acid.

Reference
Yee J, Wall SD: Infectious esophagitis, *Radiol Clin North Am* 32:1135-1146, 1994.

Cross-Reference
Gastrointestinal Radiology: THE REQUISITES, ed 2, p 14.

Comment
The presence of discrete ulcers on a background of normal mucosa separates this type of ulceration from the numerous other causes of esophageal ulceration, the most common of which is reflux esophagitis. In an immune-compromised patient the most likely diagnoses are Candida esophagitis, which is the most frequent, and a viral esophagitis. Candida esophagitis typically produces a more diffuse and fine ulceration with associated plaques, which results in a shaggy-looking mucosa. Viral esophagitis also may be diffuse but produces focal, aphthous ulceration in the esophagus as well. It is impossible to determine the type of viral agent that is to blame based solely on the appearance of the ulcer; herpesvirus, cytomegalovirus, and even human immunodeficiency virus must be considered.

Crohn's disease classically produces aphthous ulceration of the gastrointestinal tract. However, it also can produce this aphthous type of ulceration in the esophagus, as shown here, along with linear ulceration and sinus tracts in the wall. Another common entity that must be considered is medication-induced esophagitis, which can have a similar appearance. In younger patients this type of esophagitis is usually the result of tetracycline taken to treat acne, whereas in older patients this injury is usually the result of the ingestion of potassium chloride tablets for heart disease or antiinflammatory drugs for arthritic pain.

Notes

Fair Game Cases

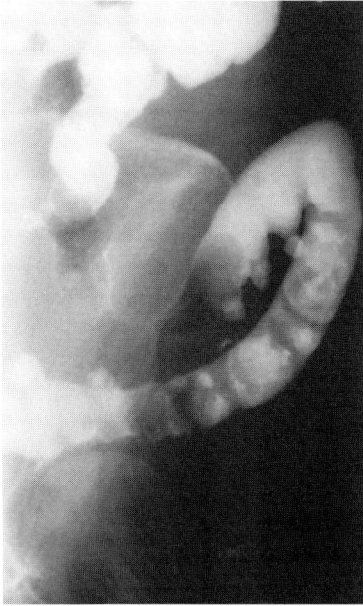

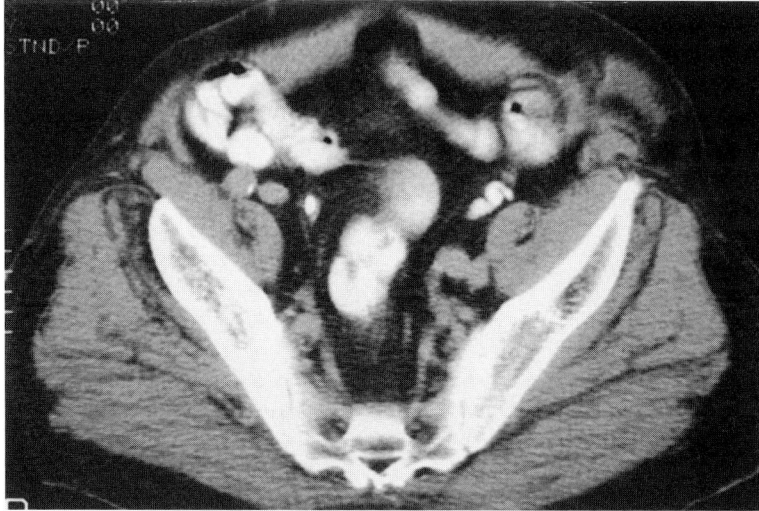

1. Through which anatomic area does this hernia pass?
2. What is meant by the term *Richter's hernia?*
3. What is the most common type of abdominal wall hernia in adults?
4. Name a type of hernia that contains a Meckel's diverticulum.

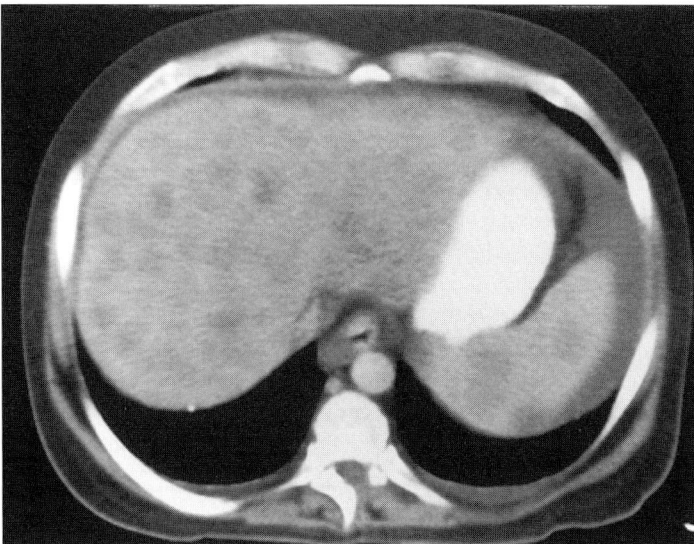

1. Name some diagnostic possibilities.
2. How often does lymphomatous involvement of the spleen appear in CT examinations?
3. What common clinical conditions have a high incidence of lymphoma as a complication?
4. What role does MRI have in staging splenic lymphoma?
5. How often does lymphoma of the liver appear without splenic involvement?

Spigelian Hernia

1. Semilunar line (linea semilunaris).

2. Only a portion of the bowel wall is contained in the hernia.

3. Incisional.

4. Littre's.

Reference

Miller PA, Mezwa DG, Feczko PJ: Imaging of abdominal hernias, *Radiographics* 15:333-348, 1995.

Cross-Reference

Gastrointestinal Radiology: THE REQUISITES, ed 2, p 278.

Comment

Numerous types of hernias can be identified along the anterior abdominal wall. With the increased use of CT, some hernias are identified in patients who have no symptoms. In the adult population, incisional hernias are by far the most common. These develop in up to 5% of patients who have abdominal operations and typically occur within the first 6 months after the surgery. Affected patients may remain asymptomatic, however. Even though laparoscopic surgery is becoming increasingly popular, hernias can still occur through those small defects in the abdominal wall because they are not surgically closed. A Richter's hernia contains only a portion of a loop of bowel wall and not the entire lumen.

Spigelian hernias are unusual. They occur in the lower abdomen, either in the right or left lower quadrant. The area through which the bowel herniates, termed the *linea semilunaris,* consists of a fibrous band of tissue joining the rectus sheath muscles with the transverse abdominal and oblique abdominal muscles. The hernia is probably the result of a weakness or defect in the union of these muscles and fibrous bands. The hernia courses obliquely between these groups of muscles and may reside between bands of muscles, making it difficult to identify on clinical examination. Often, patients with spigelian hernias have intermittent or constant pain in the lower quadrant. The hernias contain either small bowel (right) or sigmoid colon (left), depending on where they are situated. They usually have a large orifice; thus there is less likelihood of obstruction or strangulation than there is with other types of hernias. They also may spontaneously reduce. These hernias occur with similar frequency in men and women. They may be bilateral or associated with other abdominal wall defects.

Notes

Lymphoma of the Liver and Spleen

1. Lymphoma, metastases, and multiple abscesses.

2. Slightly more than half the time.

3. Acquired immunodeficiency syndrome (AIDS) and organ transplantation.

4. Very little.

5. Very rarely.

Reference

Shirkhoda A, Ros PR, Farah J, et al: Lymphoma of the solid abdominal viscera, *Radiol Clin North Am* 28:785-799, 1990.

Cross-Reference

Gastrointestinal Radiology: THE REQUISITES, ed 2, p 182.

Comment

Lymphoma can involve the spleen or liver either secondarily (as a result of systemic lymphoma) or as a primary malignancy. Primary splenic or hepatic lymphoma is fairly rare; the majority of cases involve secondary or systemic lymphoma. Lymphoma may occur spontaneously or may be a sequela of a depressed immune system, such as in patients with AIDS or in transplant recipients.

Computed tomographic imaging of splenic lymphoma is difficult, and the spleen may appear normal despite substantial lymphomatous involvement. CT findings in the spleen include homogeneous enlargement, solitary or multifocal masses, and diffuse inhomogeneous infiltration. Lymphoma is always low density compared with normal splenic tissue after intravenous injection and rarely enhances. Because lymphoma and splenic tissue have similar MR characteristics, MRI is not helpful for staging lymphoma.

Lymphoma of the liver can appear on CT as solitary or multifocal masses or diffuse infiltration. CT is much more sensitive in detecting lymphoma of the liver compared with lymphomatous involvement of the spleen. Interestingly, lymphoma of the liver usually occurs with splenic lymphoma. The presence of lesions in both the spleen and the liver is a strong indication of lymphoma. Metastases would be another consideration, but visible metastases to the spleen are much less common. Also, there is often associated adjacent adenopathy. The presence of all these findings makes lymphoma the most likely consideration.

Notes

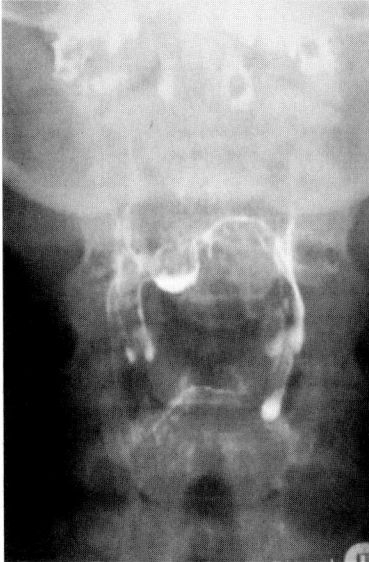

1. Besides squamous carcinoma, what is the most common tumor of the hypopharynx?
2. What is the source of cystic lesions of the hypopharynx?
3. Which branchial clefts help form the hypopharynx?
4. What other abnormalities may branchial cleft remnants produce clinically?

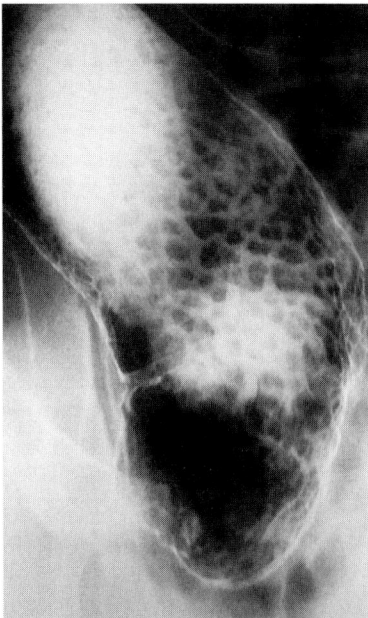

1. What is the underlying cause of this appearance?
2. What systemic condition may produce this appearance?
3. Name an infectious process known to result in this appearance.
4. What is probably the most common underlying cause of this condition?

Benign Cyst

1. Lymphoma.

2. Either branchial cleft cysts or thyroglossal duct cyst.

3. Third and fourth branchial clefts.

4. Fistulas or sinus tracts.

Reference

Low VHS, Rubesin SE: Contrast evaluation of the pharynx and esophagus, *Radiol Clin North Am* 31:1265-1291, 1993.

Cross-Reference

Gastrointestinal Radiology: THE REQUISITES, ed 2, p 3.

Comment

The majority of tumors involving the pharynx are squamous in origin. These are seen radiologically as small nodules, masses, or sometimes thickening or obliteration of the normal structures. Squamous tumors of the hypopharynx are typically seen in the vallecula, pyriform sinuses, or epiglottis. Lymphoma is more frequently seen in a posterior location, where the majority of the lymph tissue is located.

Cystic lesions in the region are invariably the result of congenital abnormalities in development, including residuals of either the branchial clefts or the thyroglossal duct. The branchial clefts are external indentations in the neck of embryos that meet with pharyngeal outpouchings and form the structure of the pharynx and head. The first and second branchial clefts help form the structures of the ear. The third and fourth help in the formation of the pyriform sinuses. If these persist beyond the embryologic stage, they may form cystic structures in the neck or base of the head. They can also persist as sinus tracts or fistulas that may arise from the pharynx. Another structure that may result in cyst formation in this region is a remnant of the thyroglossal duct, which helps in formation of the thyroid gland. In this patient the origin of the cystic structure was believed to be remnants of the thyroglossal duct.

Because these cystic lesions are submucosal in location, they are indistinguishable from other benign tumors, such as leiomyomas and other mesenchymal tumors. High resolution CT or MRI is the modality of choice in the evaluation of these structures.

Notes

Colonic "Urticaria"

1. Submucosal edema.

2. Allergic condition producing urticaria.

3. Herpes zoster infection or *Yersinia* organism infection.

4. Obstruction of the colon with proximal ischemia.

Reference

Seamen WB, Clements JL: Urticaria of the colon: a nonspecific pattern of submucosal edema, *Am J Roentgenol* 138:545-547, 1982.

Cross-Reference

Gastrointestinal Radiology: THE REQUISITES, ed 2, p 258.

Comment

This pattern of polygonal superficial lesions along the mucosa of the colon is quite rare. These plaques or reticular patterns often cover a large area of the colon and are almost always on the right side. This condition was first described in a patient who had a hypersensitivity reaction and developed these plaquelike irregularities in the colon. Because of this presentation, the authors first called the condition *urticaria of the colon.* Although the condition has since been described in association with other, nonallergic conditions, the term *urticaria of the colon* remains ingrained in the literature and is strongly associated with this distinctive entity.

The radiologic pattern present is believed to be the result of submucosal edema, which elevates the mucosa to a slight degree. Because the mucosa of the bowel is actually arranged in a honeycomb or polygonal pattern, a slight elevation allows for barium to become trapped at the edges and accentuate this appearance. More severe edema often obliterates this feature. This appearance is now considered to represent superficial edema of the colon. Pathologically, submucosal edema has been present in some specimens.

Probably the most common cause for this "urticarial" appearance is obstruction of the colon. It has been described with volvulus or obstructing cancer, and the change is probably due to chronic distention, with early ischemia developing proximally in the colon. This appearance has even been described in patients who have severe colonic ileus with cecal distention. Patients with ischemic colitis also have been known to have these changes apparent in some segments of the bowel, strengthening the relationship of this appearance to mild ischemia. Two infectious processes—herpes zoster and Yersinia colitis—cause this to change occur, although it is more strongly associated with herpes. Surprisingly the urticarial pattern is rarely seen in association with allergic or hypersensitivity reactions. The change has also been noted in patients with Crohn's disease.

Notes

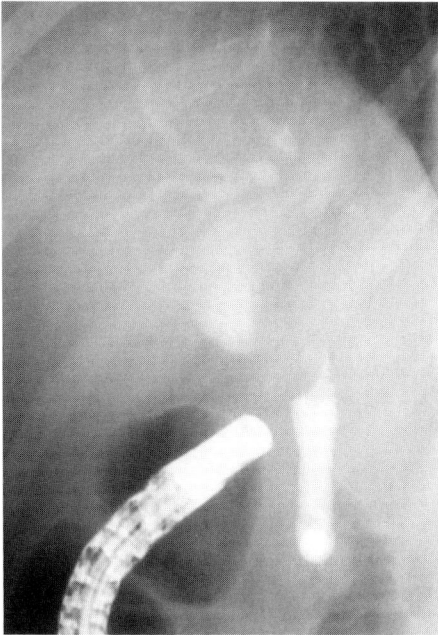

1. What is the name of this condition?
2. What underlying mechanism is producing it?
3. What condition does it mimic?
4. What major complication is associated with this condition?

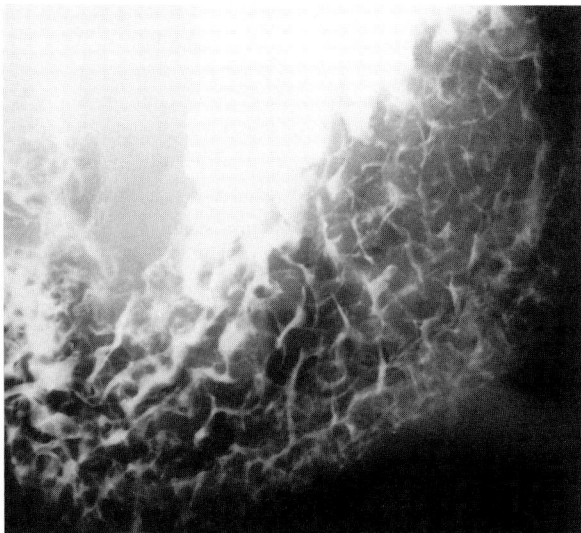
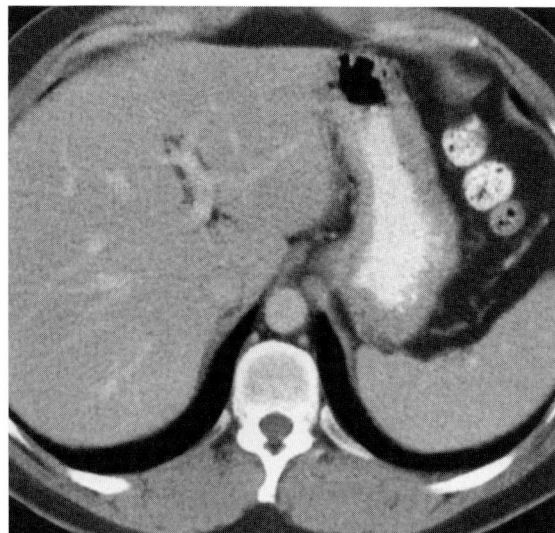

1. What is the leading cause of gastric ulcer disease in industrialized societies?
2. What is the leading cause of duodenal ulcer disease?
3. What substance does the breath test for bacterial infection in the upper gastrointestinal tract detect?
4. What is the treatment of choice for this infection?

Mirizzi Syndrome

1. Mirizzi syndrome.

2. A gallstone impacted in the cystic duct with severe local inflammation.

3. Neoplasm of the gallbladder or bile ducts.

4. Surgical ligation of the wrong ducts.

Reference

Weltman DI, Zeman RK: Acute diseases of the gallbladder and biliary ducts, *Radiol Clin North Am* 32:933-950, 1994.

Cross-Reference

Gastrointestinal Radiology: THE REQUISITES, ed 2, p 204.

Comment

This study demonstrates what is termed *Mirizzi syndrome.* This condition occurs when a stone becomes impacted in the cystic duct or neck of the gallbladder. This type of impaction is very common, but in the Mirizzi syndrome a severe local inflammatory response occurs. Of course the affected area is critical because there are several ducts and crossing vessels in the region. The inflammatory response produces a mass effect in the area. The inflammatory mass impinges on the common hepatic and bile ducts, producing varying degrees of narrowing or even obstruction. The intrahepatic bile ducts may become dilated proximal to the obstruction. There can even be secondary involvement of the major vessels in the area. There is also associated cholecystitis because the gallbladder is now obstructed.

The major concern for physicians dealing with this condition is not the inflammation itself but the difficulty in making an appropriate diagnosis and performing corrective surgery. With the inflammatory mass effect and the bile duct dilation, the condition may mimic a neoplasm of either the gallbladder or bile ducts. Adenopathy also may have a similar appearance. These changes are most confusing on endoscopic retrograde cholangiopancreatography (ERCP). Even if the correct diagnosis is made, prompt surgical intervention is typically warranted. For the surgeon the difficulty arises in identifying and isolating the correct ducts. Often the common hepatic duct is mistaken for the cystic duct, and ligation of the common hepatic duct ensues, producing disastrous complications. If possible, a stent can be placed in the extrahepatic ducts at ERCP to help identify them for the surgeon.

Notes

Helicobacter Pylori Gastritis

1. *Helicobacter pylori* infection (causes at least 50% of gastric ulcers).

2. *H. pylori* infection (causes at least 90% of duodenal ulcers).

3. Urease. It is a by-product of bacterial infection in the stomach.

4. Triple therapy (usually two antibiotics and bismuth).

Reference

Sohn J, Levine MS, Furth EE, et al: *Helicobacter pylori* gastritis: radiographic findings, *Radiology* 195:763-767, 1995.

Cross-Reference

Gastrointestinal Radiology: THE REQUISITES, ed 2, p 62.

Comment

The presence of *H. pylori* in the upper gastrointestinal tract is now believed to be the major cause of peptic ulcer disease among individuals who live in industrialized countries. The majority of gastric ulcers also are attributed to this organism, which is considered a major cause of chronic gastritis as well. Almost all duodenal ulcer patients also have *H. pylori* infection.

The radiologic abnormalities in these patients can be quite variable, and many patients have normal radiologic studies. By far the most common radiologic abnormality seen in patients with *H. pylori* infection is thickened gastric folds. The abnormality may vary from mild thickening of the folds in either the proximal stomach or antral region to bizarrely nodular folds involving a large portion of the stomach. These folds may become so thickened that they can resemble a neoplastic process, such as lymphoma. Often these fold abnormalities can be detected on CT examination. Polyps of varying sizes also have been described. Typically these are small hyperplastic polyps, although rarely a large focal polypoid mass is encountered. In many of these patients, endoscopy may be necessary to exclude malignancy. Of course, ulcers and erosions can be identified in the stomach, but this finding is less common than are the fold abnormalities. Enlarged areae gastricae also have been described, although this finding is subtle. In the duodenum, radiologic findings include ulcers, thickened folds, and narrowing or deformity.

Noninvasive techniques for detecting *H. pylori* include a breath test that detects urease activity within the upper gastrointestinal tract. Serologic tests may detect antibodies to the *H. pylori* antigen. Endoscopic studies are considered the mainstay for detection because the bacteria can be diagnosed on biopsy specimens. However, the infection itself is patchy, and multiple biopsies are often necessary to detect the organism. Treatment includes antibiotic therapy, usually involving a combination of agents, including metronidazole, tetracycline, or amoxicillin. Also, oral bismuth therapy is recommended, and histamine blockers are given to reduce acid levels.

Notes

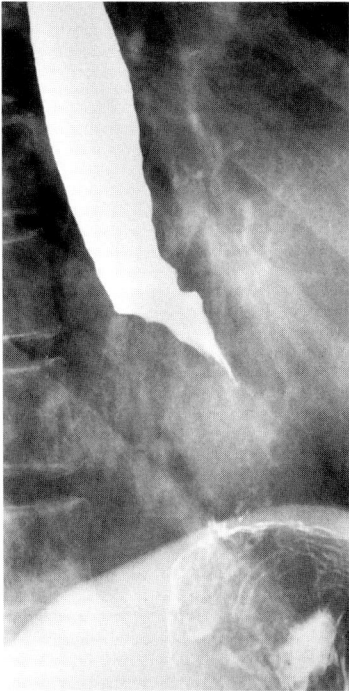

1. What organism is responsible for Chagas' disease?
2. At what age does achalasia normally present?
3. What is the cause of secondary achalasia, or pseudoachalasia?
4. What is a long-term complication of achalasia?
5. Is there a relationship between diffuse esophageal spasm and achalasia?

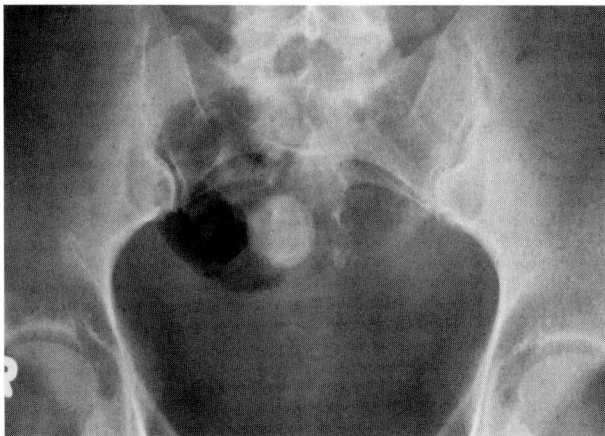

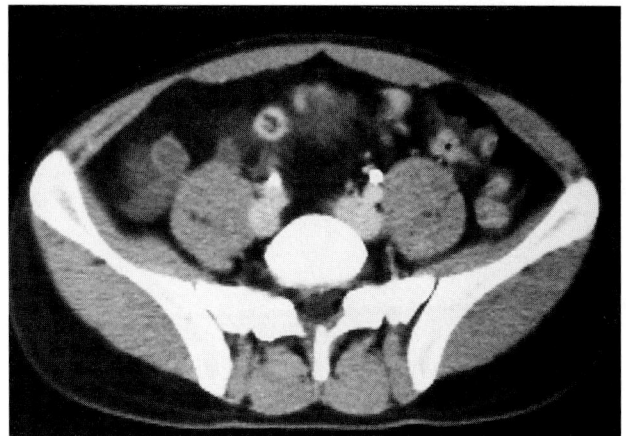

1. Where may enteroliths form in the intestines?
2. In patients with gallstone ileus, where do the calculi obstruct the lumen?
3. What is the most common congenital abnormality of the intestines?
4. What type of mucosa may be found in Meckel's diverticula?

CASE 57

Secondary Achalasia Caused by Gastric Carcinoma

1. *Trypanosoma cruzi* (a protozoan).

2. Usually between the ages of 25 and 50 years.

3. Tumor, usually a gastric carcinoma, infiltration at the gastroesophageal junction.

4. Esophageal carcinoma.

5. Some patients with diffuse esophageal spasm may later develop achalasia.

Reference
Feczko PJ, Halpert RD: Achalasia secondary to non-gastrointestinal malignancies, *Gastrointest Radiol* 10:273-276, 1985.

Cross-Reference
Gastrointestinal Radiology: THE REQUISITES, ed 2, p 21.

Comment
Achalasia is a motor disorder of the esophagus marked by aperistalsis of the esophagus, with failure of the lower esophageal sphincter to relax. This problem leads to progressive dilation of the esophagus and results in a tight, "rat tail" or "beaklike" appearance of the distal esophagus. There is a malfunction of the nervous plexus of the esophagus, but the underlying etiology is uncertain. In the early stages the patient with achalasia may appear to have diffuse esophageal spasm (i.e., coarse, nonpropulsive contractions of the distal esophagus). Achalasia is similar manometrically to diffuse esophageal spasm and has been termed *vigorous achalasia.* Over the course of several years, some patients develop the more classic form of achalasia.

Secondary achalasia, or pseudoachalasia, is caused by some underlying process producing functional changes in the esophagus that mimic or appear radiologically similar to those caused by achalasia. The most common cause is a gastric neoplasm at the cardia of the stomach, with secondary involvement of the esophagus. Lymphoma or metastases to the gastroesophageal junction region may also produce this disorder. A major differential point is that true achalasia tends to occur in younger individuals, whereas secondary achalasia caused by malignancy typically affects an older population (60 years of age and older). Rarely, secondary achalasia is a paraneoplastic condition produced by tumors remote from the gastroesophageal junction, such as tumors of the breast or lung. Chagas' disease is a parasitic infection that is common in South America. In patients with this disease a protozoan has invaded the gastrointestinal tract, destroying the ganglia of the esophagus, and the result is an achalasia-like motor disorder of the esophagus.

Notes

CASE 58

Enterolith in a Meckel's Diverticulum

1. Diverticula, appendix, and proximal to chronic strictures.

2. Terminal ileum at the ileocecal valve.

3. Meckel's diverticulum.

4. Gastric mucosa.

Reference
Pantongrag-Brown L, Levine MS, Buetow P, et al: Meckel's enteroliths: clinical, radiologic, and pathologic findings, *Am J Roentgenol* 167:1447-1450, 1996.

Cross-Reference
Gastrointestinal Radiology: THE REQUISITES, ed 2, p 128.

Comment
The presence of a large calcification in the bowel is indicative of an enterolith. Enteroliths are stones that develop as a result of the repeated deposition of calcium on a nidus of material within a luminal structure. Similar to calculi in other parts of the body, enteroliths often begin to develop within a lumen or saclike structure. The calcification appears to have formed in layers, indicating repeated episodes of calcium deposition. For an enterolith to develop in the bowel, it must be in an area of stasis, either within a saclike appendage, such as the appendix or Meckel's diverticulum, or behind a stricture.

Meckel's diverticulum is the most common congenital anomaly of the intestines, occurring in up to 3% of the population. It represents incomplete obliteration of the vitelline duct, which is an embryologic structure. Most Meckel's diverticula do not cause symptoms. However, a substantial number of these diverticula contain ectopic gastric mucosa that may be functional and may produce pain, ulceration, and bleeding. The Meckel's scan, in which technetium 99m pertechnetate is used, is taken up to the gastric mucosa and can detect areas of ectopic gastric mucosa. However, this test is not always reliable. Other complications of Meckel's diverticula include obstruction caused by either invagination and intussusception or formation of a large enterolith. Malignancy is rarely encountered.

Enteroliths are rare, forming in less than 10% of symptomatic Meckel's diverticula, and do not always calcify. When they do calcify, enteroliths may produce bleeding or obstruction. A major differential consideration is a gallstone that has eroded into the gastrointestinal tract, the so-called gallstone ileus syndrome. When these stones reach the terminal ileum, they often obstruct because they cannot pass through the ileocecal valve. It may be impossible to differentiate on plain radiographs, but CT scans may provide a clue as to the position of the enterolith.

Notes

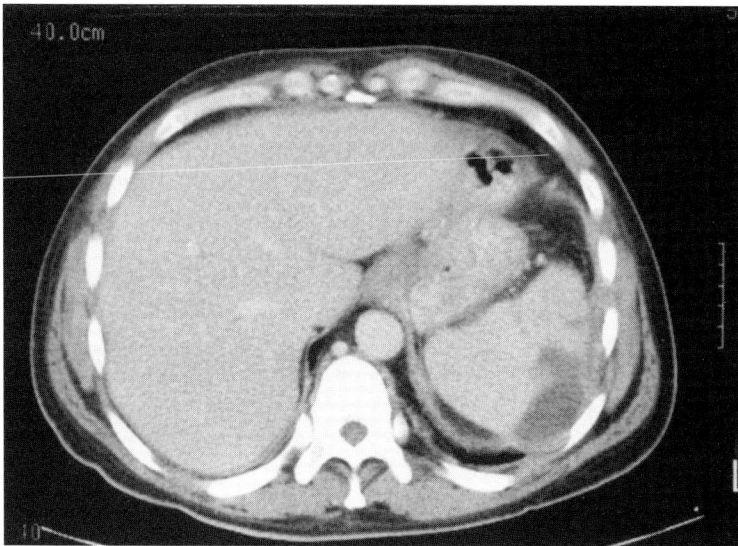

1. What are the diagnostic possibilities?
2. What clinical condition often leads to splenic abscesses?
3. What cardiac condition produces splenic abscess?
4. What local conditions are associated with the development of splenic abscess?

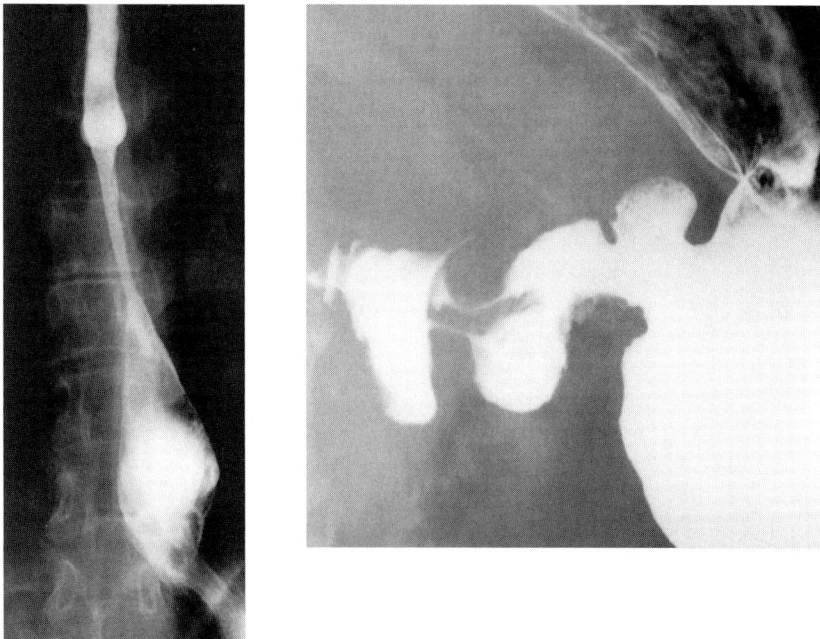

1. What are the most common radiologic findings in patients with acute caustic esophagitis?
2. Does acid ingestion affect the esophagus in a manner similar to caustic ingestion?
3. Ingestion of which product—acid or lye—involves the stomach?
4. How soon does stricture formation occur?

Splenic Abscess

1. Hematoma, abscess, infarction, lymphoma, and cyst.

2. Immunosuppression.

3. Endocarditis.

4. Pancreatitis and pyelonephritis.

Reference

Urrutia M, Mergo PJ, Ros LH, et al: Cystic masses of the spleen: radiologic-pathologic correlation, *Radiographics* 16:107-129, 1996.

Cross-Reference

Gastrointestinal Radiology: THE REQUISITES, ed 2, p 192.

Comment

Pancreatic abscesses are being encountered more frequently as a result of better diagnostic studies, such as CT and ultrasound, and the increased number of patients with immunosuppression (e.g., patients with acquired immunodeficiency syndrome, transplant recipients, and those undergoing chemotherapy). Splenic abscesses can develop in several ways, including as a result of metastatic infection from septic emboli (endocarditis), as a result of contiguous infection (pyelonephritis or pancreatitis), as a sequela of an infarct or trauma with secondary infection, and as a result of generalized immunosuppression with sepsis. A small portion of splenic abscesses develop in the absence of any underlying condition. Most infectious organisms, such as staphylococci, streptococci, and *Escherichia coli,* are aerobic. There is often a high incidence of fungal abscesses, no doubt because many of these patients are immunosuppressed.

The most common finding on plain radiography is a left pleural effusion. CT is the best modality for detecting splenic abscesses, although they also may be demonstrated by ultrasound or even MRI. The problem with CT is that many other conditions have an appearance similar to that of an abscess. Abscesses are areas of low density caused by necrotic or infected tissue. Air is rarely demonstrated but is pathognomonic of an abscess if present. A hematoma or an infarct may appear like an abscess, as would a neoplastic process, such as lymphoma. The wall of an abscess is usually thick and somewhat irregular, which may help to differentiate it from a splenic cyst. The rim of a splenic cyst enhances only when a well-defined capsule develops about the edge of the cyst, which occurs only later in the inflammatory process. Nuclear imaging may be helpful if there is concern about the nature of a splenic mass. Gallium scans and labeled white blood cell studies are active in areas of an abscess; however, lymphoma is also gallium positive. Labeled leukocyte studies always show splenic activity and may obscure an abscess.

Notes

Esophageal and Gastric Injury Resulting from Lye Ingestion

1. Motility disorders and superficial mucosal irregularity.

2. Ingestion of either product may involve the esophagus, but acid damage is often less severe.

3. Acid ingestion tends to cause more severe damage to the stomach.

4. At least 3 to 4 weeks after ingestion of the substance.

Reference

Franken EA: Caustic damage of the gastrointestinal tract: roentgen features, *Am J Roentgenol* 118:77-85, 1973.

Cross-Reference

Gastrointestinal Radiology: THE REQUISITES, ed 2, p 17.

Comment

Ingestion of alkaline (lye) or acid substances may be either intentional or accidental. Many household cleansers contain alkali or caustic substances. The degree of injury that occurs in the gastrointestinal tract is related to both the concentration and the volume of the ingested substances. The immediacy of treatment also has a significant impact regarding the sequela of this injury. Alkaline substances produce coagulative necrosis and tend to cause a more deeply penetrating injury to the bowel.

Radiologic studies can be performed as long as there are no signs of perforation, such as a widened mediastinum; soft tissue emphysema; or intraperitoneal air. Initial radiologic assessment may be performed before endoscopy is attempted and should be done with water-soluble contrast followed by thin barium. In the early stages (fewer than 12 hours after the ingestion) the only apparent problem may be a motility disorder, ranging from spasm to atony and even dilation. If there has been a severe caustic burn, superficial ulceration may be apparent in the mucosa. Over the ensuing days, the damaged mucosa sloughs and becomes edematous, with the most severe changes subsiding after several days. Radiologic examination typically is not performed during this time unless there is suspected perforation. The final phase of scarring, fibrosis, and stricture formation takes several weeks to months to develop. Not all patients develop esophageal stricturing, but it is more common in patients who ingested lye than in those who ingested acid. The strictures that are apparent can be either long and diffuse or weblike areas of narrowing.

Ingestion of both alkaline and acid substances may involve the stomach, usually in the distal antrum along the greater curvature, which is where the ingested substance often comes to rest when the patient is upright. The degree of gastric injury is usually worse with ingestion of acids. Alkaline substances may be neutralized by the gastric acidity. However, up to 20% of patients who ingested lye develop gastric injury, as seen in this patient.

Notes

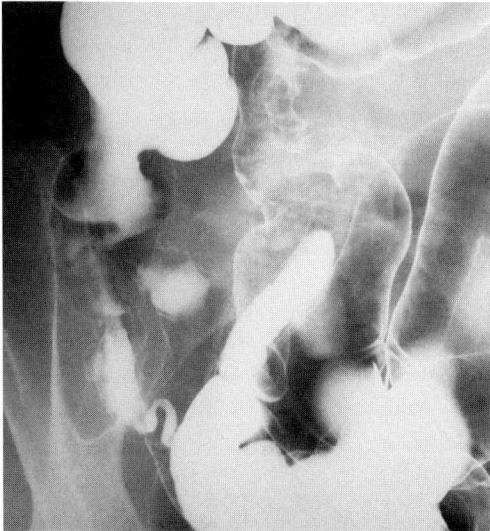

1. What neoplastic processes may produce multifocal involvement of the colon?
2. Name some infectious processes that may have this type of appearance.
3. What type of inflammatory bowel disease should be considered?
4. If the patient has pulmonary disease, what is a likely diagnosis?

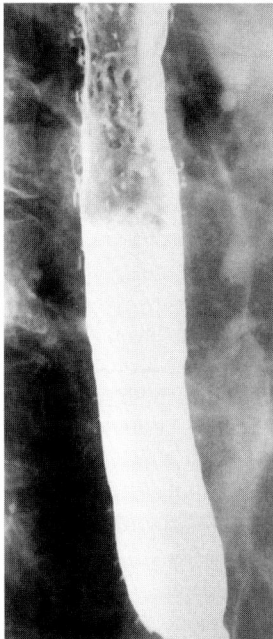

1. What structures are visible or filled by the barium?
2. Name some pathologic entities often seen in patients with this condition.
3. What common pathogen has been associated with this condition?
4. Is this pathogen ever found in a normal esophagus?

Tuberculosis of the Colon

1. Lymphoma and serosal metastases.

2. Tuberculosis and amebiasis.

3. Crohn's disease.

4. Tuberculosis.

Reference

Balthazar EJ, Gordon R, Hulnick D: Ileocecal tuberculosis: CT and radiologic evaluation, *Am J Roentgenol* 154:499-502, 1990.

Cross-Reference

Gastrointestinal Radiology: THE REQUISITES, ed 2, p 107.

Comment

The illustration in this case shows some deformity of the cecum. There is also an irregular area of narrowing in the transverse colon. This finding indicates that the process is multifocal in nature. A variety of conditions must be considered in this instance, and this patient was misdiagnosed with near disastrous consequences. One of the most common inflammatory processes of the ileocecal region is Crohn's disease. It also can affect any portion of the gastrointestinal tract, and the colon is a likely area for further involvement. Possible infectious processes include amebiasis and tuberculosis. Both of these conditions can affect the ileocecal area, as well as the rest of the colon. Of the neoplastic processes the most likely is serosal metastasis, which has an affinity for the cecal region. Lymphoma must always be considered in the differential diagnosis of multifocal gastrointestinal lesions.

The final, correct diagnosis for this patient was tuberculosis. When a chest radiograph was finally obtained, the patient had upper lobe pulmonary findings consistent with tuberculosis. However, a normal chest x-ray film should not preclude this diagnosis because intestinal tuberculosis can occur without an abnormal chest film. Most intestinal tuberculosis occurs as a result of the patient with pulmonary tuberculosis swallowing infected sputum; the intestinal tuberculosis is usually secondary. Adenopathy may occur in patients with intestinal tuberculosis but also occurs in those with Crohn's disease or lymphoma and therefore does not help differentiate the conditions. The patient was initially treated for Crohn's disease and as a result of this inappropriate therapy suffered a spread of tuberculosis.

Notes

Intramural Pseudodiverticulosis of the Esophagus

1. Dilated excretory ducts of the esophageal mucus glands.

2. Strictures (usually benign), carcinoma, inflammation, and reflux.

3. *Candida* organisms.

4. Yes, but rarely.

Reference

Levine MS, Moolten DN, Herlinger H, Laufer I: Esophageal intramural pseudodiverticulosis: a reevaluation, *Am J Roentgenol* 147:1165-1170, 1986.

Cross-Reference

Gastrointestinal Radiology: THE REQUISITES, ed 2, p 17.

Comment

Intramural pseudodiverticulosis of the esophagus is a rare condition. Anatomically it represents barium filling the excretory ducts of the mucus glands of the esophagus. These mucus glands are normal anatomic structures of the esophagus but typically are not visible on radiologic studies. However, sometimes these ducts become dilated, allowing barium to track into the ducts and glands.

Some type of inflammation must be present for these pathologic changes to occur, and the large majority of these patients have evidence of esophageal inflammation. A large proportion of patients with intramural pseudodiverticulosis also have strictures. The strictures are typically benign, but intramural pseudodiverticulosis has been reported in association with malignant strictures. *Candida* organisms have been found in patients with this condition, but the exact causal relationship is uncertain. More than likely, this finding represents a secondary infection of the glands and not a predisposing condition. Rarely this condition is found in patients with an otherwise normal esophagus.

Radiologically the intramural pseudodiverticulosis appears as small outpouchings, often with a flask shape. These outpouchings are most commonly mistaken for ulcers by those who are unfamiliar with the condition. Intramural pseudodiverticulosis may be either segmental or diffuse. Even intramural tracking and deep penetration may be evident. On CT, the condition produces changes of esophageal wall thickening and irregularity of the lumen, mimicking esophageal carcinoma. Because it is primarily a radiologic oddity, the condition's clinical course depends on treatment of the underlying condition. Often, treatment of the stricture or inflammation results in a decrease or even disappearance of the pseudodiverticulosis.

Notes

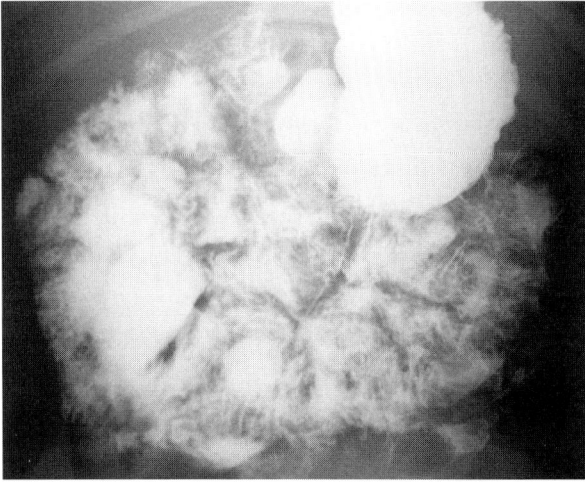

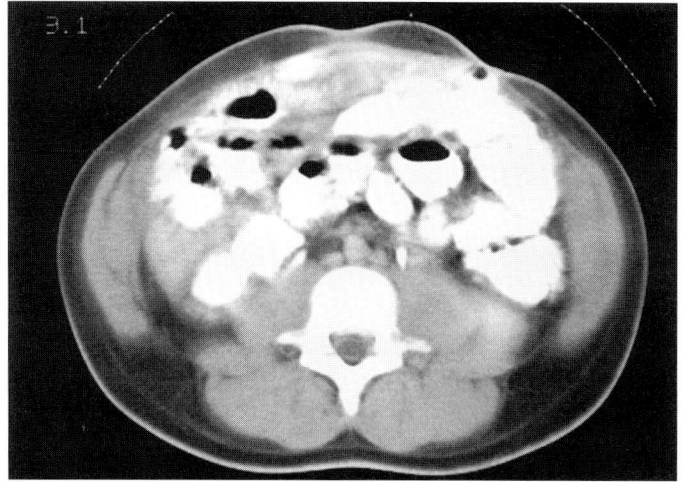

1. A dysfunction of what organ or organs may cause malabsorption?

2. What neoplasm may result in malabsorption?

3. What malabsorptive condition has associated pulmonary disease?

4. Which diseases that cause malabsorption may cause spontaneous intussusception?

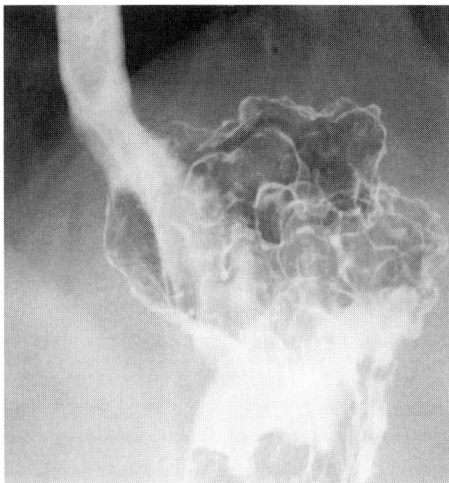

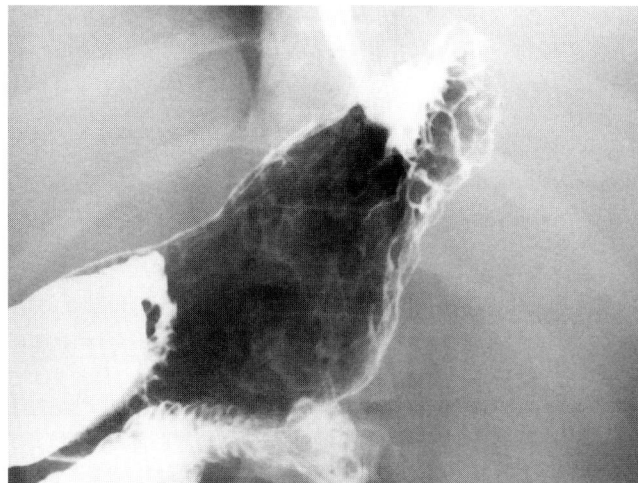

1. What neoplasm most commonly produces thickened gastric folds?

2. Name some infiltrative processes associated with thickened folds.

3. What is the cause of isolated gastric varices?

4. What is the most common infectious cause of thickened folds?

CASE 63

Malabsorption in Cystic Fibrosis

1. Pancreas and liver.

2. Gastrinoma (Zollinger-Ellison syndrome).

3. Cystic fibrosis.

4. Sprue and cystic fibrosis.

Reference

Agrons GA, Corse WR, Markowitz RI, et al: Gastrointestinal manifestations of cystic fibrosis: radiologic-pathologic correlation, *Radiographics* 16:871, 1996.

Cross-Reference

Gastrointestinal Radiology: THE REQUISITES, ed 2, p 144.

Comment

Malabsorption can be caused by numerous conditions because the proper digestion and absorption of food is a complex process. Predominantly it is the abnormal digestion of fats that leads to problems. Malabsorption may be the result of poor digestion (pancreatic insufficiency), mucosal disease (Crohn's disease or sprue), poor transport of digested materials (lymphangiectasia), or bacterial overgrowth (diverticula). Clinically these patients complain of diarrhea, steatorrhea, abdominal distention, and weight loss. Various vitamin or nutrient deficiencies can compound the problem and may be the initial complaint.

Radiologic findings can be variable, but many radiologists describe what can be termed a *malabsorptive pattern or appearance of the small bowel,* although some disagree with this categorization. Features of a small bowel examination that suggest malabsorption are dilation of the small bowel loops, thickening of the valvulae or folds, and evidence of increased fluid in the bowel lumen. Transit time is variable but tends to be prolonged. Flocculation (clumping or precipitation) of the barium is rare with the new barium suspensions.

Cystic fibrosis is a congenital defect resulting in the thickening of secretions from various organs. With modern medical care, many patients with cystic fibrosis now live into adolescence and even adulthood. The majority have malabsorption at some time during their life. The cause of the malabsorption is a combination of factors. Mainly there is progressive pancreatic dysfunction, particularly involving exocrine glands. The pancreatic secretions are low in bicarbonate and enzymes, which leads to malabsorption. Pancreatic enzymes may be given orally to help alleviate this problem. In addition, there is a disturbance of absorption at the mucosal level as a result of inspissation of secretions in the mucosal glands. Slow transit time and bacterial overgrowth also may contribute to the malabsorption.

Notes

CASE 64

Gastric Varices

1. Lymphoma.

2. Eosinophilic gastritis, sarcoidosis, Crohn's disease, Ménétrier's disease, and amyloidosis.

3. Thrombosis of the splenic vein.

4. *Helicobacter pylori.*

Reference

Fishman EK, Urban BA, Hruban RH: CT of the stomach: spectrum of disease, *Radiographics* 16:1035, 1996.

Cross-Reference

Gastrointestinal Radiology: THE REQUISITES, ed 2, p 60.

Comment

It is extremely common to find thickened gastric folds on upper gastrointestinal examinations. The width of the gastric folds is usually less than 5 mm in the distal stomach and less than 8 mm proximally. Normal gastric folds tend to run parallel to the lumen, whereas folds that are irregularly thickened, nodular, or serpiginous in appearance are usually considered abnormal. Associated gastric wall thickening also may be visible on CT examination.

The presence of thickened rugal folds, gastric wall thickening, or both is a nonspecific finding. A variety of diseases may produce this radiologic finding, which can even be seen in healthy patients. The most common cause is some type of gastritis, such as alcoholic gastritis. *H. pylori* infection of the stomach is now recognized as an extremely common cause of inflammatory disease of the stomach and is by far the most common infectious process of the upper gastrointestinal tract. Zollinger-Ellison syndrome (gastrinoma) should always be considered, although it is quite rare. Numerous benign infiltrating processes, including eosinophilic gastritis, sarcoidosis, amyloidosis, Crohn's disease, and Ménétrier's disease, also may produce fold thickening. Of the neoplastic processes, lymphoma most typically presents as thickened folds. Adenocarcinoma and even metastases also must be considered but are less common.

Varices of the stomach usually have associated esophageal varices and are related to increased portal venous pressure resulting from a variety of causes. Isolated gastric varices, however, are a specific condition associated with splenic vein occlusion. The spleen normally drains via the splenic vein, but if it occludes, there are short gastric veins that act as collateral circulation. These veins course over the proximal stomach and connect to the coronary vein, which then flows into the portal circulation. Splenic vein thrombosis is usually the sequela of pancreatitis or pancreatic carcinoma and less commonly the result of retroperitoneal processes, surgery, or hypercoagulability state.

Notes

A

B

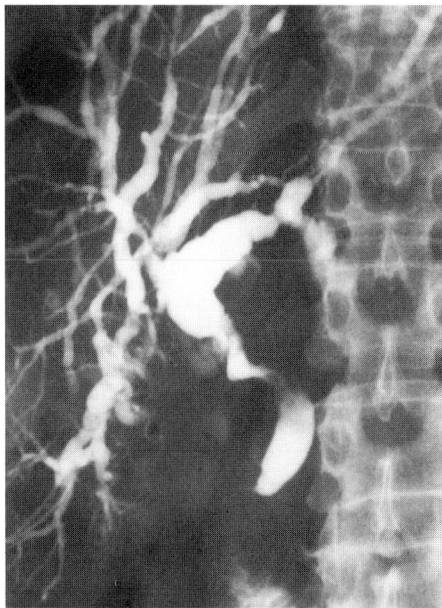

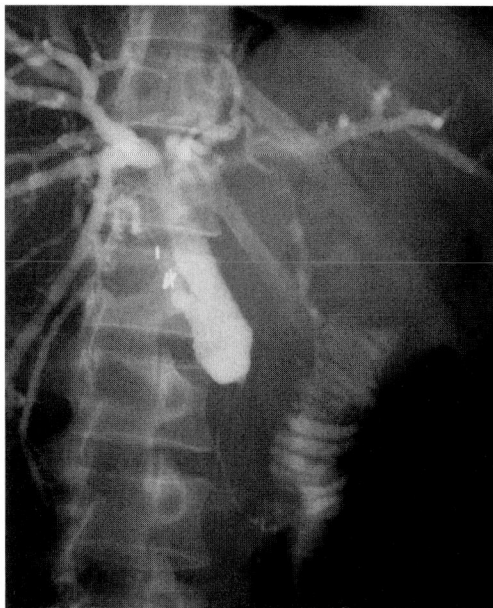

1. What is the most likely cause of the narrowing seen in the figure on the left?
2. What can produce the narrowing seen in the figure on the right?
3. What entity can produce narrowing in both these areas?
4. Name possible causes of narrowing at the liver hilus.

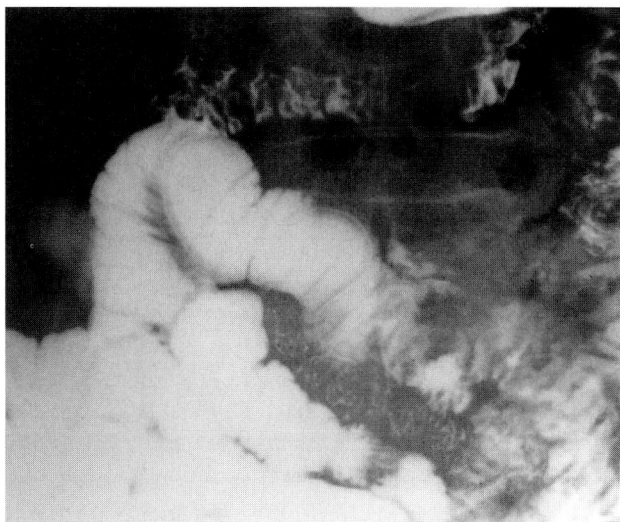

1. What is this parasitic infection called?
2. What is its prevalence?
3. What is a common complication of this parasitic infection?
4. What changes may it produce in the chest?

CASE 65

Lymph Nodes Compressing a Duct (A) and Pancreatitis (B)

1. Lymph nodes in the porta hepatis.

2. Pancreatitis or pancreatic carcinoma.

3. Cholangiocarcinoma.

4. Enlarged lymph nodes, cholangiocarcinoma, gallbladder inflammation, or tumor.

Reference

Fulcher AS, Turner MA, Capps GW: MR cholangiography: technical advances and clinical applications, *Radiographics* 19:25-41, 1999.

Cross-Reference

Gastrointestinal Radiology: THE REQUISITES, ed 2, p 206.

Comment

Evaluation of narrowing of the extrahepatic biliary tree is quite simple if the anatomy is studied and the pathologic possibilities occurring at the level of the stricture are considered. It is best to divide the extrahepatic bile ducts into the pancreatic portion, suprapancreatic portion, and region of the bifurcation.

Narrowing of the common bile duct as it passes through the pancreatic parenchyma is most often caused by pancreatic disease. Both pancreatitis and pancreatic carcinoma may produce narrowing of the ducts, and it is often impossible to differentiate between the two conditions by evaluating the ducts. Cholangiocarcinoma may occur anywhere in the ducts and must be considered as well.

Narrowing of the duct above the pancreatic parenchyma is most often the result of adenopathy compressing the ducts. The adenopathy may be caused by tumors of the stomach or pancreas or even lymphoma. Less commonly, extraabdominal malignancies, such as breast or lung cancer and melanoma, produce metastatic adenopathy in this region. Again, cholangiocarcinoma can produce narrowing in this area.

Narrowing near the hepatic bifurcation or the common hepatic duct region can result from numerous causes. Adenopathy in the region can be the result of the aforementioned lesions. Also, it is a good location for cholangiocarcinoma, particularly the so-called Klatskin tumor. In this area, diseases of the gallbladder produce ductal narrowing. This narrowing can be inflammatory in nature (Mirizzi syndrome) or the result of secondary invasion by carcinoma of the gallbladder.

Notes

CASE 66

Ascariasis of the Small Bowel

1. Ascariasis.

2. It is the most common intestinal parasitic infection, affecting up to a quarter of the world's population.

3. Migration into the biliary system.

4. Pulmonary hypersensitivity with bronchospasm, infiltrates, and eosinophilia.

Reference

Cevallos AM, Farthing MJG: Parasitic infections of the gastrointestinal tract, *Curr Opin Gastroenterol* 9:96-102, 1993.

Cross-Reference

Gastrointestinal Radiology: THE REQUISITES, ed 2, p 122.

Comment

One of the most common parasitic infections is produced by the nematode, *Ascaris lumbricoides.* It infects a major proportion of the world's population. With the ease of worldwide travel, as well as immigration, this parasite is encountered in all areas of the world. The pathway of infection is quite complicated. The eggs of this parasite are ingested when infected water or food is consumed. In the gastrointestinal tract (small bowel) the larvae hatch and burrow through the intestinal wall. From there, they reach the portal venous system and travel to the liver and the lungs. The larvae then reach the bronchial system, where they can be found in the sputum, and reach the intestines by being swallowed in the sputum. Once they again reach the intestines, they grow into adult worms, which are quite large.

The parasite produces diseases in many ways. The larvae may produce a local hypersensitivity reaction, which is particularly evident when they are in the lungs. When they are in the intestines, the worms produce nutritional deficiencies. As the worms grow, the large mass of the worms can produce obstruction and even appendicitis. Perforation of the intestines with peritonitis can even occur. Often the patient's symptoms are quite vague, with occasional pain and diarrhea. The worms can also migrate into the biliary system, where they can produce cholangitis or pancreatitis because of their size, as well as a local inflammatory response.

Radiologically the worms are visible on barium studies because they are so large. There may be a single worm, or they may occur in large masses. A hallmark of these worms is that they ingest the barium during the examination, and then barium outlines the intestinal tract of the worms, as is evident in this image.

Notes

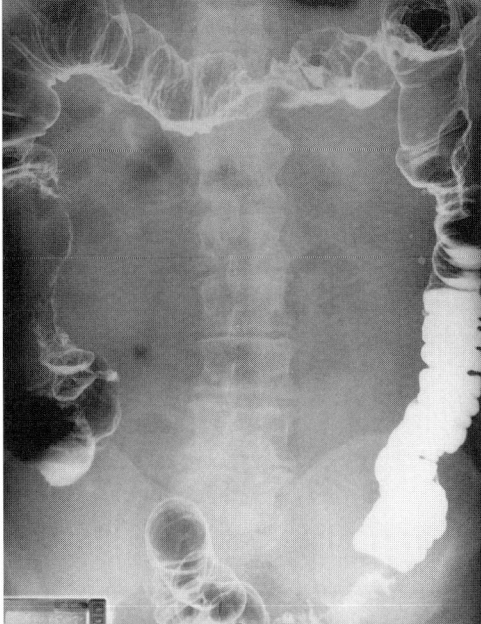

1. What may be producing this appearance?
2. What is the most common source of these lesions?
3. What is the method of spread?
4. What other areas also may be involved?

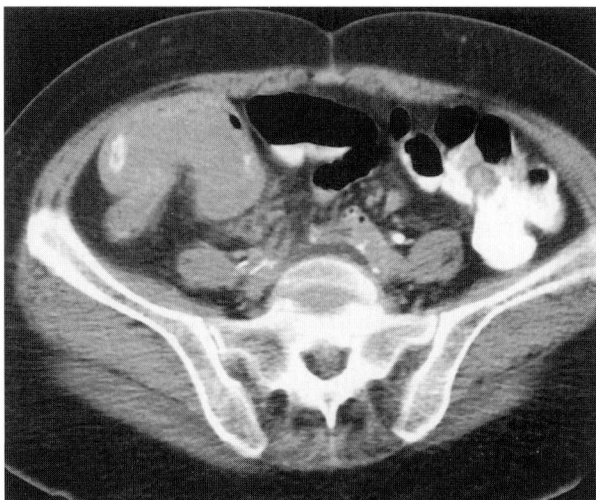

1. What is the most likely diagnosis?
2. In an adult, what would be the most likely underlying cause?
3. What would be the treatment for an adult with this problem?
4. Besides obstruction, what other complications may occur?

C A S E 6 7

Serosal Metastases to the Colon

1. Serosal metastases.

2. Ovarian cancer in women, followed by colonic, gastric, and pancreatic neoplasms.

3. Flow of ascitic fluid.

4. Anterior wall of the rectum, distal ileum, and right paracolic gutter.

Reference

Rubesin SE, Levine MS: Omental cakes: colonic involvement by omental metastases, *Radiology* 154:593-596, 1985.

Cross-Reference

Gastrointestinal Radiology: THE REQUISITES, ed 2, p 274.

Comment

Tumor may spread to the colon by way of serosal metastases, direct contiguous invasion, or hematogenous metastases. Serosal metastases occur when a tumor has access to the peritoneum. Tumor cells are shed into the peritoneal cavity and distributed according to the flow of the ascitic fluid. The flow of this fluid has been well described. The flow extends along the small bowel mesentery to the right lower quadrant. From there, it reaches the pelvis, and then tracks laterally up the lateral paracolic gutters. At areas where there is stasis or pooling of the ascitic fluid, tumor cells are likely to reside and begin to grow.

Common areas in which the development of serosal metastases is seen include the anterior rectum (pouch of Douglas), sigmoid mesentery, distal ileum, cecum, and right and left paracolic gutters. Any intraabdominal tumor may produce these peritoneal metastases. In women the most common cause is ovarian cancer. However, any gynecologic tumor or colonic, gastric, or pancreatic malignancy may result in the development of this type of lesion. In addition, any extraabdominal tumor that metastasizes to the abdomen may eventually produce peritoneal metastases.

The radiologic appearance of serosal metastases is fairly similar among all the malignancies. Initially, only a slight mass effect or the lack of distention in a segment of bowel may be visible. As the tumor invades the muscular layers, there may be a desmoplastic reaction. The development of transverse stripes as a result of this muscular invasion has been described. This development can progress to spiculation of the contours of the bowel, kinking of the bowel, angulation of the bowel, and finally obstruction of the lumen.

Notes

C A S E 6 8

Intussusception of the Bowel

1. Intussusception.

2. Mass or other intraluminal object.

3. Surgery.

4. Ischemia or bleeding.

Reference

Bar-Ziv J, Solomon A: Computed tomography in adult intussusception, *Gastrointest Radiol* 10:355-357, 1985.

Cross-Reference

Gastrointestinal Radiology: THE REQUISITES, ed 2, p 278.

Comment

Intussusception is the telescoping of one bowel segment inside the lumen of the adjacent segment. In children this condition is most often idiopathic in nature and can be reduced by the pressure of an enema. Adults are a different consideration, however. Intussusception in the adult is most often (in at least 90% of cases) caused by a leading point, that is, an object in the lumen of the bowel that is propelled down the lumen as a result of peristaltic activity. Typically this object is a tumor of some type. Often it is a large polypoid mass, which may be malignant, or sometimes it is just a benign tumor, such as a lipoma. Either way, adult intussusception is not often amenable to decompression by an enema, although sometimes it can be accomplished. Even if it is decompressed, the mass producing the intussusception must be dealt with, requiring surgery. Also the vascular supply to the intussusceptum is often compromised, and the risk of ischemia and perforation is great.

Computed tomography is increasingly used to diagnose abnormalities of the abdomen, particularly the acute abdomen. Sometimes the intussusception is first diagnosed by CT. Signs of intussusception on CT include a target sign, a mass within the bowel lumen with layers of variable density around it, and a kidney-shaped mass distending the lumen with proximal obstruction. The last presentation is supposed to have the worst prognosis because it is often associated with ischemia. The case illustrated here falls in this last category.

Notes

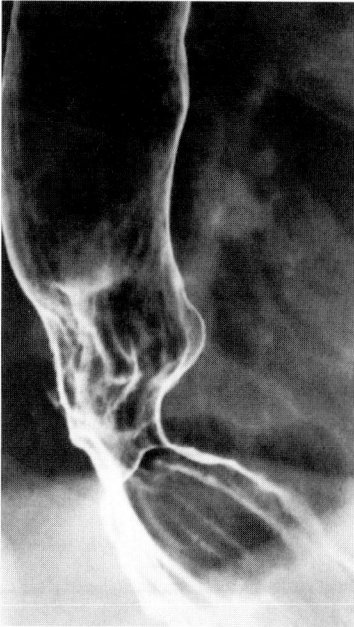

1. What radiologic findings suggest the diagnosis?
2. What is the etiology of Barrett's metaplasia?
3. Name some clinical conditions that are associated with an increased incidence of carcinoma, particularly adenocarcinoma of the esophagus.
4. What is the main difference between the spread of squamous carcinoma and the spread of adenocarcinoma of the esophagus?

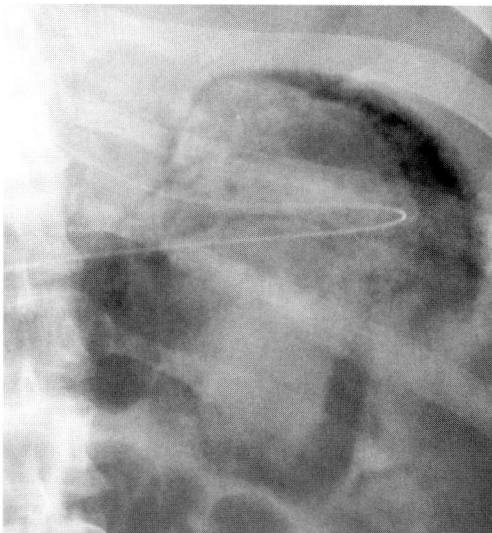

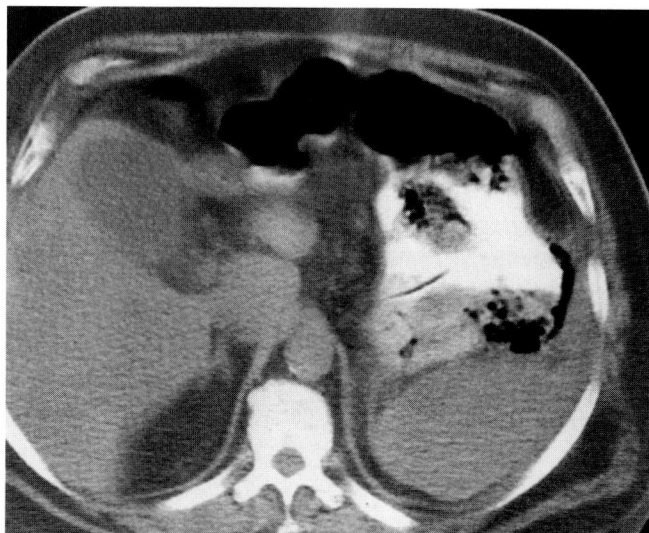

1. What common organisms produce this abnormality?
2. Ingestion of what type of substance may cause this problem?
3. What aspect of the patient history is pertinent when this finding is discovered?
4. What other conditions can be associated with this finding?

CASE 69

Barrett's Esophagus and Adenocarcinoma Occurring in Chronic Reflux Esophagitis

1. The major finding is stricture, usually proximally, and plaquelike mucosal irregularities.

2. Long-standing gastroesophageal reflux.

3. Chronic reflux, scleroderma, achalasia, and lye strictures.

4. Adenocarcinoma tends to readily cross the gastroesophageal junction into the stomach.

Reference

Chen MYM, Frederick MG: Barrett esophagus and adenocarcinoma, *Radiol Clin North Am* 32:1167-1182, 1994.

Cross-Reference

Gastrointestinal Radiology: THE REQUISITES, ed 2, p 16.

Comment

Barrett's esophagus is actually a metaplastic transformation of the normal squamous mucosa of the esophagus into columnar epithelium, similar to the stomach. Although it was initially believed to be a congenital abnormality, it is now recognized as an acquired condition secondary to long-standing gastroesophageal reflux disease. It can be encountered in young patients as a result of prolonged nasogastric intubation, but in older patients it is often associated with hiatal hernia and reflux.

The most important feature of Barrett's metaplasia is that it is the leading cause of primary adenocarcinoma of the esophagus. The majority of adenocarcinomas arising in the esophagus probably occur because of the presence of Barrett's metaplasia. Thus patients who have a predisposition to chronic reflux are at an increased risk for developing adenocarcinoma. The largest group includes those with hiatal hernias or severe reflux. Another group is composed of scleroderma patients, who are known to develop esophageal strictures as a result of chronic reflux. Achalasia patients who have had repeated dilations or myotomies also may develop this condition.

Radiologically, Barrett's mucosa should be considered in any patient who has a benign-appearing stricture of the esophagus, usually caused by reflux. The more proximal the stricture, the more the diagnosis should be considered. Also, small plaquelike irregularities of the mucosa in the region of a stricture also indicate possible Barrett's metaplasia. This finding can be seen only when the high-quality double-contrast technique is used. Malignant degeneration may be difficult to detect because stricturing and mucosal irregularity mask the early malignant changes.

Notes

CASE 70

Emphysematous Gastritis Caused by Infection

1. Hemolytic streptococci, *Clostridia* species, and coliform bacteria.

2. Corrosives.

3. Recent endoscopy or surgical procedure.

4. Peptic ulcer disease, gastric outlet obstruction, and pulmonary disease.

Reference

Feczko PJ, Mezwa DG, et al: Clinical significance of pneumatosis of the bowel wall, *Radiographics* 12:1069-1078, 1992.

Cross-Reference

Gastrointestinal Radiology: THE REQUISITES, ed 2, p 70.

Comment

The finding of air in the wall of the stomach is frequently an ominous sign. Although air in the stomach wall can be a sequela of recent endoscopy or gastric surgery, it is a rare complication. Despite the thousands of endoscopic procedures performed, a radiologist rarely encounters air in the gastric wall as a result of them.

Most commonly the occurrence of air in the wall represents a severe infection of the stomach, a type of phlegmonous gastritis. Although many organisms have been isolated in these infections, the most common are hemolytic streptococci, *Clostridia welchii,* and coliform bacteria. Infection does not appear to have a strong association with diabetes, although the condition can be a contributing factor. Infection has been identified in otherwise healthy patients, as well as in those with a variety of chronic, debilitating conditions (e.g., transplant recipients, postoperative patients, those with AIDS). The process by which the infection develops is uncertain, but it is believed that ulcers or other breaks in the mucosa allow bacteria access to the submucosal tissue, with resultant spread of infection. Discovery of phlegmonous gastritis probably indicates impending necrosis of the gastric wall. Prompt therapy, including gastrectomy and antibiotics, is necessary because the mortality is quite high.

Emphysematous gastritis also can be encountered in patients with gastric outlet obstruction, in whom elevated intraluminal pressures may force air into the gastric wall. Rarely the condition is seen in patients with pulmonary disease who also develop pneumatosis in other parts of the gastrointestinal tract. Patients who ingest corrosive agents in an attempt to commit suicide also can develop this complication, which heralds necrosis of the gastric wall. As is true of other radiologic findings, the clinical history is the most important factor in establishing the correct diagnosis.

Notes

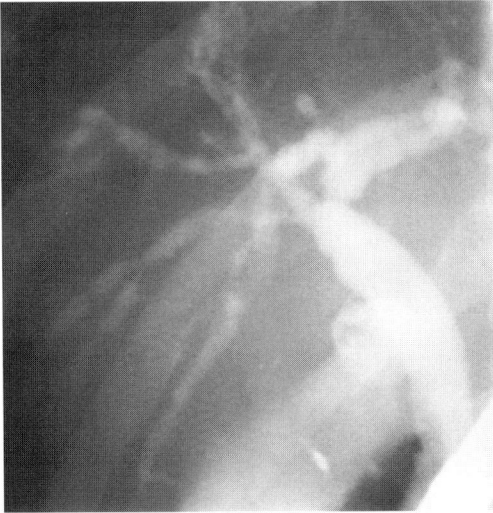

1. What infectious processes may produce this appearance?
2. What underlying condition may the patient have?
3. What parasites frequently involve the biliary system?
4. What infectious processes produce hepatitis in patients with AIDS?

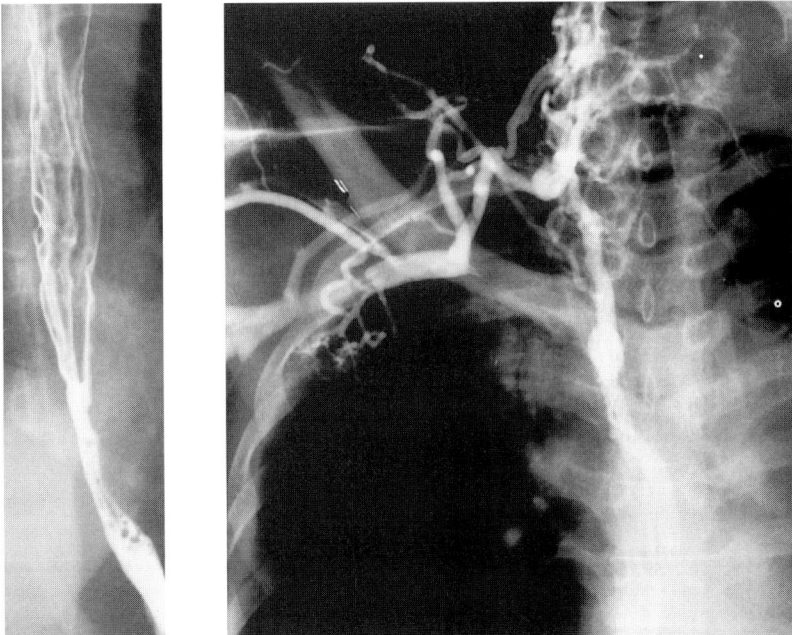

1. What clinical symptoms may this patient exhibit?
2. What structure must be obstructed for "downhill" varices to occur?
3. What pathologic condition most commonly produces this finding?
4. What other conditions may cause this abnormality?

CASE 71

AIDS-Associated Cholangitis

1. Ascending bacterial cholangitis, cytomegalovirus (CMV), and cryptosporidiosis.

2. Human immunodeficiency virus (HIV) infection.

3. *Ascaris* species and *Clonorchis sinensis.*

4. CMV and pneumocystic infection.

Reference

Feczko PJ: Gastrointestinal complications of human immuno-deficiency virus (HIV) infection, *Semin Roentgenol* 29:275-287, 1994.

Cross-Reference

Gastrointestinal Radiology: THE REQUISITES, ed 2, p 203.

Comment

Abnormal results of liver function tests are common among patients infected with HIV. Liver failure is a frequent source of morbidity and even mortality in these patients. Numerous possibilities must be considered. First, the at-risk population for HIV also has a high incidence of conventional hepatitis. In addition, these patients are prone to developing diffuse liver infections as a result of CMV or pneumocystic organisms. Systemic fungal infections also can involve the liver. The most frequent source of abnormal liver enzymes in these patients is probably opportunistic infection of the biliary system. The bile ducts are infected with organisms, usually CMV or crypto-sporidiosis, that are common pathogens in the gastrointestinal tract of the AIDS patient. With repeated episodes of biliary system infection, the ducts develop inflammation and fibrosis, resulting in multiple areas of irregularity or narrowing.

Ultrasound is the best modality for the identification of acute infection in these patients. There may be gallbladder wall thickening as seen in cholecystitis, or actual echogenic material may be present in the ducts as a result of the cellular debris. On imaging studies the best way to diagnose the biliary tract changes is by direct injection. Usually the extrahepatic ducts are not significantly affected. However, the intrahepatic ducts show narrowing and attenuation. There may be focal areas of dilation between the strictures. The changes are indistinguishable from those associated with sclerosing cholangitis as seen in patients with inflammatory bowel disease. Only the appropriate history can help differentiate the two diseases.

Notes

CASE 72

"Downhill" Varices Resulting from Lung Carcinoma

1. Venous distention in the neck, facial swelling, and arm swelling. These patients are often asymptomatic, however.

2. Superior vena cava (SVC).

3. Lung carcinoma with extension into the mediastinum.

4. Mediastinal fibrosis resulting from previous irradiation or infection, adenopathy resulting from lymphoma or other metastatic disease, substernal goiter, or thrombus resulting from indwelling catheters.

Reference

Levine MS: *Radiology of the esophagus,* Philadelphia, 1989, WB Saunders, p 200.

Cross-Reference

Gastrointestinal Radiology: THE REQUISITES, ed 2, p 8.

Comment

Typically, varices of the esophagus course in what is termed an *uphill direction.* That is, they start in the abdomen, extend along the gastric veins, and then run into the esophageal veins, where the blood reenters the systemic circulation at the point where the azygos vein drains into the SVC. The most common cause for this type of varices is underlying liver disease, typically alcoholic liver cirrhosis in the United States. In other countries, infectious causes are often the source of liver cirrhosis.

Venous structures of the head and neck must drain back to the heart via the SVC. If that structure becomes blocked, the collateral flow must be via intercostal vessels and mediastinal veins. These structures then drain into the venous plexus surrounding the esophagus. The blood thus drains in a "downhill" direction, from the head toward the heart. If the azygos vein is still patent, the collateral flow is directed back into the systemic circulation at the azygos level. Thus the varices are visible only in the upper third of the esophagus. If the process involves both the SVC and the azygos vein, the downhill varices continue down the entire extent of the esophagus to the coronary veins of the upper abdomen and then into the portal circulation. In this instance the varices are seen throughout the entire esophagus.

By far the most common cause of SVC obstruction is lung carcinoma that either directly invades the SVC or compresses it with adenopathy. Any process that produces bulky mediastinal adenopathy can also produce downhill varices. Also, fibrosis of the mediastinum causes gradual compression of the SVC, with resultant obstruction. Occasionally, patients with indwelling catheters of long duration may develop a thrombus in the SVC, which could lead to eventual occlusion. Given the high flow state of the SVC, this complication is rare.

Notes

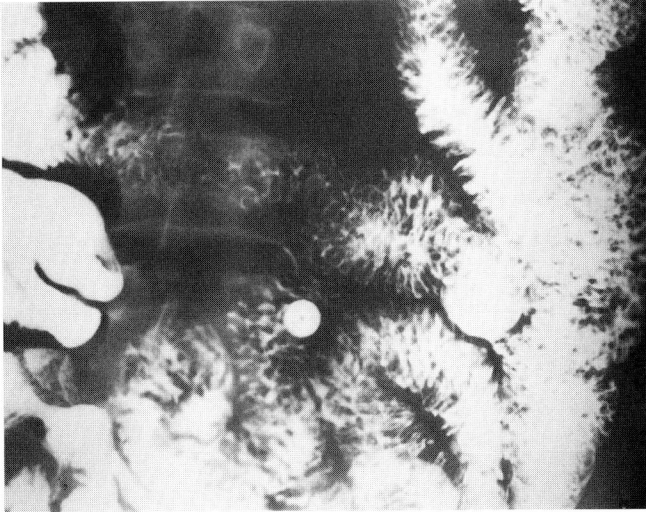

1. What diffuse small bowel conditions may produce adenopathy?
2. What clinical group is affected by Whipple's disease?
3. What condition is also known as *pseudo-Whipple's disease?*
4. What other organs can be involved in Whipple's disease?
5. What is the causative agent of Whipple's disease?

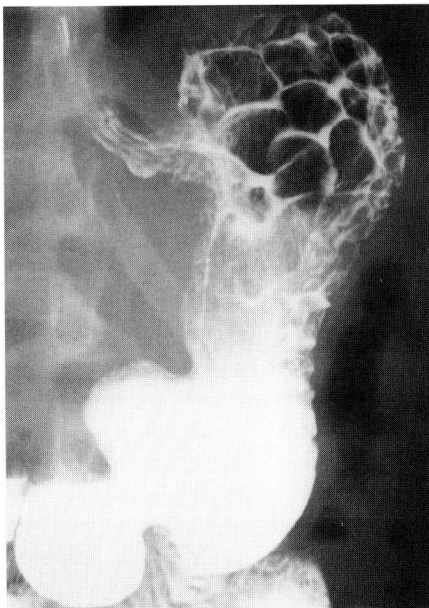

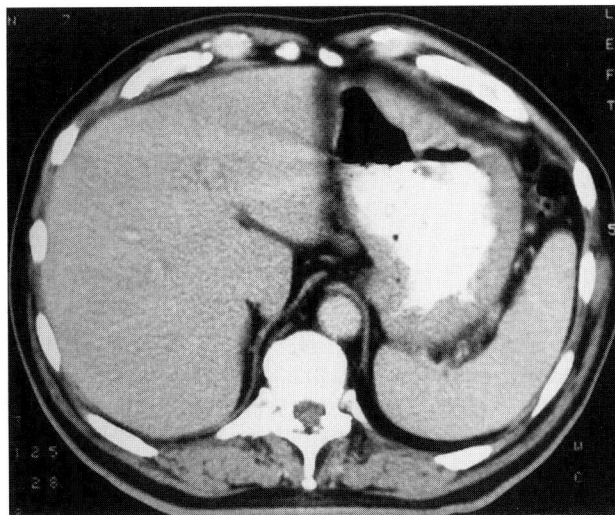

1. Do patients with eosinophilic gastroenteritis develop a peripheral eosinophilia?
2. What portions of the stomach are involved by Ménétrier's disease?
3. What are the manifestations of sarcoidosis of the stomach?
4. Which of these conditions respond to steroids?

C A S E 7 3

Whipple's Disease

1. Crohn's disease, lymphoma, Whipple's disease, *Mycobacterium* species infection, and sprue.

2. Middle-aged men.

3. *Mycobacterium avium-intracellulare* infection.

4. Joints, heart valves, and the central nervous system.

5. Whipple's bacilli.

Reference

Horton KM, Fishman EK: Uncommon inflammatory diseases of the small bowel: CT findings, *Am J Roentgenol* 170:385-391, 1998.

Cross-Reference

Gastrointestinal Radiology: THE REQUISITES, ed 2, p 111.

Comment

Whipple's disease is a rare clinical condition produced by small bowel infection with Whipple's bacilli. The organism primarily involves the small bowel mucosa but can also infect the joints, central nervous system, and even heart valves. Diagnosis is made by biopsy of the proximal small bowel mucosa. Biopsy shows that the lamina propria is filled with macrophages that stain periodic acid-Schiff (PAS) positive. The fragments of the bacilli in the macrophages retain the stain.

Whipple's disease predominantly affects middle-aged men. Clinical symptoms include diarrhea and steatorrhea caused by malabsorption, fevers, arthralgias, and nervous system complaints. These latter symptoms may actually precede the gastrointestinal complaints. There are reports of a mild immune deficiency associated with this condition. Although the disease once had a fatal course, it is now easily treated with a several-month course of antibiotics.

On small bowel examination, there may be a mild degree of thickening of the valvulae of the small bowel, perhaps as a manifestation of mild lymphangiectasia, which often develops in this condition. A more subtle finding, which can best be seen on enteroclysis, is a fine micronodular pattern (1- to 2-mm elevations) on the small bowel mucosa. An unusual finding is the presence of low density mesenteric lymph nodes as seen on CT examination. The Whipple's bacillus extends into the lymphatic system, causing mild lymphangiectasia and fat deposition in the lymph nodes. Fold thickening and low density lymph nodes are also seen in patients with *Mycobacterium avium-intracellulare* infection of the bowel, which is why it is often termed *pseudo-Whipple's disease.*

Notes

C A S E 7 4

Ménétrier's Disease of the Stomach

1. Nearly always, and typically the eosinophilia is 10% or greater.

2. Although classically described as proximal, the disease can also involve the antrum in up to one half of patients.

3. Slight nodularity to thickened folds. In advanced cases the thickening of the wall resembles a scirrhous process.

4. Eosinophilic gastritis and sarcoidosis respond well to steroids; Ménétrier's disease does not.

Reference

Furth EE, Rubesin SE, Levine MS: Pathologic primer on gastritis: illustrated sum and substance, *Radiology* 197:693-699, 1995.

Cross-Reference

Gastrointestinal Radiology: THE REQUISITES, ed 2, p 65.

Comment

Thickened gastric folds are a common radiologic finding that can be produced by a number of unusual disorders. The imaging finding itself is so nonspecific that all of the various disorders cannot be distinguished by their radiologic appearance. In a patient with peripheral eosinophilia and thickened gastric folds, eosinophilic gastritis should be strongly considered. There is often associated small bowel disease in patients with fold thickening. Sarcoidosis of the stomach may be more common than first appreciated; according to some reports the condition can be identified in up to 10% of gastric biopsies. There is always associated pulmonary disease, and other portions of the gastrointestinal tract may be involved. Both of these conditions respond dramatically to steroids, as do few other gastric conditions.

Ménétrier's disease is a rare condition in which marked glandular hypertrophy of the stomach develops without any underlying cause. There is associated enlargement of the gastric rugae, hypochloremia, and hypoproteinemia. Despite the fact that there is often increased mucous secretion in the stomach, gastric acid output is reduced, which differentiates the disease from other hypertrophic gastritis in which acid output is often elevated. Protein-losing enteropathy is another distinguishing characteristic of Ménétrier's disease. Patients often have pain, weight loss, vomiting, and diarrhea. According to the classic description of the disease the hypertrophic fold changes occur only in the proximal stomach, but it is now known that the thickened folds can be seen throughout the stomach, even the antrum. Spontaneous remission can occur, but often Ménétrier's disease is a chronic recurrent illness that responds poorly to various therapies (e.g., antibiotics and H_2 blockers). In severe instances, gastric resection may be required. Controversy remains regarding whether the condition is premalignant.

Notes

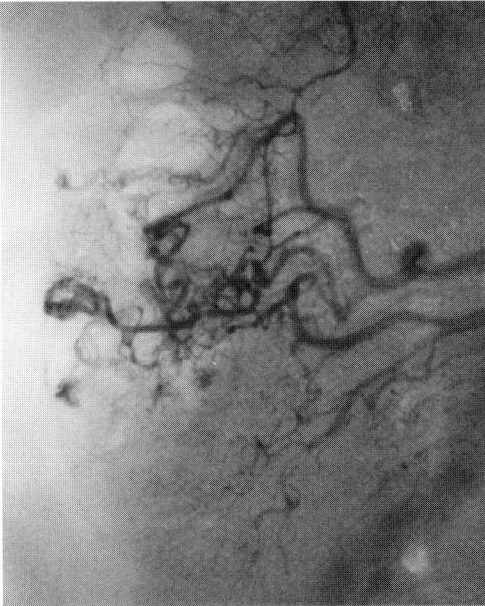

1. What is the most common cause of lower gastrointestinal bleeding in adults?
2. What is the distinctive angiographic abnormality in this patient?
3. What is the most common location for this abnormality?
4. In what age group is this abnormality seen?

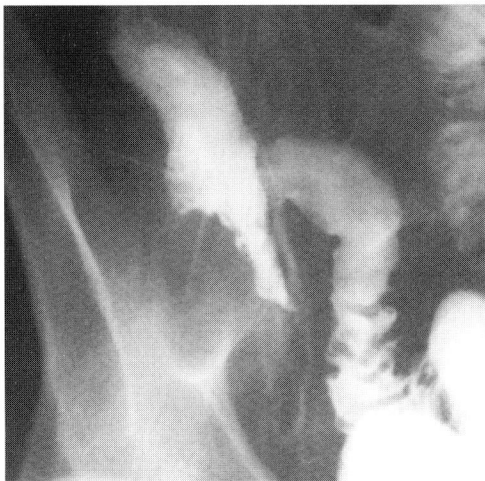

1. Name conditions that produce a coned cecum and terminal ileal disease.
2. What infectious condition in that region typically spares the terminal ileum?
3. Ulcerative colitis typically produces what change in the terminal ileum?
4. What fungal infection may produce this abnormality?

Vascular Ectasia (Angiodysplasia) of the Colon

1. Diverticula.

2. Early draining vein.

3. Right colon.

4. Elderly.

Reference

Miller KD, Tutton RH, Bell KA, et al: Angiodysplasia of the colon, *Radiology* 132:309-313, 1979.

Cross-Reference

Gastrointestinal Radiology: THE REQUISITES, ed 2, p 312.

Comment

Severe bleeding from the lower gastrointestinal tract is a common clinical dilemma. The most common cause is bleeding from diverticula. Tumors rarely present with severe, profuse gastrointestinal bleeding. The other abnormality that should be considered in such cases is angiodysplasia of the colon. Angiodysplasia is a generic term describing vascular malformations in the bowel wall. These malformations are not congenital in nature, but are believed to be acquired abnormalities, perhaps resulting from repeated venous obstruction caused by contraction of the bowel wall. Repeated muscular contraction of the wall is believed to produce venous obstruction with distention of capillaries and veins and lead to the eventual development of a vascular malformation. This theory is somewhat speculative, however. Angiodysplasias predominantly affect the elderly. There is a loose association with aortic stenosis.

Angiography is the primary method of defining the lesions. If they are close to the mucosal surface of the bowel, the lesions also may be identifiable on colonoscopy. At angiography, there may be a slightly dilated feeding artery, although this is not a constant finding. Only larger malformations are visible angiographically as a tuft of vessels or a small blush of contrast localized to one area. The hallmark of angiodysplasia is its venous drainage. There is often a slightly dilated vein draining the lesion, which is often more densely opacified as well. Also, it typically fills earlier than the other veins. This early draining, slightly enlarged vein may be the only finding to help identify the lesion. It is recommended that the arterial injection be of short duration (<4 seconds) so that the early draining vein can be easily identified. Sometimes the artery and the vein are simultaneously opacified, resulting in a railroad track appearance.

Most angiodysplasias are seen in the right colon, although a small percentage of them are found in the left colon. Treatment is typically surgical in nature, although it is important that the lesion be identified as the site of bleeding. Many of these abnormalities are just incidental findings in older patients.

Notes

Amebiasis of the Cecum

1. Tuberculosis and Crohn's disease.

2. Amebiasis.

3. Dilated terminal ileum (backwash ileitis).

4. Blastomycosis.

Reference

Gardiner R, Smith C: Infective enterocolitides, *Radiol Clin North Am* 25:67-78, 1987.

Cross-Reference

Gastrointestinal Radiology: THE REQUISITES, ed 2, p 265.

Comment

The coned appearance of the cecum is produced by several diseases, most of which are inflammatory in nature. In determining the exact cause, the radiologist must make a proper evaluation of the region. The most common causative condition encountered in industrialized societies is Crohn's disease. Tuberculosis can present with an appearance virtually identical to that of Crohn's disease, with a coned cecum and inflammation of the terminal ileum. Adjacent inflammatory conditions, such as appendicitis and diverticulitis, are considerations. Neoplasms, such as adenocarcinoma and lymphoma, are also in the differential diagnosis. Long-standing ulcerative colitis may produce a coned cecum but often with a dilated terminal ileum, the so-called backwash ileitis. Other rare conditions that can produce this appearance include anisakiasis, blastomycosis, and *Yersinia* species infection.

Amebiasis is an infection of the bowel produced by the protozoan *Entamoeba histolytica.* It is acquired by ingestion of infected water or soil that contains the cysts. When infection occurs, it can range from very mild or indolent to severe, acute colitis. When cysts spread to the liver or lungs, they can produce abscesses. Changes in the colon include ulceration, which can be either diffuse granularity, collar-button ulcers, or aphthous ulcers. The colon may have skip lesions, with intervening areas of normal bowel, and thus may resemble Crohn's disease. Focal severe inflammation may mimic annular carcinomas. There also may be pronounced granulation tissue formation, leading to protuberant lesions called *amebomas,* which can also mimic neoplasia.

The cecum is invariably infected in amebiasis, and the classic appearance is that of the coned cecum. This abnormality is often seen in the chronic stages of colitis. One strong differential consideration is that amebiasis does not affect the terminal ileum, as does Crohn's disease and tuberculosis. However, amebiasis is seen predominantly in underdeveloped countries and should be considered only if the history is appropriate.

Notes

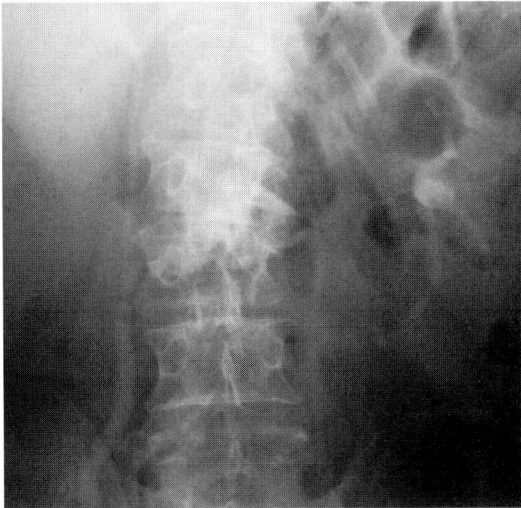

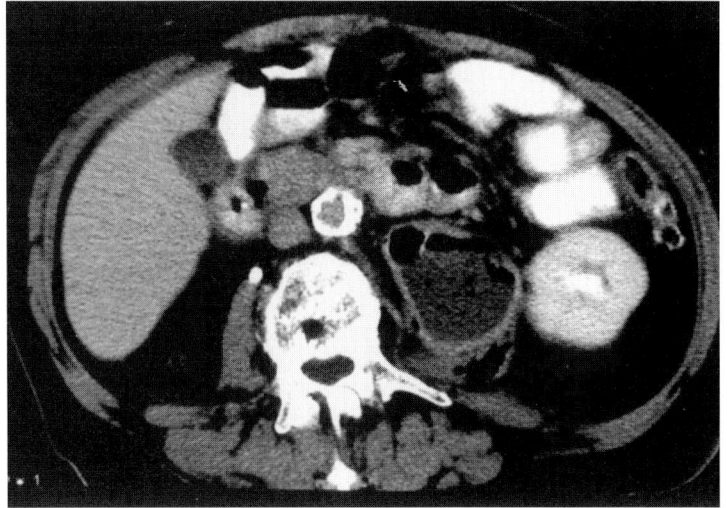

1. What is the most likely diagnosis?
2. What is the primary symptomatology?
3. What is the source of the abnormality?
4. What is the best therapeutic approach?

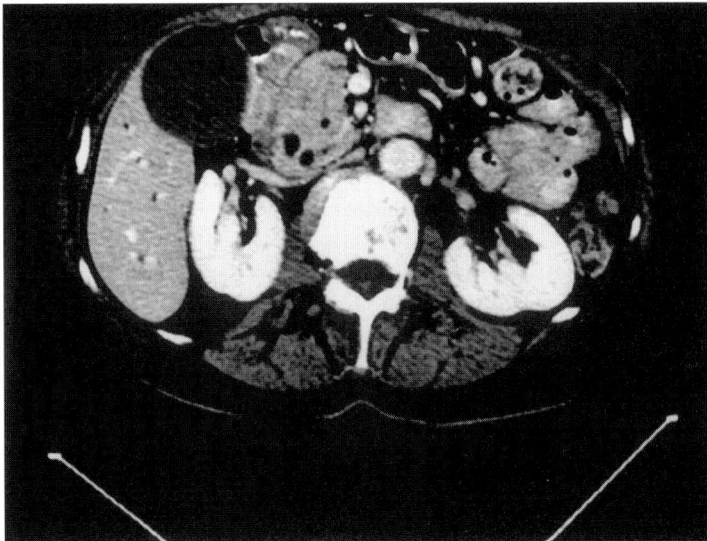

1. What is this sign called?
2. What pancreatic diseases could produce this appearance?
3. What biliary disease could produce this appearance?
4. What duodenal diseases should be considered?

Psoas Abscess

1. Psoas abscess.

2. Flank pain.

3. Adjacent infection from the kidneys or spine, surgery, colon abnormalities, or hematogenous spread from another source (drug addicts).

4. Percutaneous catheter drainage.

Reference

Gazelle GS, Mueller PR: Abdominal abscess: imaging and intervention, *Radiol Clin North Am* 32:913-931, 1994.

Cross-Reference

Gastrointestinal Radiology: THE REQUISITES, ed 2, p 302.

Comment

This patient had flank pain and was initially believed to have a kidney stone, hence the resultant intravenous pyelogram. An astute radiologist noticed the linear collections of air along the paraspinal region and ordered a CT examination that served to confirm the diagnosis of psoas abscess, which is quite evident on the CT study. Psoas abscesses were once quite common, often being the sequela of adjacent inflammatory processes in the kidneys or spine (tuberculosis). Today the abscess may be the result of a surgical procedure. They are also encountered in immunosuppressed patients and are often caused by bacteria spread via the blood stream. Psoas abscesses are a common complication of intravenous drug use. Pathologic conditions of the colon may spread to the adjacent psoas muscle, resulting in an abscess. This process can be occur with diverticulitis, Crohn's disease, appendicitis, or perforating neoplasm. In this patient the abscess was the result of diverticulitis in the sigmoid colon that spread along the psoas muscle.

This abscess, along with many other abdominal abscesses, is amenable to treatment by percutaneous catheter drainage. Shortly after the CT scan, a drainage catheter was placed through the patient's back and into the abscess. This action along with aggressive antibiotic therapy allowed the patient to leave the hospital after several days. At a later date, once the inflammation had subsided, the diverticulitis was surgically treated.

Notes

Double-Duct Sign

1. Double-duct sign.

2. Pancreatitis or pancreatic carcinoma.

3. Stone impacted in the ampulla, or cholangiocarcinoma.

4. Duodenal or ampullary carcinoma.

Reference

Zeman RK, Silverman PM, Ascher SM, et al: Helical CT of the pancreas and biliary tract, *Radiol Clin North Am* 33:887-901, 1995.

Cross-Reference

Gastrointestinal Radiology: THE REQUISITES, ed 2, p 207.

Comment

Simultaneous dilation of the pancreatic and biliary tracts often indicates disease in the area where both ducts are anatomically close or joined together. The term *double-duct sign* refers to narrowing of both ducts in the head of the pancreas, where they are close together, or with regard to cross-sectional imaging it indicates dilation of both pancreatic and bile ducts. Basically, diseases that involve the pancreatic head or ampullary region can produce this abnormality.

The double-duct sign was initially described in relation to pancreatic carcinoma; narrowing of both the pancreatic duct and the common bile duct in the head was indicative of pancreatic carcinoma. However, it soon became apparent that pancreatitis could produce a similar abnormality of the ducts, and based on this finding it was often difficult to distinguish the etiology. Some feel that the closer the involved ducts are, the more likely it is that the narrowing is caused by carcinoma.

Lesions in the ampullary region of the ducts also can produce simultaneous dilation. Thus a stone impacted in the ampulla may produce this appearance. A ductal neoplasm of the distal ducts near the ampulla could also obstruct both ducts. Finally, lesions of the duodenum, either duodenal carcinoma or a neoplasm of the papilla, can simultaneously obstruct both ducts.

Notes

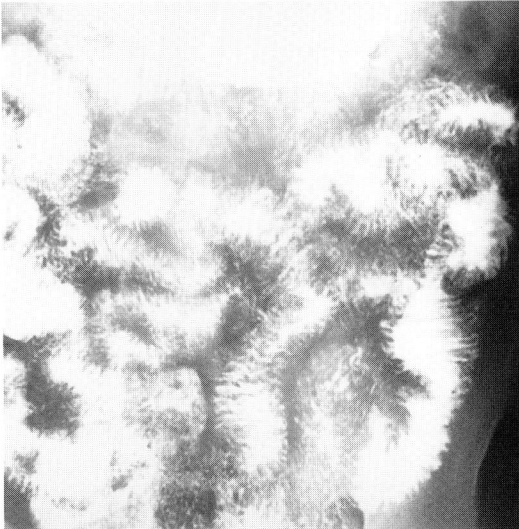

1. What protozoan parasitic infection occurs in sporadic outbreaks as a result of contaminated water?
2. What infection is caused by the ingestion of raw, infected fish?
3. How is giardiasis best diagnosed?
4. What organism produces Chagas disease, which destroys the ganglion cells of the bowel?

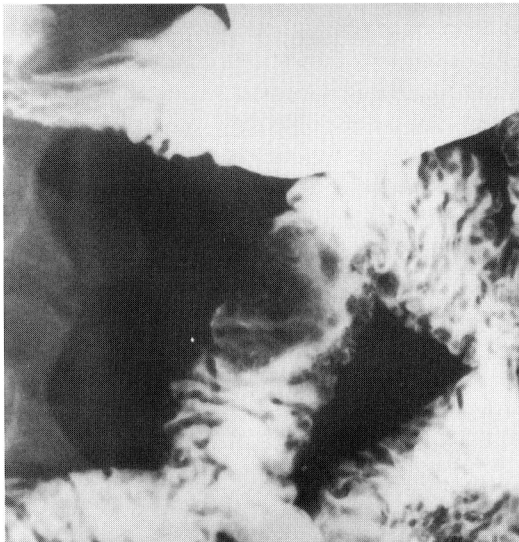

1. Histologically, of what tissue type do most duodenal polyps consist?
2. Where do most villous adenomas of the duodenum occur?
3. What is the most common cause of polypoid lesions at the base of the duodenal bulb?
4. What is the incidence of duodenal polyps in patients with familial polyposis coli?

CASE 79

Giardiasis of the Small Bowel in a Patient with Immunoglobulin Deficiency

1. Giardiasis or cryptosporidiosis.

2. Anisakiasis.

3. Small bowel biopsy or aspiration.

4. *Trypanosoma cruzi.*

Reference

Brandon J, Glick SN, Teplick SK: Intestinal giardiasis: the importance of serial filming, *Am J Roentgenol* 144:581-584, 1985.

Cross-Reference

Gastrointestinal Radiology: THE REQUISITES, ed 2, p 309.

Comment

Giardia lamblia is a flagellated protozoan. It occurs endemically in many parts of the world, and many people harbor the organism yet remain asymptomatic. It is estimated that more than 1% of the U.S. population carries the organism. It is best known, however, as a pathogen that produces sporadic outbreaks of diarrhea through contamination of the water supply. However, it readily afflicts immunocompromised individuals. Infections occur when an individual drinks the contaminated water, and *G. lamblia* is one of the causes of traveler's diarrhea.

Once ingested, the organism resides in the duodenum and jejunum, where it exists as a motile flagellated protozoan. The organism binds to the brush border of the epithelial cells, where an antibody response occurs. Because the organism resides in the mucosa, the infection can be diagnosed by duodenal or small bowel biopsies or aspiration. Giardiasis also produces cysts that travel down the bowel lumen and are then expelled in the feces. When the infected feces contact water, contamination occurs. These cysts may be evident in the stool but are often difficult to diagnose, which is why the small bowel biopsy is the best method for diagnosis.

Radiologically these patients may have thickened folds in the proximal small bowel as a result of the inflammatory response. Infection appears to be confined to the duodenum and jejunum. In severe cases the bowel may have a spruelike appearance, but this is rare. Information regarding the patient's immune status is clinically important when making the diagnosis. Giardiasis is common among patients with immunoglobulin deficiencies. Also, it affects transplant recipients, patients undergoing chemotherapy, and patients with acquired immunodeficiency syndrome.

Notes

CASE 80

Villous Adenoma of the Duodenum

1. Adenomatous polyps.

2. Periampullary region.

3. Prolapse of gastric mucosa or a gastric polyp.

4. More than half of these patients develop duodenal polyps.

Reference

Delpy JC, Braneton JN, Drouillard J, et al: Non-Vaterian duodenal adenomas: report of 24 cases and review of the literature, *Gastrointest Radiol* 8:135-142, 1983.

Cross-Reference

Gastrointestinal Radiology: THE REQUISITES, ed 2, p 88.

Comment

Since the advent of the biphasic upper gastrointestinal examination, the occurrence of solitary polyps in the duodenum has been found to be more common than once thought. In contrast to the stomach, where most polyps are hyperplastic, in the duodenum, solitary polyps are most frequently adenomas. Hyperplastic polyps of the duodenum are rare, despite the inflammatory changes that occur there. As is true of colonic polyps, the larger the adenoma, the more likely it is to be malignant.

The location of the polyp may be a helpful distinguishing feature. A polypoid filling defect in the bulb may be a gastric polyp, prolapsing mucosa, a Brunner's gland adenoma (not a true adenomatous polyp), another type of tumor (leiomyoma, metastasis, etc.), an adenoma, or an ectopic pancreatic rest. The more distal the polyp is in the duodenum, the more likely it is to be an adenoma or villous adenoma. Villous adenomas are particularly common in the periampullary region. Leiomyomas and ectopic pancreatic rest can occur anywhere but are more common in the proximal half of the duodenum. As a general rule of thumb, the more distal the lesion is in the duodenum, the more likely it is to be clinically important.

Duodenal polyps are seen with increased frequency in the patient with virtually any of the polyposis syndromes. In the patient with familial polyposis coli, the growths may be either adenomas or hyperplastic polyps. Patients with Gardner's syndrome or familial polyposis coli have a high incidence of periampullary malignancies, particularly those with Gardner's syndrome.

Notes

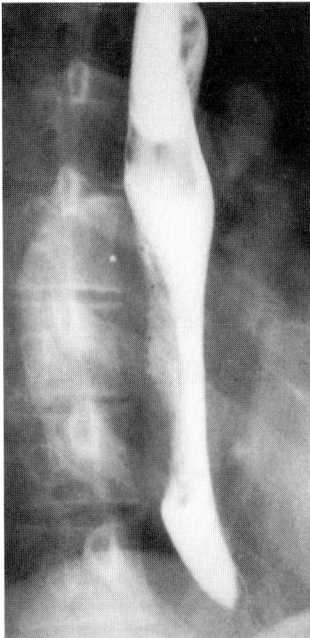

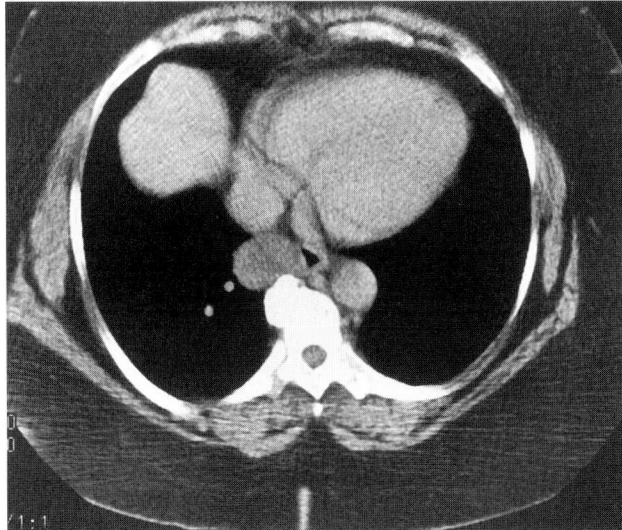

1. What are the most common benign tumors of the esophagus?
2. What type of cells line a duplication cyst of the esophagus?
3. Do duplication cysts of the esophagus communicate with the lumen?
4. What is the difference between a duplication cyst and a retention cyst?

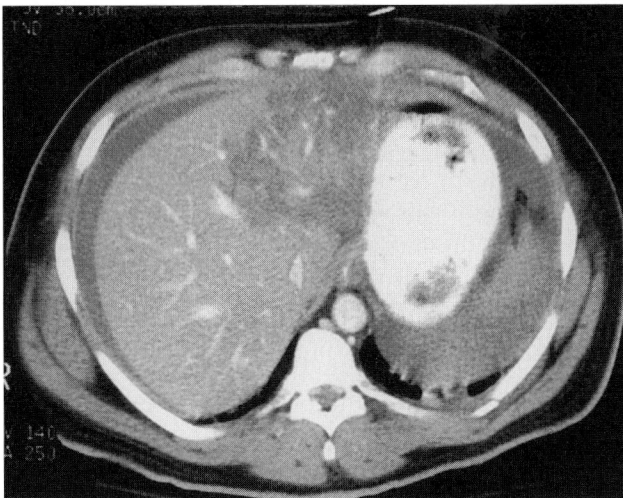

1. What is the most common cause of liver hematomas?
2. What nonneoplastic condition may be associated with spontaneous liver hemorrhage?
3. What vascular structures are most often injured in blunt hepatic trauma?
4. What is the best treatment for liver hemorrhage?

Duplication Cyst of the Esophagus

1. Leiomyomas, neurofibromas, granular cell tumors, and lipomas.

2. Usually ciliated columnar-lined epithelium.

3. Occasionally, although most present as submucosal masses.

4. Retention cysts are postulated to be acquired as a result of obstructed glands, whereas duplication cysts are a congenital development.

Reference
Levine MS: *Radiology of the esophagus,* Philadelphia, 1989, WB Saunders, p 127.

Cross-Reference
Gastrointestinal Radiology: THE REQUISITES, ed 2, p 8.

Comment
A submucosal mass of the esophagus with obtuse margins should lead to the consideration of a benign tumor of the esophagus. Most benign tumors (e.g., leiomyomas, lipomas, and neurofibromas) arise from tissues that are present in the wall of the esophagus. These lesions occur far more frequently than do duplication cysts.

Duplication cysts are congenital developments. Embryologically the pulmonary system arises as buds from the primitive gut. The tracheobronchial tree arises from the upper portion of the esophagus. Occasionally, aberrant buds of tissue arise from other portions of the esophagus, leading to duplication cysts or bronchopulmonary sequestrations. Interestingly the tissue lining the esophageal duplication cyst is ciliated columnar epithelium and not squamous epithelium. Thus the esophageal duplication cyst more closely resembles a bronchogenic cyst and may be difficult to differentiate pathologically. Although this particular lesion was completely within the wall of the esophagus, the pathologist described it as a bronchogenic cyst because of its cellular lining.

Most duplication cysts are found incidentally during routine radiologic studies. Rarely they produce symptoms of dysphagia. Sometimes the duplication cysts communicate with the lumen of the esophagus, usually because of ulceration of the overlying mucosa, probably a result of trauma caused by ingested food. A retention cyst is an acquired lesion. The exact mechanism by which they are acquired is uncertain, although some believe that retention cysts may be caused by obstruction of esophageal glands, with mucous retained in the submucosa.

Notes

Liver Laceration Resulting from an Automobile Accident

1. They are usually iatrogenic; most are caused by biopsies.

2. Pregnancy-induced hypertension, or eclampsia, and childbirth.

3. Hepatic veins.

4. Catheter embolization.

Reference
Federico JA, Horner WR, Clark DE, et al: Blunt hepatic trauma, *Arch Surg* 125:905-909, 1990.

Cross-Reference
Gastrointestinal Radiology: THE REQUISITES, ed 2, p 174.

Comment
Trauma to the liver is a fairly common finding in industrialized societies. The major cause of hepatic trauma and its complications of bleeding and hematoma is iatrogenic, usually the result of biopsies and other percutaneous passage of devices into the liver. The second most common cause is blunt trauma, usually associated with automobile accidents or other deceleration injuries. This case is a classic example of liver injury caused by impact with a steering wheel. Spontaneous hepatic hematomas and extracapsular hemorrhage also can occur in patients with tumors such as hepatic adenomas and hepatomas. Pregnant women are prone to spontaneous liver hemorrhage without any other underlying conditions; sometimes this hemorrhage is related to pregnancy-induced hypertension, but it may occur spontaneously.

A complex classification has been devised for the staging of liver trauma. This system is based on the size and depth of liver lacerations, the size of the hepatic hematoma, the location of the hematoma, and possible vascular injury, such as active bleeding or evidence of devascularization. Hepatic injuries also are associated with a high incidence of splenic injuries and rib or pelvic fractures. The most common vessels injured in blunt trauma are the hepatic veins, which usually avulse from their attachment to the inferior vena cava. Portal vein and hepatic artery injuries are fairly rare.

The best method for the assessment of hepatic injury is CT examination. Liver lacerations are marked by linear or branching areas of low density in the hepatic parenchyma. They do not have to extend out to the capsule. These fractures follow the distribution of the venous system on occasion. Sometimes the only finding is some periportal low density, which is actually hemorrhage. Hematomas may be hyperdense on noncontrast studies but hypodense after the administration of contrast. Poor prognostic signs include deep perihilar lacerations, evidence of vascular injury, and active bleeding. Posttraumatic complications include pseudoaneurysms, abscesses, and bilomas.

Notes

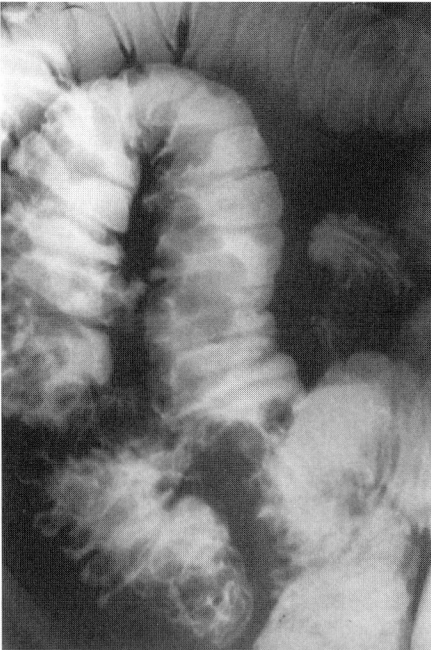

1. What is Cowden disease?
2. What are the features of Cronkhite-Canada syndrome?
3. What disease may cause cutaneous masses and small bowel tumors?
4. What histologic type of polyps occur in patients with Peutz-Jeghers syndrome?

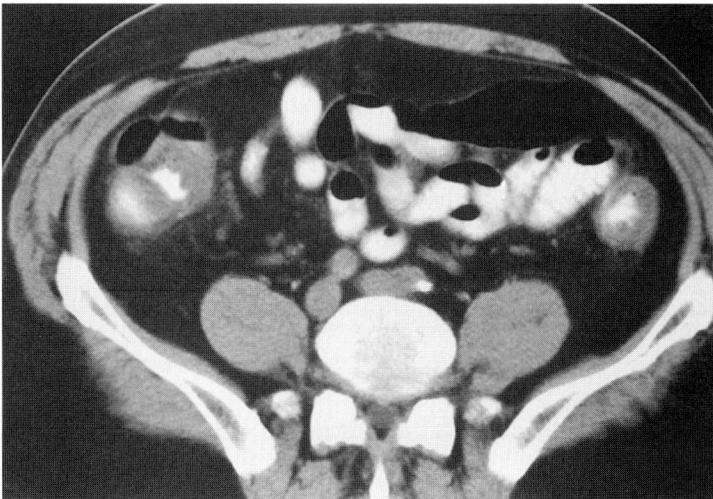

1. What is the predisposing factor for the development of this condition?
2. What organism is responsible?
3. How often is there rectal sparing in this condition?
4. What is the treatment?

Peutz-Jeghers Syndrome

1. Disorder causing hamartomas of the small bowel, hyperkeratosis, and thyroid and breast abnormalities.

2. Multiple intestinal hamartomas, alopecia, anorexia, and weight loss.

3. Neurofibromatosis.

4. Hamartomas.

Reference

Sener RN, Kumcuoglu Z, Elmas N, et al: Peutz-Jeghers syndrome: CT and US demonstration of small bowel polyps, *Gastrointest Radiol* 16:21-23, 1991.

Cross-Reference

Gastrointestinal Radiology: THE REQUISITES, ed 2, p 120.

Comment

Multiple polyps of the small bowel occur in a number of conditions, and it is not always possible to differentiate the etiology. Sometimes certain features, particularly clinical features, can help to establish the diagnosis.

The most well-known small bowel polyposis syndrome is Peutz-Jeghers syndrome. This disorder is characterized by multiple hamartomatous polyps of the gastrointestinal tract and mucocutaneous melanotic pigmentation, particularly in the oral cavity. The polyps are usually hamartomas and occur predominantly in the jejunum and less frequently in the ileum, stomach, and colon. It is an autosomal dominant inheritance with variable penetrance, and there is no gender or racial predilection. Polyps are usually apparent by the second or third decade of life. The syndrome is associated with a slightly increased risk of malignancy involving the gastrointestinal tract and extraintestinal area. However, the increased risk is believed to be a genetic predisposition unrelated to the hamartomatous polyps.

Cowden disease is also a multiple hamartomatous condition. It includes hamartomas of the gastrointestinal tract, breast, and thyroid. Hyperkeratosis of the skin also occurs. Cowden disease is a rare condition, and little is known of it. Cronkhite-Canada syndrome is another rare small bowel intestinal syndrome. In patients with this syndrome there is a diffuse intestinal polyposis involving not only the small bowel but the stomach and colon as well. The polyps are inflammatory. The major features are protein-losing enteropathy and malabsorption, which result in nail dystrophy, alopecia, and some pigmentary changes. It is a nonfamilial occurrence, and its etiology is uncertain. Patients with neurofibromatosis also can develop multiple neurofibromas of the gastrointestinal tract, predominantly in the stomach and small bowel. These growths may bleed or intussuscept.

Notes

Pseudomembranous Colitis

1. Consumption of antibiotics.

2. *Clostridium difficile.*

3. Often (in 20% to 70% of cases).

4. Discontinuation of antibiotics; sometimes vancomycin is prescribed.

Reference

Ros PR, Buetow PC, Pantongrag-Brown L, et al: Pseudomembranous colitis, *Radiology* 198:1-12, 1996.

Cross-Reference

Gastrointestinal Radiology: THE REQUISITES, ed 2, p 281.

Comment

Pseudomembranous colitis is frequently encountered. It actually represents an infection with the *Clostridium difficile* bacillus, although the relationship is variable. *C. difficile* can be found in many healthy patients (20% of the population), in whom it does not produce extensive colonization. Under certain circumstances (e.g., during the course of antibiotic therapy or chemotherapy), an overgrowth of this bacterium may develop, which is why this condition is often called *antibiotic-associated colitis.* However, many episodes of diarrhea associated with antibiotic use are not caused by *C. difficile* infection; probably only the most severe cases are caused by this bacterium. The relationship is even more difficult to establish in that the onset of symptoms may occur anywhere from a few days to 8 weeks after antibiotics have been initiated, although typically it takes fewer than 2 weeks.

C. difficile produces several endotoxins, some of which are detectable with laboratory assays. These toxins produce an inflammatory and necrotic change in the mucosa, with subsequent loss of fluid through the wall of the bowel. On sigmoidoscopy there are small, raised, yellowish plaques; cellular debris; and mucus, hence the term *pseudomembranous colitis.* The inflammatory process may involve the whole colon, but in a substantial number of patients the rectum is spared or only segments of the colon are involved.

Radiologically, in severe cases the abnormalities may be apparent on plain abdominal films. The findings include thickening of the haustral folds, thickening of the bowel wall, and a shaggy appearance of the mucosa. The changes may mimic ischemia. Barium studies are usually not indicated but show the thickened folds and irregular margins to the barium. Toxic megacolon can occur in patients with this condition. CT is probably the best modality for evaluation of severe cases because the thickened bowel is readily apparent and the study does not precipitate any complications. Treatment is discontinuation of the antibiotics, sometimes use of vancomycin, and supportive therapy.

Notes

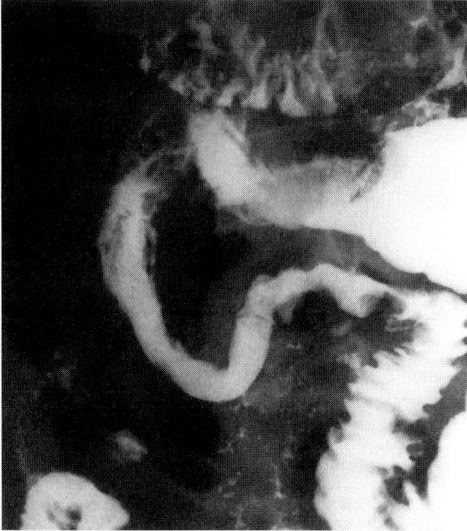

1. What conditions may produce focal strictures of the small bowel?
2. Use of what illegal drugs may produce ischemic changes in the intestines?
3. Hypercoagulable states may produce what type of changes in the intestines?
4. What layer of bowel is least affected by the vascular supply?

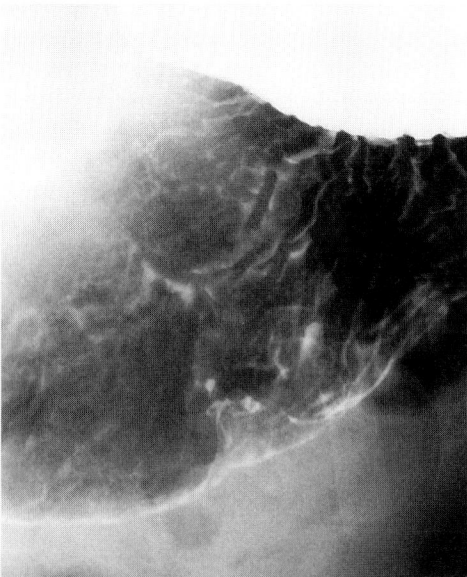

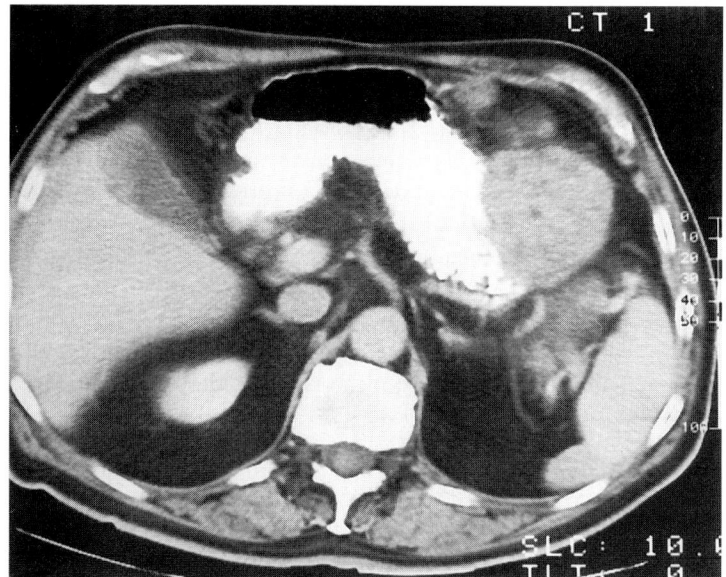

1. What neoplasms of the stomach grow exophytically?
2. What is the most common benign submucosal tumor of the stomach?
3. How is a leiomyoma distinguished from a leiomyosarcoma?
4. What congenital abnormality may mimic a leiomyoma?

Ischemic Stricture of the Small Bowel

1. Crohn's disease, certain infections, radiation therapy, and ischemia.

2. Cocaine or amphetamines.

3. Venous ischemic changes.

4. Serosal layer.

Reference
Scholz FJ: Ischemic bowel disease, *Radiol Clin North Am* 31: 1197-1217, 1993.

Cross-Reference
Gastrointestinal Radiology: THE REQUISITES, ed 2, p 107.

Comment
Bowel ischemia can be caused by a variety of processes. The disease may result from major arterial occlusion, or the arterioles alone may be affected by some process. Often, ischemia may not be accompanied by any obvious vascular obstructive process, making diagnosis difficult.

Radiologically the earliest change in the bowel is thickening of the mucosal folds. The involved segments may be hyperperistaltic. However, within hours, as the ischemia progresses, the bowel usually becomes atonic. The bowel wall may become edematous as cells lose their integrity, and hemorrhage into the bowel wall may occur. These pathologic abnormalities produce further fold thickening and even effacement of the fold pattern. Separation of the bowel loops also is evident as a result of the thickening of the bowel wall. If the ischemia progresses, the bowel wall may become necrotic. This necrosis may be manifested by air developing in the bowel wall. However, air in the wall also may be a result of loss of mucosal integrity and may not always indicate complete bowel necrosis. In certain instances, bowel has recovered despite the presence of pneumatosis in conjunction with the ischemia. If the ischemic changes can be reversed and blood flow can be reestablished, the bowel will survive. However, there may be residual scarring and fibrosis of the involved segments of intestine. These ischemic strictures may appear as rigid, nonmotile segments on small bowel examination because of the fibrosis that ensued. The mucosa may be featureless or diminished, as in this patient. Once this appearance develops, it may remain with the patient for the rest of his or her life.

Notes

Leiomyosarcoma of the Stomach

1. Generally, tumors of spindle cell origin, such as leiomyosarcomas, leiomyomas, and leiomyoblastoma, and rarely, neurofibromas or even lymphomas.

2. Leiomyoma.

3. Mitotic activity evident on pathologic examination (or the presence of metastases).

4. Ectopic pancreatic rest or duplication cyst.

Reference
Fishman EK, Urban BA, Hruban RH: CT of the stomach: spectrum of disease, *Radiographics* 16:1035, 1996.

Cross-Reference
Gastrointestinal Radiology: THE REQUISITES, ed 2, p 71.

Comment
Smooth muscle or spindle cell tumors are among the more commonly encountered tumors of the stomach. They account for almost half of all benign stomach tumors. Only a small percentage (<10%) are malignant in nature. Benign leiomyomas occur equally among men and women, whereas malignant leiomyosarcomas are more common in men. There tends to be a slight increase in the number of tumors with increasing age.

It is difficult to radiologically distinguish between leiomyomas, leiomyosarcomas, and other submucosal tumors. The benign leiomyoma can be found anywhere in the stomach, whereas its sarcomatous counterpart is usually more proximal. The pattern of growth is variable. The majority of both types of lesions grow endogastrically, or into the lumen. However, a small percentage grow exogastrically, or into the abdominal cavity, creating only a mild extrinsic mass impression on the stomach. This growth is fairly unique and should be considered whenever a large intraabdominal mass with growth into the abdominal cavity is encountered. The tumors that grow into the lumen may ulcerate and can be large or even multiple. Because these tumors are vascular in nature, the ulceration may lead to catastrophic hemorrhage.

Distinguishing benign from malignant smooth muscle tumors is difficult even for the pathologist. The classic criterion has been the number of mitoses visible per high power field (>10 for leiomyosarcomas). However, the nature of the histologic activity of the tumor is variable in different parts, and sampling can have a significant impact on the mitotic activity and pleomorphism viewed by the pathologist. Some believe that size of the tumor is just as important. Tumors less than 5 cm in diameter are more likely to be malignant. Finally, the absolute criterion is evidence of metastatic disease. If the lesion is indeterminate based on pathologic findings, CT is often necessary to determine the exact nature of the tumor.

Notes

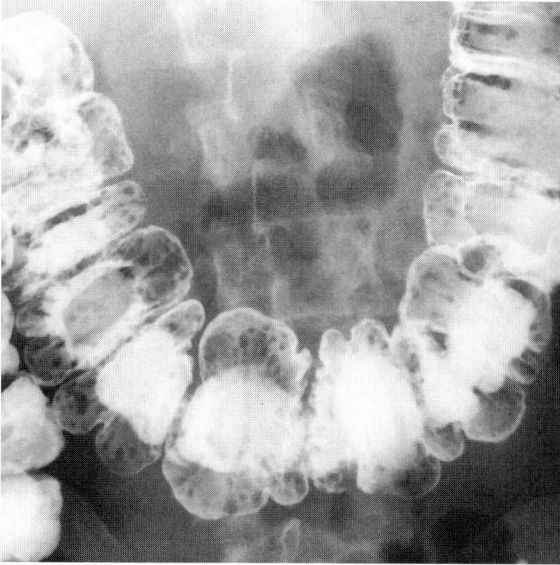

1. What is the inheritance pattern of most colonic polyposis syndromes?
2. What bony abnormalities are seen in patients with adenomatous polyposis syndrome?
3. What syndrome develops central nervous system tumors?
4. What thyroid abnormality may develop in patients with this condition?

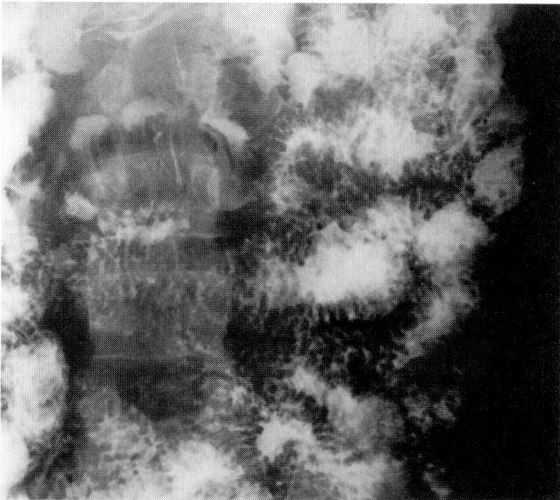

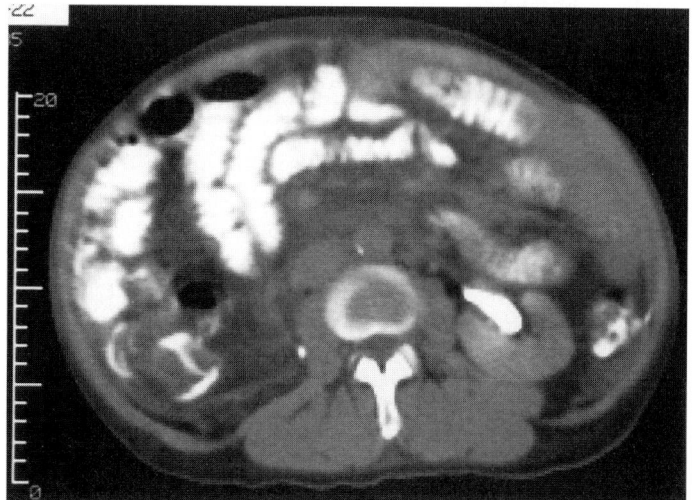

1. Below what level must serum albumin fall to produce edema?
2. What congenital problem may produce this appearance?
3. Failure of which two organs can also produce these changes?
4. Blockage of what structure may induce similar changes?

CASE 87

Familial Adenomatous Polyposis Syndrome

1. Autosomal dominant.

2. Osteomas and cortical hyperostosis.

3. Turcot's syndrome.

4. Thyroid carcinoma.

Reference

Harned RK, Buck JL, Olmsted WW, et al: Extracolonic manifestations of the familial adenomatous polyposis syndrome, *Am J Roentgenol* 156:481-485, 1991.

Cross-Reference

Gastrointestinal Radiology: THE REQUISITES, ed 2, p 253.

Comment

Numerous adenomatous polyps of the colon, particularly in a young adult, usually indicate the presence of a polyposis syndrome. For decades, these polyps were classified as familial polyposis coli or Gardner's syndrome. Patients with the latter condition were believed to develop the extracolonic manifestations. These conditions are inherited as autosomal dominant traits (although a certain proportion are spontaneous) and cause the formation of numerous adenomatous colonic polyps. Many now believe that these two conditions represent variable penetrance of the same genetic defect and classify these entities as familial adenomatous polyposis syndrome (FAPS).

In patients with FAPS, polyps may occur outside the colon, usually in the stomach. These growths usually are hyperplastic polyps or so-called fundic gland polyps. Adenomas also occur with slightly increased frequency in the stomach and duodenum, and there is an increased incidence of periampullary carcinoma (the second most frequent malignancy after colonic carcinoma) among these patients. In some studies the incidence of small bowel adenomas has been notably increased.

Extraintestinal manifestations include bony abnormalities. Osteomas, although classically associated with Gardner's syndrome, occur in up to 50% of patients. There also is an increased incidence of cortical hyperostosis and dental abnormalities associated with FAPS. Epidermal cysts have been described, as have pigmented lesions of the retina. The incidence of thyroid carcinoma also is believed to be increased, particularly in women. Large intraabdominal fibrous tumors, mesenteric fibromatosis, and desmoid tumors occur sporadically. Some believe that there is a slight increase in the incidence of pancreatic carcinoma and benign liver tumors. Tumors of the central nervous system (glioblastomas and medulloblastomas) are generally associated with Turcot's syndrome, but many claim that the incidence of these tumors is increased in patients with FAPS as well, and Turcot's is just another variation of FAPS.

Notes

CASE 88

Bowel Wall Edema

1. 2 g.

2. Lymphangiectasia.

3. Liver or kidneys.

4. Lymph ducts draining the intestines.

Reference

Stevens RL, Jones B, Fishman EK: CT halo sign: new finding in intestinal lymphangiectasia, *J Comput Assist Tomogr* 21:1005-1011, 1997.

Cross-Reference

Gastrointestinal Radiology: THE REQUISITES, ed 2, p 110.

Comment

Edema of the bowel can develop as a result of a variety of conditions and thus can present frequently in a practice in which there are a number of patients with long-standing debilitating diseases. The two groups of patients that most commonly develop this condition are those with failure of the liver and those with failure of the kidneys. Kidney failure may lead to retention of fluid, with resultant exudation into the tissues. This process can occur throughout the body, involving many organs, and the small bowel is affected in a manner similar to other structures. Because of the use of dialysis, this problem is now rarely encountered. End-stage liver failure is probably the more common source of small bowel edema. The edema occurs mainly as a result of the hypoalbuminemia that occurs in patients with this condition. Patients with long-standing cirrhosis often develop low albumin levels. As the albumin level drops below 2 g, bowel wall edema tends to develop. Also complicating liver disease is the presence of portal hypertension, which impairs venous flow from the intestines, and possible elevation of pressure in the lymphatic channels; both of these complications diminish the body's ability to remove excess fluid from the tissues.

Other conditions also may produce these changes. Any disorder that produces obstruction of the lymphatic channels of the bowel can produce intestinal edema. This edema may be present in patients with extensive adenopathy at the root of the mesentery or the porta hepatis and is typical among patients with lymphoma or metastatic disease. Also, patients who have had radiation for a neoplasm could develop fibrosis and obstruction of lymphatic channels. A rarer causative condition is intestinal lymphangiectasia, which is a congenital defect in the lymphatic channels draining the bowel. Angioneurotic edema, which is also an inherited disorder, has been known to cause edema of the intestines.

Notes

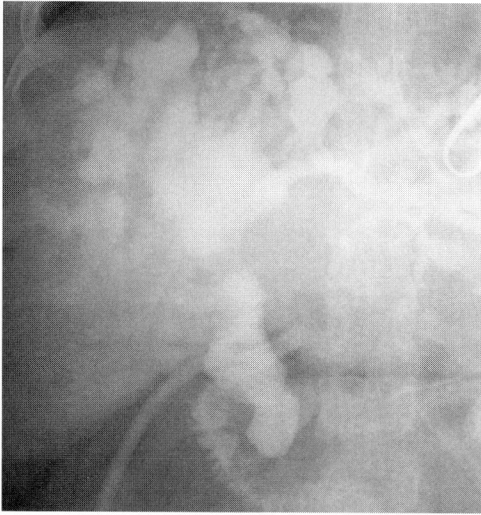

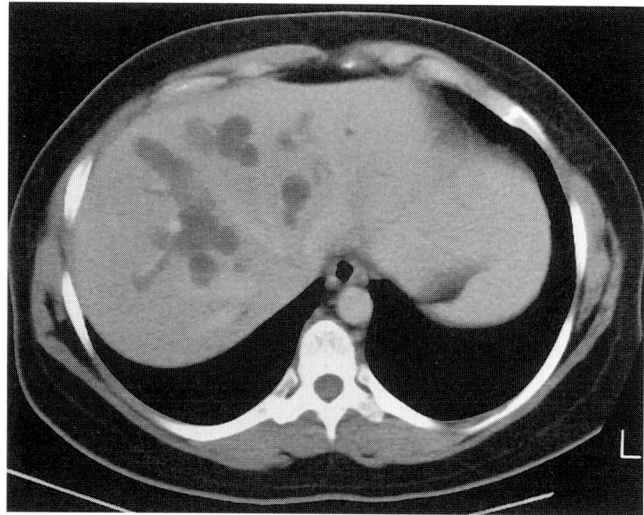

1. What is the most likely diagnosis?
2. How often do hepatic cysts communicate with the biliary system?
3. When do the pathologic changes begin to occur?
4. What are the major complications?

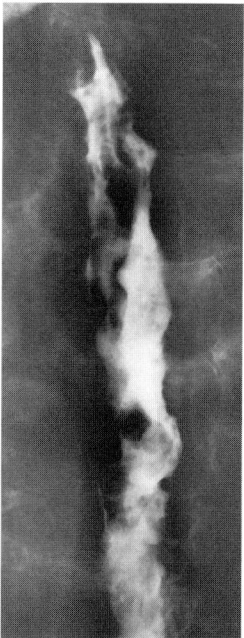

1. Do varices ever occur in the absence of a predisposing condition?
2. What parasite is the world's most common cause of portal hypertension and varices?
3. What layer of bowel is normally lacking in the esophagus?
4. Why do "jump" metastases occur in esophageal carcinoma?

CASE 89

Caroli's Disease (Type V Choledochal Cyst)

1. Caroli's disease.

2. Rarely.

3. During childhood, but they usually do not present clinically until adulthood.

4. Cholangitis, fibrosis, portal hypertension, and cholangiocarcinoma.

Reference

Rizzo RJ, Szucs RA, Turner MA: Congenital abnormalities of the pancreas and biliary system, *Radiographics* 15:49-68, 1995.

Cross-Reference

Gastrointestinal Radiology: THE REQUISITES, ed 2, p 209.

Comment

Caroli's disease is considered a rare type of congenital biliary cystic disease or choledochal cyst (type V). It is also termed *communicating cavernous ectasia of the bile ducts.* It represents a cystic dilation of some of the intrahepatic branches and ectasia of the ducts. There may be associated dilation of the extrahepatic biliary system, resembling a choledochal cyst in appearance. The disease is congenital in nature, but its development is poorly understood. There may be associated cystic disease of the kidneys (usually medullary sponge kidney), but there is no strong association with polycystic kidney disease. Also, there does not appear to be a strong familial association.

Patients with this disorder begin to develop the pathologic dilation in infancy or childhood but often do not present clinically until adulthood. Because of the dilation, patients have a strong predilection toward the development of stones, infection, and abscesses. There is one type or variant of the disease in which progressive hepatic fibrosis with eventual cirrhosis and portal hypertension develops. These patients do very poorly and die quickly unless treated by liver transplantation. Most of the complications can be treated as they occur, although the prognosis depends on the type and number of complications that develop. As is true of most choledochal cyst patients, there is a markedly increased incidence of cholangiocarcinoma in patients with Caroli's disease.

On ultrasound or CT the multiple fluid-filled structures resemble multiple hepatic cysts. However, hepatic cysts rarely communicate with the biliary system. It is only after imaging of the biliary system by direct injection that the true nature of this disease is discovered.

Notes

CASE 90

Varicoid Carcinoma of the Esophagus

1. Yes, they are termed *idiopathic varices.*

2. *Schistosoma* species.

3. Serosal layer.

4. Lymphatic plexus of the esophagus extends longitudinally.

Reference

Wolfman NT, Scharling ES, Chen MYM: Esophageal squamous carcinoma, *Radiol Clin North Am* 32:1183-1201, 1994.

Cross-Reference

Gastrointestinal Radiology: THE REQUISITES, ed 2, p 21.

Comment

Esophageal carcinoma can appear in many different forms. The most common is that of a stricture, usually irregular in nature. It also may be an eccentric mass or even a polypoid mass within the lumen. It may ulcerate, with resultant bleeding. The anatomy of the esophagus is somewhat different from that of the remainder of the gastrointestinal tract, which results in the rapid spread of the neoplasm and the resultant poor prognosis.

Unlike the rest of the gastrointestinal tract, there is no serosal layer in the esophagus, and neoplasms are known to directly invade the adjacent structures, resulting in high morbidity. Also, the lymphatic drainage of the esophagus is complex. There is an extensive network of lymphatic channels in all layers of the esophagus. This characteristic results in metastases spreading circumferentially and to adjacent lymph node groups in the mediastinum. The tumor may "jump" or disseminate throughout the length of the esophagus via these channels. There may be intervening normal mucosa between these areas of tumor. This pattern of spread is believed to result in the varicoid appearance of esophageal carcinoma.

Varicoid carcinoma is an unusual variant of esophageal carcinoma. The tumor spreads submucosally down the length of the esophagus, producing thickened folds. The appearance may mimic esophageal varices, hence the name. Because of this pattern of spread, dysphagia is usually a late symptom, and the disease has usually had spread extensively before being detected. Thus the patient with this form of esophageal neoplasm has a poor prognosis.

Notes

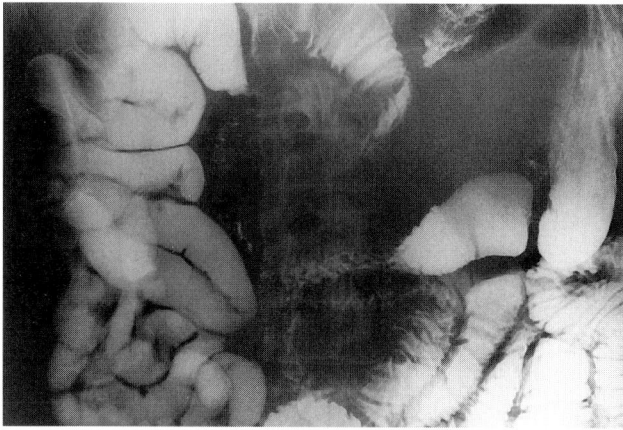
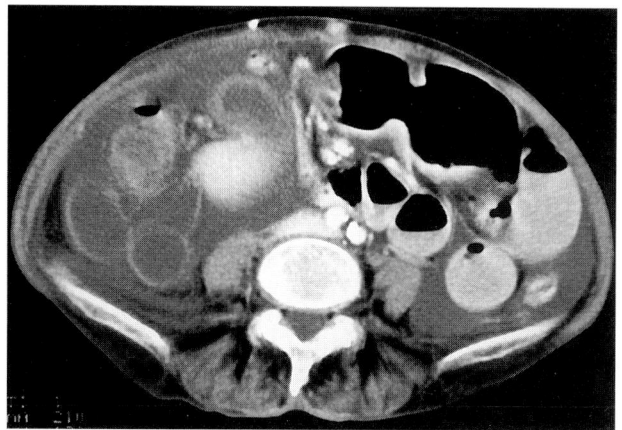

1. What is the most common internal hernia?
2. Where is the defect in patients with these types of hernias?
3. Through which fossae do these hernias pass?
4. Which type of paraduodenal hernia is most common?

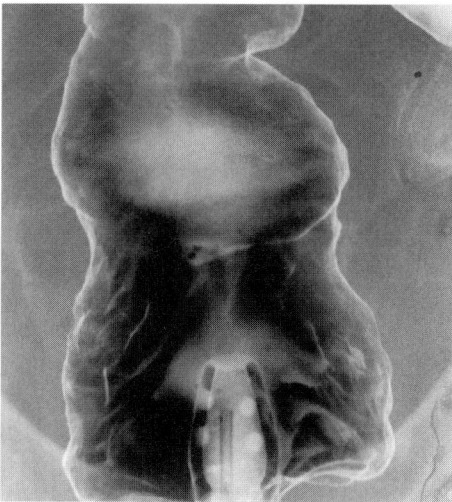
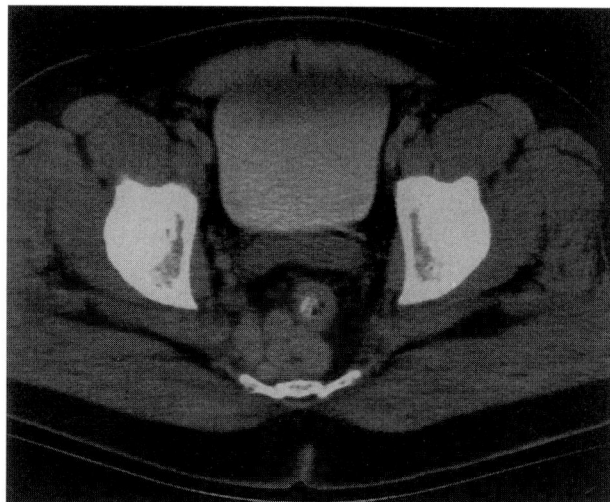

1. What is the most likely diagnosis?
2. What underlying conditions may produce this abnormality?
3. What is the treatment?
4. How is this condition related to rectal hemorrhoids?

CASE 91

Right Paraduodenal Hernia

1. Paraduodenal hernia.

2. Mesocolon.

3. Left, fossa of Landzert; right, fossa of Waldeyer.

4. Left.

Reference
Warshauer DM, Mauro MA: CT diagnosis of paraduodenal hernias, *Gastrointest Radiol* 17:13-15, 1992.

Cross-Reference
Gastrointestinal Radiology: THE REQUISITES, ed 2, p 298.

Comment
Numerous hernias and malpositions of the intestines may occur internally in the abdominal cavity without any external evidence or even symptomatology. These hernias were once considered quite rare, but with the increase in CT of the abdomen, they are recognized more often. The paraduodenal hernias are the most common internal hernia. Other less common internal hernias include paracecal, lesser sac, and transmesenteric hernias. Almost all internal hernias originate from some developmental anomaly that results in structures developing improperly, being malpositioned, or having defects.

There are two different types of paraduodenal, or mesocolic, hernias—left and right. They are often termed *mesocolic hernias* because they represent an anomaly of the transverse mesocolon embryologically and are lined by the mesocolon. As the transverse mesocolon develops, loops of intestine become entrapped. A right paraduodenal hernia lies behind the hepatic flexure and extends through what is termed the *fossa of Waldeyer.* This hernia may be associated with abnormal fixation of the cecum and even Ladd's bands between the liver and intestines. Portions of the mesentery and vessels extend to the right upper quadrant.

A left paraduodenal hernia extends through the fossa of Landzert. Usually a group of jejunal loops enter the left upper quadrant and displace the stomach and splenic flexure. Left mesocolic hernias increase in size and become symptomatic more often than do right paraduodenal hernias, which may be why they are considered more common. The major complications of these hernias include obstruction, which often develops later in life. Also, ischemia may develop as the blood supply to these loops becomes compromised. CT is by far the best modality to demonstrate the anatomy, although hernias can be demonstrated by small bowel examination. Surgery is the only method of treatment.

Notes

CASE 92

Rectal Varices

1. Rectal varices.

2. Portal hypertension, inferior vena cava obstruction, severe abdominal adhesions, and other venous obstruction.

3. Only the underlying condition can be treated.

4. Two different entities; unrelated to one another.

Cross-Reference
Gastrointestinal Radiology: THE REQUISITES, ed 2, p 259.

Comment
The presence of numerous serpiginous filling defects in the rectum is unusual. However, if such defects appeared in the esophagus or proximal stomach, the likely diagnosis would be varices. This case is atypical in that these thickened, serpiginous folds are in the rectum. Varices of the rectum are quite uncommon even when there are varices in the esophagus and other areas. These defects are unrelated to internal hemorrhoids; however, the unsuspecting clinician may erroneously diagnose rectal varices as hemorrhoids. Internal hemorrhoids present as filling defects at the anal verge.

The rectum is an area in which connections between portal venous flow and systemic venous flow can occur. Rectal venous flow may go through the pelvis and into the systemic circulation, and upper rectal flow often goes into the portal system. If there is portal venous obstruction, there may be shunting of blood through other pathways and into the systemic circulation. Portal hypertension usually takes pathways through the esophagus and spleen and rarely through the rectum. However, thrombosis of the superior mesenteric vein may lead to collateral flow through the rectum. Typically, rectal varices are much more uncommon than varices in other locations.

If pelvic venous drainage is obstructed as a result of inferior vena cava obstruction, systemic circulation could shunt through the rectum, into the portal system, and then back to the heart. Although rare, this process is another way that rectal varices can develop.

Notes

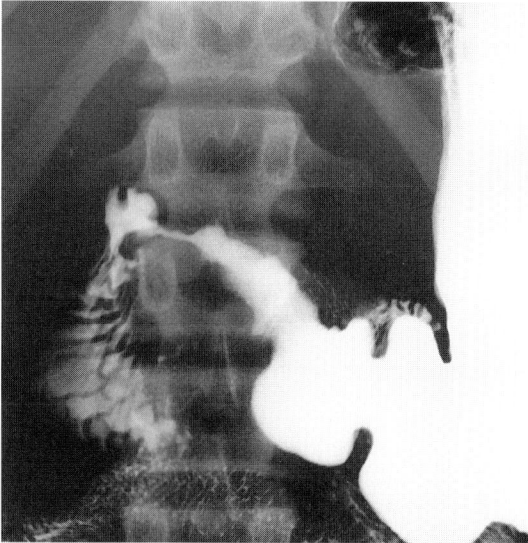

1. What is the most common cause of gastric erosions?
2. In patient's with Crohn's disease, what area of the stomach is most commonly involved?
3. Does Crohn's disease of the stomach occur as an isolated finding?
4. What is meant by the "ram's horn" sign?

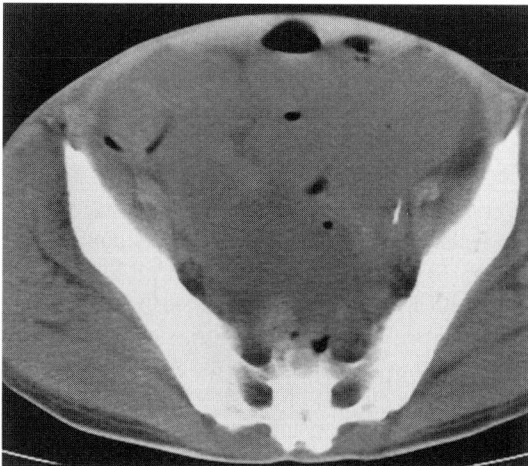

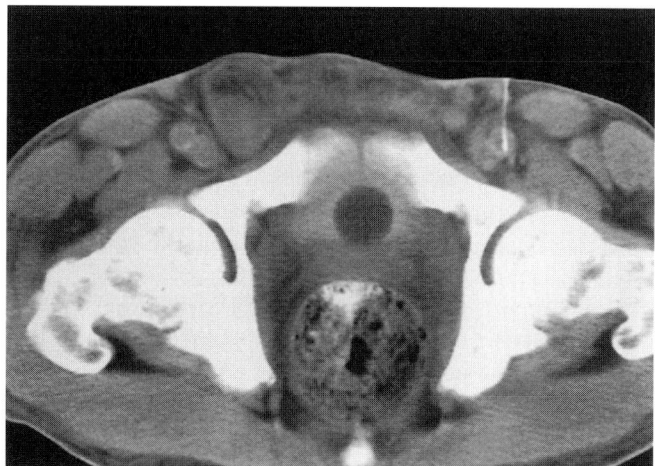

1. What is the origin of air in dilated bowel in a patient with obstruction?
2. What is the most common cause of small bowel obstruction?
3. In differential air-fluid levels, what difference in height would favor the diagnosis of obstruction rather than ileus?
4. What is the most specific modality for demonstrating mechanical obstruction?

Crohn's Disease of the Stomach

1. Peptic ulcer disease.

2. Antrum.

3. Almost always occurs in conjunction with ileal or colonic Crohn's disease.

4. Concomitant involvement of the duodenum with narrowing and scarring.

Reference

Levine MS: Crohn's disease of the upper gastrointestinal tract, *Radiol Clin North Am* 25:79-92, 1987.

Cross-Reference

Gastrointestinal Radiology: THE REQUISITES, ed 2, p 58.

Comment

Crohn's disease of the stomach is nearly always found in the distal aspect of the organ. The antrum is first to become involved, and the disease may spread more proximally. Rarely is the fundus ever involved by Crohn's disease. Many patients also have associated involvement of the duodenum. Rarely is the stomach the only part of the gut that is involved by Crohn's disease; most often there is ileal or colonic Crohn's disease as well, and it should be assumed that there will be disease in other portions of the gastrointestinal tract, too. As a corollary, the incidence of Crohn's disease involving the stomach can range between 5% and 40% of cases.

The most common presentation of Crohn's disease in the stomach is that of gastric erosions. These erosions are identical to other types of erosions in the stomach, and there is no way to radiologically distinguish them. As the disease progresses the severity of the inflammation may increase, and ulcers may become confluent and linear or stellate in configuration. As with other portions of the gastrointestinal tract, the inflammation is transmural, resulting in fibrosis and scarring. Typically (according to some reports in more than half of the cases of gastric Crohn's disease) there is involvement of the adjacent duodenum. When Crohn's disease is long-standing, the antrum and duodenum become a featureless rigid tube; this presentation is called the *pseudo-Billroth I sign* or *ram's horn sign* and may be so severe that it resembles a scirrhous carcinoma.

Fistulas are a rare complication of gastric Crohn's disease but can develop into the transverse colon. However, postinflammatory polyps may develop as a sequela of Crohn's disease of the stomach.

Notes

Mechanical Obstruction of the Small Bowel Caused by Right Inguinal Hernia

1. Swallowed air.

2. Fibrous adhesions.

3. 3 cm or more.

4. CT.

Reference

Maglinte DDT, Reyes BL, Harmon BH, et al: Reliability and role of plain film radiography and CT in the diagnosis of small bowel obstruction, *Am J Roentgenol* 167:1451-1455, 1996.

Cross-Reference

Gastrointestinal Radiology: THE REQUISITES, ed 2, p 100.

Comment

One of the problems most frequently evaluated by the radiologist (and surgeon) is suspected bowel obstruction. This evaluation is particularly difficult in the patient who develops distention after a surgical procedure. The main differential concern is whether a true mechanical obstruction has developed or whether the bowel dilation is secondary to an adynamic ileus.

Most mechanical obstructions occur as the result of fibrous adhesions, which develop within days after surgery. Often, it takes months or years before these obstructions become symptomatic. Other causes include hernias, either in the abdominal wall or internally. Fibrous bands also may lead to volvulus or closed loop–type obstructions. Ischemia is another potential cause of postoperative obstruction that would require immediate therapy. An adynamic ileus is a disorder of intestinal motility that results in diminished motility and subsequent dilation of the bowel. Surgery may induce this condition as a result of manipulation of the bowel. Medications, particularly those taken to relieve pain, can cause intestinal hypomotility. Inflammation or hemorrhage into the intestinal cavity can result in adynamic ileus. Finally, systemic problems, such as electrolyte imbalance, sepsis, and shock, also can cause adynamic ileus.

For decades, contrast examination of the small bowel, along with plain film radiography, has been the standard for evaluation of the patient with suspected obstruction. Enteroclysis has been shown to be of somewhat greater benefit but often is impractical for the postoperative patient. Many now advocate the use of CT, which can assess the site of obstruction and possible underlying causes of the problem. It is as sensitive as the other modalities and can be quite specific for determining the cause of the problem, which is most helpful for clinicians.

Notes

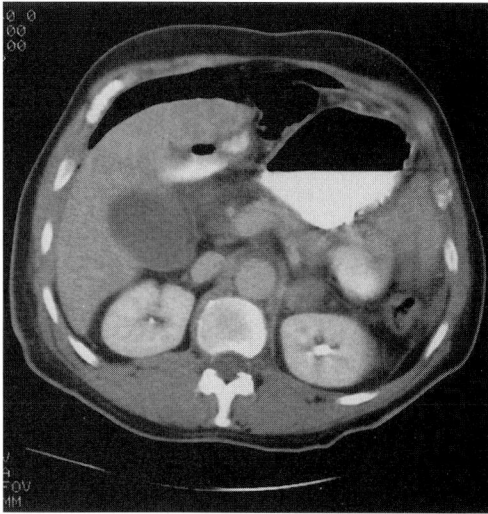

1. What modality is the most sensitive for detecting free intraperitoneal air?
2. What is the likely diagnosis in this case?
3. Where do perforating ulcers most commonly occur?
4. What other diagnostic studies should be performed?

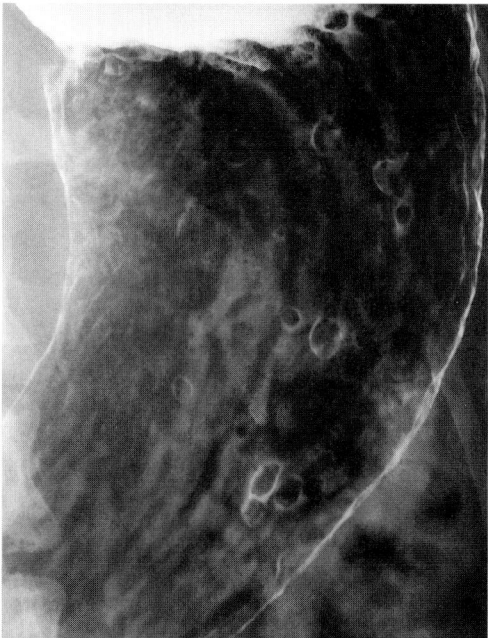

1. What is the most common cause of multiple gastric polyps?
2. What type of polyposis may produce gastric polyps?
3. What histologic type of tissue comprises the polyps in Cronkhite-Canada syndrome?
4. What other lesions are found in patients with Cowden disease?

Perforated Duodenal Ulcer

1. CT.

2. Perforated ulcer.

3. Anterior aspect of stomach or duodenal bulb.

4. None.

Reference

Glick SN: Duodenal ulcer, *Radiol Clin North Am* 32:1259-1274, 1994.

Cross-Reference

Gastrointestinal Radiology: THE REQUISITES, ed 2, p 299.

Comment

The CT scan shown here demonstrates small amounts of free intraperitoneal air. CT may demonstrate as little as 1 to 2 ml of free intraperitoneal air. Studies have shown that upright or decubitus radiographs also may demonstrate similarly tiny amounts of free intraperitoneal air. However, in practice, CT has proved more sensitive than other modalities in demonstrating free intraperitoneal air. Also, patients are often too sick to obtain adequate positional views for abdominal studies, and the CT demonstration of free intraperitoneal air is not dependent on adequate positioning or technique. Also noted in this case is the presence of a triangular collection of contrast inferior to the liver. This triangular collection would be unusual within bowel. Most likely it is obtaining its configuration as the contrast collects along the inferior edge of the liver and conforms to its borders.

A perforated ulcer can be difficult to diagnose, and diagnosis is often made at the time of surgery. Plain radiographs of the abdomen reveal only the presence of free intraperitoneal air, which is a nonspecific finding. However, with the increased use of CT in the emergency setting, the detection of contrast leaking into the peritoneal cavity, as well as the presence of free intraperitoneal air, has become possible. The small collection of contrast along the inferior edge of the liver strongly suggests the diagnosis of perforated duodenum. However, if the contrast were in the lesser sac or left side of the abdomen, it would favor the diagnosis of perforation of the stomach. Given the aforementioned findings, it is not necessary to perform further studies, and surgery should be performed promptly.

Notes

Multiple Gastric Polyps Associated with Cronkhite-Canada Syndrome

1. Inflammation producing hyperplastic polyps.

2. Familial polyposis, including Gardner's syndrome, Peutz-Jeghers syndrome, Cronkhite-Canada syndrome, Cowden disease, and juvenile polyposis.

3. Inflammatory or juvenile hamartomatous type.

4. Circumoral papillomatosis, skeletal malformations, and tumors of the gastrointestinal tract, skin, breast, and thyroid.

Reference

Feczko PJ: Incidental filling defects (polyps) in the stomach. In Thompson W, editor: *Common problems in gastrointestinal radiology,* Chicago, 1989, Year Book.

Cross-Reference

Gastrointestinal Radiology: THE REQUISITES, ed 2, p 70.

Comment

With the advent of biphasic upper gastrointestinal examination, it is not uncommon to encounter multiple small polyps within the gastric lumen. These growths are often found throughout the body and in the proximal stomach. For the most part these small polyps are the sequela of previous inflammation of the stomach and histologically are hyperplastic or inflammatory polyps. On occasion, they are due to metastases, and rarely they indicate the presence of a polyposis syndrome of the gastrointestinal tract.

Almost all of the polyposis syndromes may cause polyps to develop in the stomach. Patients with familial polyposis (or Gardner's syndrome) have a high incidence of gastric polyps. Unlike their adenomatous counterparts in the colon, gastric polyps can be either adenomatous or hyperplastic. Although adenomatous polyps are potentially premalignant, they are believed to be much less likely to develop into gastric carcinoma. Patients with Peutz-Jeghers syndrome develop hamartomatous lesions in the stomach with no malignant potential. Juvenile polyps also are hamartomas and may occur sporadically or as part of a diffuse juvenile polyposis syndrome.

Cronkhite-Canada syndrome is a nonfamilial polyposis syndrome. It is associated with a group of skin abnormalities, including alopecia, onychodystrophy, and hyperpigmentation. Clinically these patients also have weight loss and protein and electrolyte depletion. It is this last group of symptoms that may be life-threatening. The condition usually occurs in middle-aged patients and sometimes in the elderly. The polyps are inflammatory or hamartomatous and have no malignant potential. Typically the growths are quite small. Cowden disease is a rare cause of hamartomatous polyps in the stomach; this disorder is hereditary and results in formation of diffuse hamartomatous and ectodermal abnormalities throughout the body.

Notes

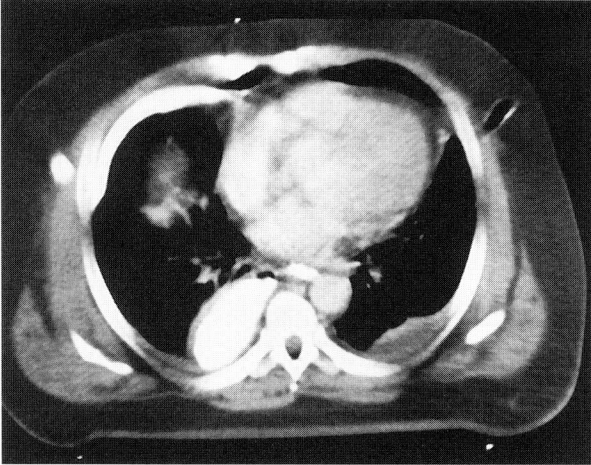

1. What is the most common cause of esophageal perforation?
2. What is the mechanism of esophageal rupture in blunt trauma?
3. What mechanisms other than vomiting may produce spontaneous esophageal rupture?
4. What contrast material demonstrates small esophageal perforations best?

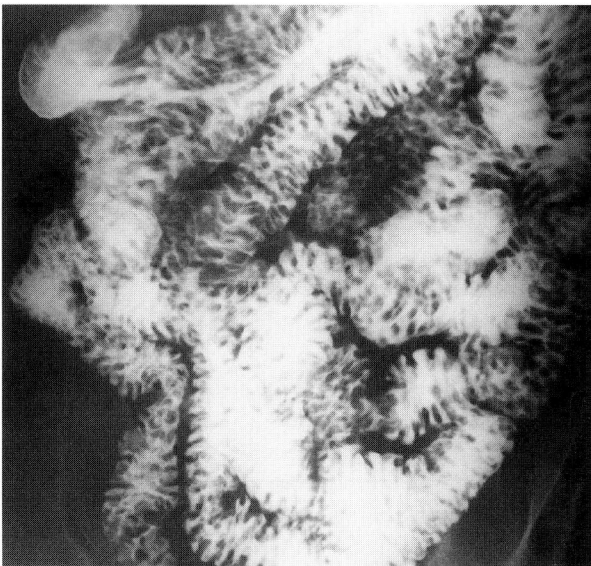

1. What diseases may produce diffuse small bowel granularity?
2. What is the most common site of bowel involvement in patients with systemic amyloidosis?
3. What is the most common radiologic finding of the small bowel in patients with amyloidosis?
4. What conditions are known to result in the deposition of amyloid in the bowel?

Boerhaave's Syndrome

1. Endoscopic procedure.

2. Sudden elevation of intraluminal esophageal pressure.

3. Seizures, coughing, asthma, childbirth, severe straining, and blunt trauma.

4. Barium.

Reference

Buecker A, Wein BB, et al: Esophageal perforation: comparison of use of aqueous and barium-containing contrast media, *Radiology* 202:683-687, 1997.

Cross-Reference

Gastrointestinal Radiology: THE REQUISITES, ed 2, p 19.

Comment

Perforation or rupture of the wall of the esophagus is a severe condition with extremely high mortality if not discovered quickly. Its occurrence is most often related to some type of medical procedure, either endoscopy or passage of some instrument or tube via the mouth or nose.

Spontaneous rupture of the esophagus, or Boerhaave's syndrome, involves a full-thickness esophageal tear, usually in the lower third of the esophagus, related to vomiting or retching. It also may be produced by other conditions, such as blunt trauma and all causes of excessive straining, that can result in a sudden rise of intraluminal esophageal pressure. Typically the rupture occurs in the left side of the lower esophagus because the right side is supported by the aorta. Radiologically a left-sided pleural effusion is often visible on chest radiographs. There also may be mediastinal widening or emphysema. The clinical history often provides important clues regarding the development of the condition, which should be suspected in the patient with a history of vomiting or straining and associated changes in the lower mediastinum and lower left side of the chest.

Historically, water-soluble contrast agents have been preferable for the detection of esophageal perforation. The contrast is easily absorbed from the mediastinum and pleural spaces, whereas barium remains in those areas, producing granulomas and possibly fibrosis. In cases of suspected esophageal perforation a water-soluble agent should be the first contrast material used for evaluation. However, numerous authors have shown that many small esophageal perforations are not detected radiologically by the water-soluble contrast. It is now recommended that the normal water-soluble esophagram be followed by a low density barium study, which will detect small areas of perforation and sinus tracts that are not detected by the water-soluble material. In addition, the complications of barium in the mediastinum are believed to be less severe than originally thought.

Notes

Amyloidosis of the Small Bowel

1. Crohn's disease and amyloidosis.

2. Small bowel, followed by the colon and the stomach.

3. Fine mucosal granules or nodules.

4. Multiple myelomas, rheumatoid arthritis, chronic inflammatory conditions, and aging.

Reference

Tada S, Iida M, Matsui T, et al: Amyloidosis of the small intestine: findings on double-contrast radiographs, *Am J Roentgenol* 156:741-744, 1991.

Cross-Reference

Gastrointestinal Radiology: THE REQUISITES, ed 2, p 114.

Comment

Amyloidosis is a condition involving the abnormal deposition of extracellular hyaline fibrils in various organs of the body and sometimes diffusely. Because this process may occur with aging, it should be considered common, yet it produces symptoms in only a few individuals. There is a primary form of amyloidosis that occurs without predisposing factors; it may be familial in nature or just a sporadic event. Secondary amyloidosis occurs as a result of some predisposing condition. The predisposing condition is often a chronic inflammatory state, such as rheumatoid arthritis, inflammatory bowel disease, autoimmune disease, or chronic infection. Probably the most well-known form of the disease is the amyloid deposition that occurs in patients with multiple myelomas. Amyloidosis can involve various organs, particularly the skin, liver, spleen, gastrointestinal tract, kidneys, and heart.

Amyloidosis of the intestinal tract usually produces symptoms of diarrhea, malabsorption, pain, and other vague complaints, resembling numerous other diseases that also produce malabsorption. The entire gastrointestinal tract can be involved by amyloidosis, but the small bowel is believed to be the most frequent site of involvement. Rectal involvement also is quite common, and the diagnosis can be made by rectal biopsy. The radiologic findings in the small bowel have been classically described as thickening of the valvulae of the intestines. However, use of double-contrast techniques has proved fine granularity of the mucosa of the small bowel to be a more frequent finding. Another common abnormality is multiple fine nodules, measuring 1 to 2 mm in size. Sometimes they can be larger and present as actual polyps or polypoid protrusions in the lumen. Pathologically this granularity is fine amyloid deposition in the mucosa, whereas the nodules or polyps are areas of confluent amyloid deposition.

Notes

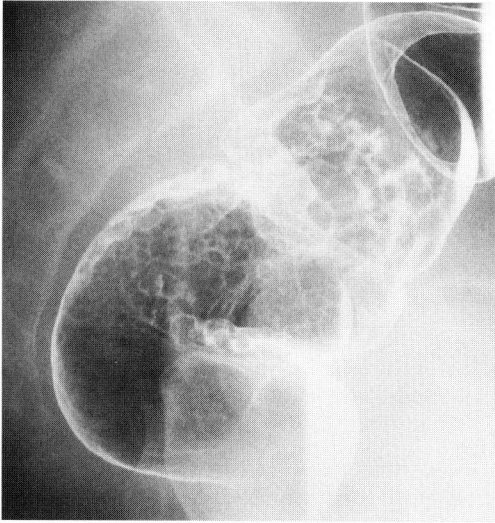

1. Where does this lesion most typically occur?
2. What is the most frequent histologic diagnosis?
3. What is the incidence of carcinoma in villous adenomas?
4. What condition has a similar appearance in the ascending colon and cecum?

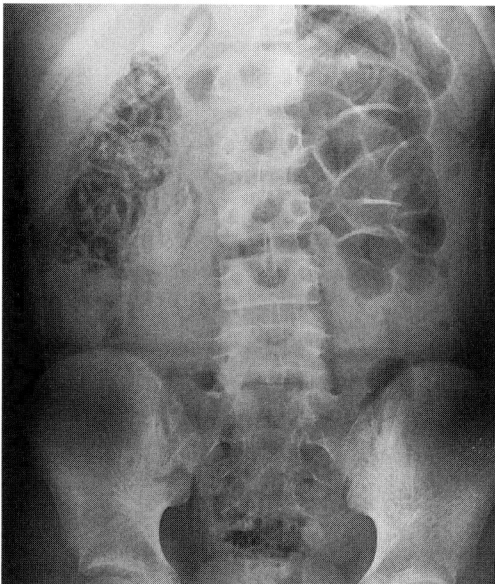

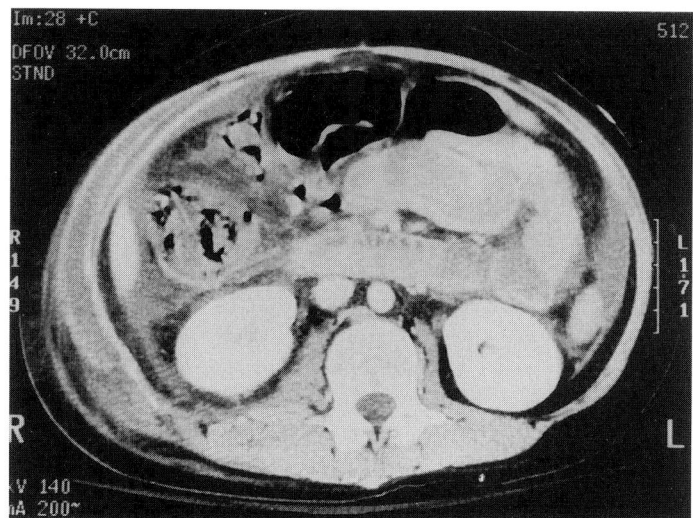

1. What are some possible causes of pneumatosis of the colon?
2. In the pediatric age group, what are the most likely causes?
3. What possible underlying medical conditions may this patient have?
4. Is the course of treatment for this condition surgical or medical?

CASE 99

Carpet Lesion of the Colon

1. Either the rectum or the ascending colon or cecum.

2. Villous adenoma.

3. 20% to 40%.

4. So-called urticaria of the colon.

Reference
Rubesin SE, Saul SH, Laufer I, et al: Carpet lesions of the colon, *Radiographics* 5:537-552, 1985.

Cross-Reference
Gastrointestinal Radiology: THE REQUISITES, ed 2, p 240.

Comment
Neoplastic lesions of the colon usually present as polypoid protuberances into the lumen of the bowel. On occasion they grow superficially or even infiltrate through the wall of the bowel. The "carpet" lesion of the colon results when a neoplastic growth develops superficially along the mucosa rather than growing in a polypoid fashion. This growth produces a subtle irregularity of the mucosal surface, and the barium that becomes entrapped within the interstices of the lesion has the appearance of shag carpet, hence the terminology. Tumors that develop in this fashion typically occur in areas of the colon where the diameter is quite large. Most are found in the rectum and cecum and to a lesser extent in the ascending colon. These areas are where peristaltic activity is least likely to push an intraluminal lesion distally, which may promote intraluminal growth as seen in other areas.

Pathologically these tumors tend to be either villous adenomas or tubulovillous adenomas. Rarely are they just simple adenomas. The lesions typically are larger than 3 cm because they are often difficult to diagnose when they are small. Lacking the intraluminal component, only with good double-contrast technique can the subtle mucosal irregularity be appreciated. It is a well-known fact that the incidence of carcinoma in colonic adenomas increases with increasing size as well as with histologic findings. Villous adenomas more frequently have carcinoma than do simple adenomas. Despite their large size and villous histologic features, the presence of carcinoma in these lesions is not that frequent, which is surprising because many of these lesions are 5 cm or larger at the time of diagnosis. However, surgical resection is often necessary to deal with these lesions. They are often too large to be removed endoscopically and because of their lack of intraluminal component are not amenable to endoscopic removal.

The major differential lesion that may mimic the carpet lesion is termed *urticaria of the colon.* This lesion is an area of submucosal edema of the colon.

Notes

CASE 100

Neutropenic Colitis (Typhlitis) of the Right Colon

1. Ischemia, colitis (inflammatory bowel disease), enterocolitis (infectious), steroid use, endoscopic procedures, and obstructive pulmonary disease.

2. Neutropenic colitis, endoscopic procedures, obstructive pulmonary disease (asthma), and steroid use.

3. Neutropenic colitis is seen in patients with leukemia, lymphoma, and sometimes acquired immunodeficiency syndrome.

4. Medical management is the primary treatment.

Reference
Merine DS, Fishman EK, Jones B, et al: Right lower quadrant pain in the immunocompromised patient, *Am J Roentgenol* 149:1177-1179, 1987.

Cross-Reference
Gastrointestinal Radiology: THE REQUISITES, ed 2, p 281.

Comment
Neutropenic colitis, or typhlitis, is an inflammatory condition of the right side of the colon that occurs in patients undergoing treatment for leukemia, lymphoma, and sometimes other malignancies. Typically this condition affects the pediatric population, but in some instances it has been encountered in the adult population. The clinical findings include fever, abdominal pain, and sometimes diarrhea. CT is the diagnostic modality of choice, demonstrating thickened bowel wall (sometimes with pneumatosis) and pericolic inflammatory changes in the mesenteric fat. These changes in the bowel are the result of a combination of edema, hemorrhage, and inflammatory exudate. Neoplastic involvement is not really a feature of the disease.

In the pediatric age group, pneumatosis frequently is a result of conditions such as asthma or is a sequela of a surgical or endoscopic procedure. If the patient has been taking steroids to treat any medical condition, the medication could be the cause of the pneumatosis. The history of a compromised immune system immediately makes neutropenic colitis the primary diagnostic consideration, however. Interestingly the treatment of neutropenic colitis is primarily aggressive antibiotic treatment. Surgery is necessary for only those patients with obvious rupture and abscess development. Despite the pneumatosis and pericolonic inflammatory changes, the patient shown in this case responded well to the antibiotics and did not require surgery.

Notes

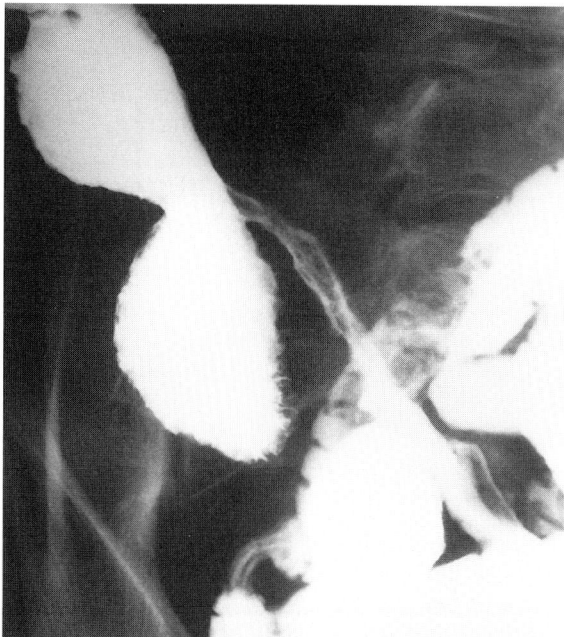

1. What infectious agents most commonly involve the terminal ileum?
2. What inflammatory conditions may be accompanied by adenopathy?
3. How often is intestinal tuberculosis accompanied by pulmonary tuberculosis?
4. What rare anaerobic bacterium is known to involve the terminal ileum?

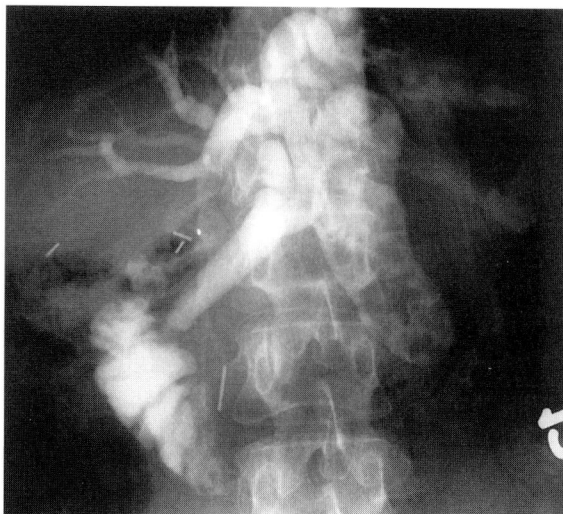

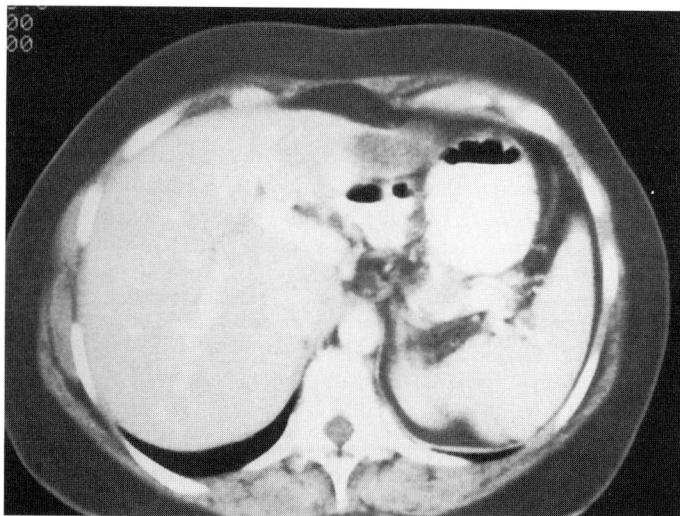

1. What abnormality is notable?
2. What underlying condition is often present?
3. Are there associated anomalies?
4. Is this abnormality associated with a higher incidence of any diseases?

C A S E   1 0 1

Tuberculosis of the Ileum

1. *Mycobacterium tuberculosis* and *Yersinia enterocolitica.*

2. Crohn's disease, tuberculosis, and *Yersinia* species infection.

3. Approximately half the time, although this is variable.

4. *Actinomyces israelii.*

Reference

Gardiner R, Smith C: Infective enterocolitides, *Radiol Clin North Am* 25:67-78, 1987.

Cross-Reference

Gastrointestinal Radiology: THE REQUISITES, ed 2, p 107.

Comment

Inflammatory changes in the terminal ileum are common because this segment of intestine is the most frequently involved by infectious processes. Unfortunately, the changes that occur in the terminal ileum—narrowing, bowel wall thickening, ulceration, and even adenopathy—are nonspecific as far as identifying the organism involved.

When considering the population of the entire world, tuberculosis is by far the most common infectious organism of the small bowel. This disease involves primarily the ileocecal region and less commonly the proximal small bowel and colon. In economically depressed areas, tuberculosis can be almost endemic. In these areas the tuberculous infection is often primary, being transmitted by the ingestion of infected food. The organism that most commonly causes tuberculosis is *M. bovis,* which is transmitted when a person drinks infected milk from cows that harbor the organism. In more developed countries the incidence of tuberculous infection of the intestine is markedly decreased but still is encountered. In industrialized nations, tuberculosis of the intestines is often contracted from pulmonary tuberculosis and the resultant ingestion of infected sputum into the gut. However, only approximately half of the patients with intestinal tuberculosis have radiologic evidence of pulmonary tuberculosis. The absence of abnormalities on chest radiographs does not exclude the possibility of intestinal tuberculosis.

Differentiating tuberculosis from Crohn's disease is often difficult because the same radiologic appearances and complications, such as fistulas and adenopathy, occur in both diseases. Biopsy of the terminal ileum is often necessary to confirm the diagnosis. Differentiation is crucial because the treatment for Crohn's disease is often immunosuppressive in nature (steroids), and if this type of medication is given to someone with intestinal tuberculosis, the tuberculosis will spread.

Notes

C A S E   1 0 2

Ectopic Gallbladder

1. Gallbladder displaced to the left.

2. Gallbladder is often on a mesentery, or there may be left lobe disease.

3. Rarely; it is usually an isolated finding.

4. No.

Reference

Rizzo RJ, Szucs RA, Turner MA: Congenital abnormalities of the pancreas and biliary tree in adults, *Radiographics* 15:49-68, 1995.

Cross-Reference

Gastrointestinal Radiology: THE REQUISITES, ed 2, p 230.

Comment

Embryologically the gallbladder develops as a bud off of the biliary system. Although classically it lies along the inferior margin of the right lobe of the liver, the gallbladder can occupy some very unusual positions, which is not surprising given the numerous anomalies that occur in the biliary system. However, anomalous position of the gallbladder usually is not associated with a higher incidence of related anomalies and is typically an isolated finding. Intrahepatic location of the gallbladder is a common variant of position. Alternatively the gallbladder can be located on a mesentery, causing it to lie quite low along the right flank or even be retrohepatic. The gallbladder also has been known to be suprahepatic or retroperitoneal in location or even located in the transverse mesocolon or abdominal wall. Ectopic gallbladders produce difficulties in diagnosis when inflammation occurs. It is doubtful that patients with ectopic gallbladders have a significantly higher incidence of disease.

A gallbladder that crosses the midline often is associated with the left lobe of the liver. It may be on a mesentery and may be herniating through the foramen of Winslow into the lesser sac. When the gallbladder is in this position, there is often a higher association with atrophy or some disease of the left lobe. This anomaly produces the malposition of the gallbladder.

Notes

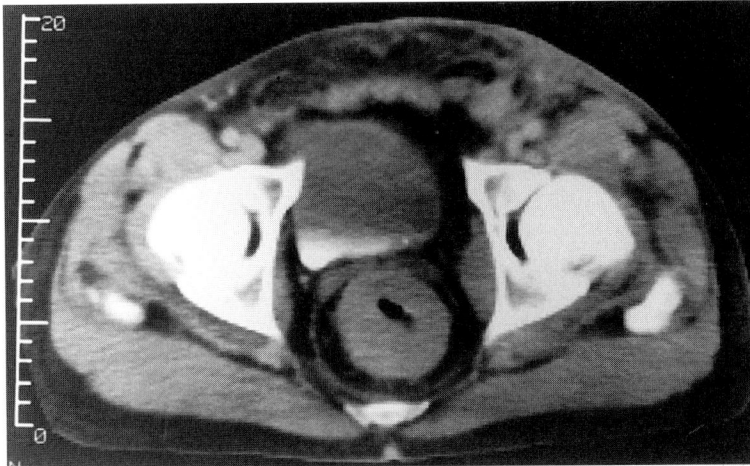

1. What can produce this appearance?
2. What possible underlying conditions can produce this appearance?
3. Name possible causes for this condition.
4. Is there any increased incidence of malignancy associated with this condition?

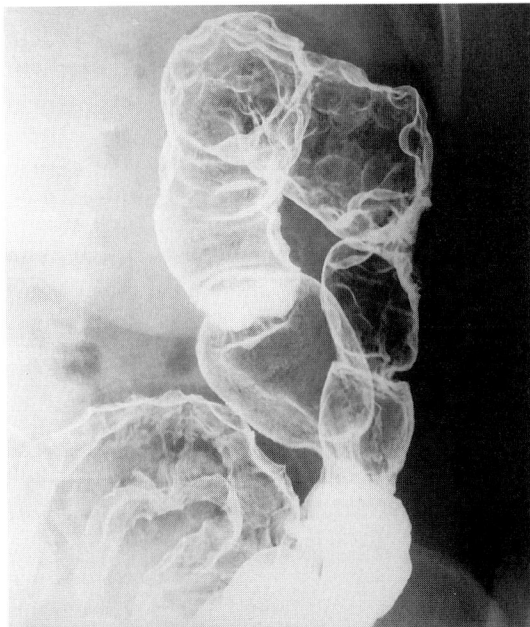

1. What is the histologic nature of the polyps in Gardner's syndrome?
2. What size are most lymphoid follicles in the colon?
3. The presence of polyps in the small bowel excludes the diagnosis of what colonic polyposis syndrome?
4. How often does lymphoma affect the colon?

CASE 103

Proctitis Associated with AIDS

1. Rectal inflammation, or proctitis.

2. Human immunodeficiency virus (HIV) infection, immunosuppression, and ulcerative colitis.

3. Viral or bacterial infection.

4. Usually not.

Reference

Feczko PJ: Gastrointestinal complications of human immuno-deficiency virus, *Semin Roentgenol* 29:275-287, 1994.

Cross-Reference

Gastrointestinal Radiology: THE REQUISITES, ed 2, p 283.

Comment

Computed tomography of the rectum demonstrates symmetric rectal wall thickening. The various portions of the rectal wall are not readily distinguishable, however. This appearance can be caused by inflammation of the rectum. There are numerous causes for rectal inflammation. One of the more common causes is proctitis, as seen in ulcerative colitis or nonspecific proctitis. This condition can produce similar findings. The bowel can have a target-like appearance because the different layers have different densities. This appearance is lacking in this patient, although it does not exclude the diagnosis.

One of the more common etiologies for proctitis is HIV infection. There are numerous causes for proctitis in these patients. Sometimes the inflammation is caused by a sexually transmitted disease (e.g., gonorrhea, lymphogranuloma venereum, herpes). Other times the inflammation represents an opportunistic infection (e.g., cytomegalovirus, *Salmonella* organisms). The radiologic changes that occur do not help distinguish the underlying etiology. The rectal wall is typically thickened in a diffuse fashion. Perirectal inflammatory changes may or may not be present, although they may be more evident near the anus. This appearance of rectal wall thickening may persist for quite some time in these patients and is sometimes a long-term finding. Resolution may be quite slow because of the underlying immunologic problems.

Notes

CASE 104

Lymphoma: Multinodular Appearance

1. Adenomatous.

2. Typically less than 5 mm in diameter in normal patients.

3. Almost none; small bowel polyps have been reported with varying frequency in almost all the polyposis syndromes.

4. At least 10% of the time.

Reference

Williams SM, Berk RN, Harnet RK: Radiologic features of multinodular lymphoma of the colon, *Am J Roentgenol* 143:87-91, 1984.

Cross-Reference

Gastrointestinal Radiology: THE REQUISITES, ed 2, p 259.

Comment

The presence of multiple polyps in the colon raises several possibilities. A polyposis syndrome of the bowel should be considered of course. Most polyps involve the colon, but a substantial number also have some type of small bowel involvement. Because it is now appreciated that most of the hereditary polyposis syndromes can affect both small and large bowel, the area affected is no longer a differential point. Postinflammatory polyps resulting from inflammatory bowel disease are another consideration and are found in patients with ulcerative colitis or Crohn's disease. Lymphoid follicles of the colon can be mistaken for a polyposis syndrome, but typically they are smaller than 5 mm in diameter, although some have been noted to be larger, even in unaffected individuals.

Non-Hodgkin's lymphoma frequently affects the gastrointestinal tract. Although series vary, the incidence of colon involvement in patients with lymphoma ranges from 10% to 24%. Primary lymphoma of the colon is relatively rare and usually involves other portions of the gastrointestinal tract or is systemic in nature. Lymphoma can have a varied radiologic appearance, including that of an intraluminal mass, endo-exoenteric mass, mural infiltration, mesenteric disease, or multiple polyps. Typically, when lymphoma presents as multiple nodules, the tumors begin to grow in the lymphatic tissue near the muscularis propria. Thus lymphoma can affect the motility of the bowel. Lymphoma also tends to distort the haustra more than a polyposis syndrome would. This characteristic may make lymphoma mimic inflammatory bowel disease or even ischemia of the colon. If the nodules remain small, they may be difficult to distinguish from lymphoid follicles. Some state that as lymphoid follicles begin to exceed 5 mm in size the possibility of lymphoma or Crohn's disease must be considered. The small polyps of lymphoma can develop central umbilication, which is similar in appearance to Crohn's disease or lymphoid follicles, making differentiation difficult.

Notes

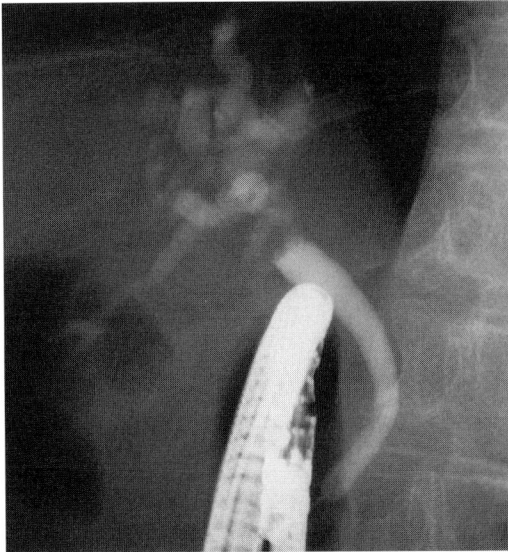

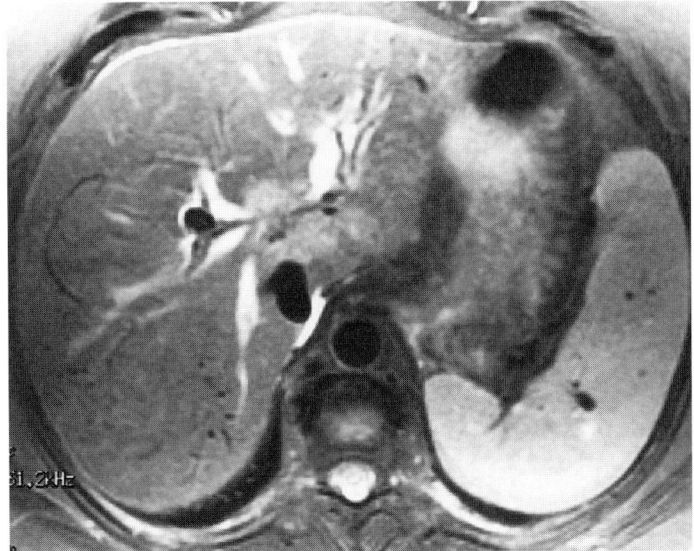

1. What is the most likely diagnosis?
2. What is this condition called?
3. What conditions predispose a patient to cholangiocarcinoma?
4. In what forms can this tumor appear?

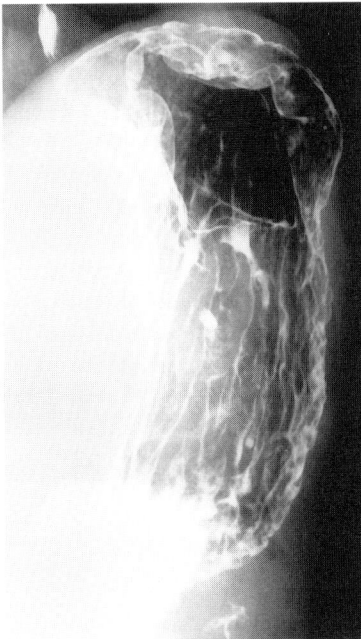

1. What is the most likely cause of this gastric abnormality?
2. What tumors may appear in this manner?
3. What primary gastric tumor should be considered?
4. What other imaging findings may be noted in patients with Kaposi's sarcoma?

CASE 105

Cholangiocarcinoma (Klatskin Tumor)

1. Cholangiocarcinoma.

2. Klatskin tumor.

3. Sclerosing cholangitis, choledochal cyst, congenital hepatic fibrosis, and recurrent parasitic infection.

4. Strictures, polyps, and liver masses.

Reference

Choi BI, Lee JH, Han MC, et al: Hilar cholangiocarcinoma: comparative study with sonography and CT, *Radiology* 172:689-692, 1989.

Cross-Reference

Gastrointestinal Radiology: THE REQUISITES, ed 2, p 205.

Comment

Cholangiocarcinomas are an adenomatous type of tumors that arise from the lining of the bile ducts. Because they can arise from any portion of the biliary system (even the tiniest branches in the liver), the appearance of cholangiocarcinomas can be quite variable. They most often form strictures, which are termed *scirrhous.* They also may form polypoid masses that project into the lumen of the ducts. In the liver parenchyma itself, cholangiocarcinomas are often identified as liver masses and are indistinguishable from other liver tumors. Those patients in whom these growths arise in the extrahepatic bile ducts have the best prognosis. Cholangiocarcinomas may produce jaundice or other symptoms before they spread to adjacent structures. Cholangiocarcinoma is often fatal because it invades adjacent critical structures in the region, such as the bile ducts and portal vein. Distant metastases are not common.

Injection of the bile ducts may reveal an area of narrowing or a polypoid lesion in the duct lumen. Proximal ductal dilation is often evident. On CT examination the tumors themselves are typically evident only when they are in the liver parenchyma and mass effect is visible. Approximately one third of cholangiocarcinomas present as liver masses because they grow exophytically into the liver parenchyma.

The type of cholangiocarcinoma that arises at the confluence of the right and left bile ducts is termed a *Klatskin tumor.* This tumor is typically a scirrhous type of cholangiocarcinoma that grows along the ducts, producing thickening of the wall of the ducts and progressive narrowing of the lumen. As the tumor grows, focal lobar atrophy may become evident. CT may demonstrate a mass in the region. The condition is almost invariably fatal because critical structures in the region, such as the portal vein, are often invaded. Enlarged lymph nodes in the porta hepatis and Mirizzi syndrome caused by an impacted stone in the cystic duct may mimic this condition.

Notes

CASE 106

Metastatic Kaposi's Sarcoma to the Stomach in Patients with AIDS

1. Metastasis.

2. Metastatic Kaposi's sarcoma, melanoma, and lung carcinoma.

3. Leiomyoma.

4. Small bowel tumors, adenopathy, and hemorrhage.

Reference

Wall SD, Friedman SL, Margulis AR: Gastrointestinal Kaposi's sarcoma in AIDS: radiographic manifestations, *J Clin Gastroenterol* 6:165-171, 1984.

Cross-Reference

Gastrointestinal Radiology: THE REQUISITES, ed 2, p 73.

Comment

Although considered a rare tumor, Kaposi's sarcoma is a well-known complication of acquired immunodeficiency syndrome (AIDS). This tumor is particularly common among the male homosexual population and is seen less frequently in other groups at high risk for AIDS, although the reason is unknown. The tumor has a particular predilection for metastases to the abdomen and gastrointestinal tract. The most well-known presentation of these metastases is a mural polyp or mass, often with central ulceration, the so-called "bull's eye" lesion. This growth is typically found in the stomach. In this case the tumor could be considered a classic "bull's eye" lesion. For some uncertain reason, in the small bowel, Kaposi's sarcoma tends to be a diffusely infiltrating process, often with associated hemorrhage. The appearance in the small bowel is frequently that of hemorrhage, with regular thickened folds (resembling a stack of coins). In this patient the "bull's eye" lesions in the stomach and small bowel hemorrhage are strongly indicative of metastatic Kaposi's sarcoma.

Other lesions that should be considered in this patient include metastatic disease from either melanoma or lung carcinoma. Stromal cell tumors of the stomach also have central ulceration, but they are rarely multiple in nature.

Notes

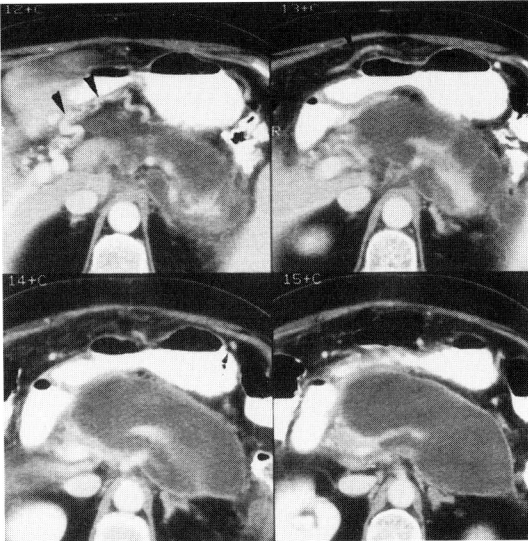

1. What is this appearance called?
2. Of what condition is it a sequela?
3. What other condition may have this appearance?
4. What is a major complication of this condition?

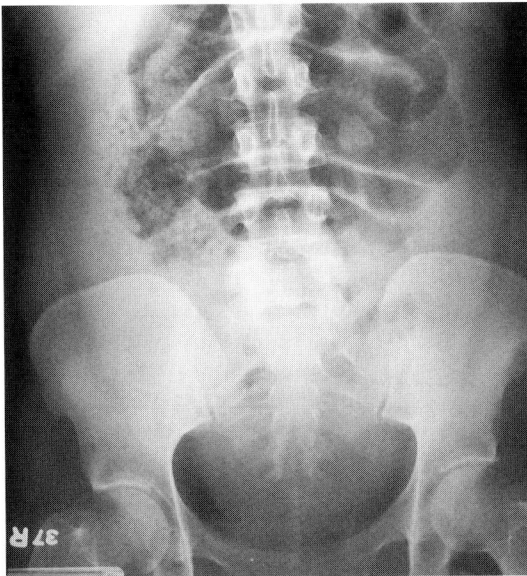

1. What is probably present in the abdomen?
2. What solid organ is most commonly injured by blunt trauma?
3. If the patient has a positive pregnancy test, what is the diagnosis?
4. What renal abnormality could cause this appearance?

CASE 107

Pancreatic Phlegmon

1. Phlegmon.

2. Acute pancreatitis.

3. Hemorrhagic pancreatitis.

4. Abscess or infection.

Reference

Ros PR, Hamrick-Turner JE, Chiechi MV, et al: Cystic masses of the pancreas, *Radiographics* 12:673-686, 1992.

Cross-Reference

Gastrointestinal Radiology: THE REQUISITES, ed 2, p 143.

Comment

Various fluid collections develop about the pancreas during episodes of acute inflammation. Some of these collections are within the pancreas, and others are in the peripancreatic tissues. Usually the fluid collections are more focal and may or may not be well defined. Most resolve within a few weeks. In severe cases the entire pancreas may be involved with inflammatory changes and fluid in a diffuse fashion. There may be associated massive enlargement of the pancreatic region by this inflammatory tissue (to the point that it may be clinically palpable). This condition is termed a *phlegmon.* It represents diffuse inflammation of the gland with fluid collections in and about the pancreas. The pancreas itself may be indiscernible, being replaced by all the inflammatory tissue. This condition may lead to complete necrosis of the gland. In some instances, diffuse hemorrhagic pancreatitis may have a similar appearance.

The phlegmon may resolve over the next few weeks, although the possible complications of necrosis, hemorrhage, and infection must be carefully watched for. Patients with this condition are particularly prone to these complications. If the phlegmon fails to respond, one of the aforementioned complications could be to blame or there could be some underlying condition, such as a bile duct stone, producing this situation.

Notes

CASE 108

Hemoperitoneum Caused by Ruptured Ectopic Pregnancy

1. Fluid.

2. Spleen.

3. Ruptured ectopic pregnancy.

4. None, kidneys are retroperitoneal.

Reference

Federle MP, Jeffrey RB: Hemoperitoneum studied by computed tomography, *Radiology* 148:187-192, 1983.

Cross-Reference

Gastrointestinal Radiology: THE REQUISITES, ed 2, p 125.

Comment

The radiograph shows evidence of free fluid within the abdominal cavity. Findings include increased density in the pelvis in a V-shaped configuration and fluid between the ascending and descending colon and the flank stripes. Fluid within the peritoneal cavity can represent ascites, inflammation, blood, or urine. The appropriate history should be obtained in this situation. Ascites can be the result of a variety of causes and is by far the most common cause of long-standing fluid accumulation in the abdomen.

In the setting of severe symptomatology or trauma, all of the diagnostic possibilities must be considered. Hemoperitoneum is the most likely cause. In patients who have sustained blunt trauma, the fluid could be the result of laceration of the spleen or the liver. Laceration of bowel or mesentery is less common. Other acute but nontraumatic causes include a ruptured ectopic pregnancy and ruptured blood vessel. A perforated viscus caused by ulceration, inflammation, or trauma usually produces ascitic fluid with little hemorrhage. Urine is another consideration in the setting of trauma, but the only cause is rupture of the bladder. Severe injury to a retroperitoneal structure almost never causes intraperitoneal bleeding unless it is penetrating. Pancreatitis is the only condition affecting a retroperitoneal structure that produces free intraperitoneal fluid, and this finding occurs only in the setting of acute pancreatitis.

Notes

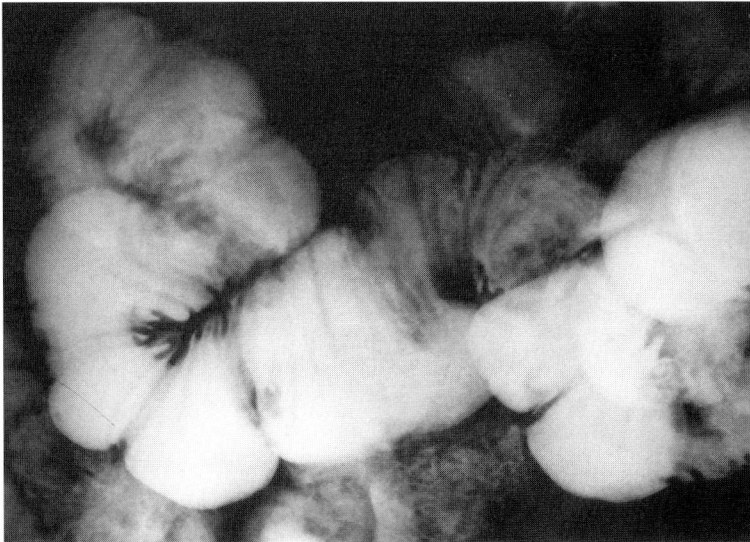

1. Of what disorders does CREST syndrome consist?
2. In mixed connective tissue disease, what intestinal organ is most commonly involved?
3. What underlying pathologic changes does the bowel undergo as a result of scleroderma?
4. What is meant by the term *hidebound* in reference to the appearance of the bowel?

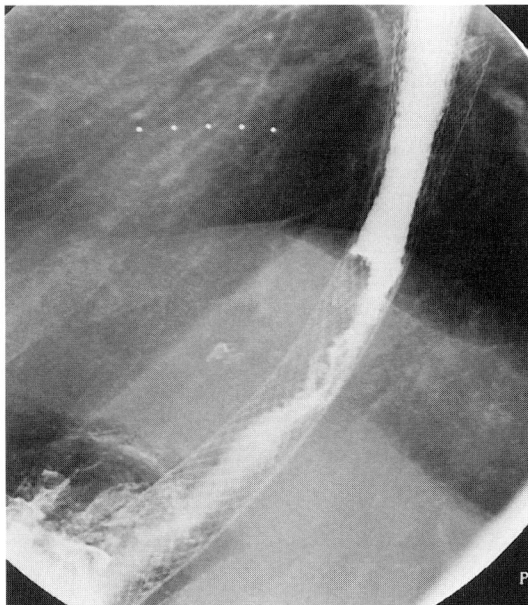

1. How is this device most commonly used in the esophagus?
2. A mass at the end of the stent is usually due to what problem?
3. Where does bleeding or a fistula often develop?
4. Can these stents be moved by electromagnetic forces within an MR scanner?

CASE 109

Scleroderma of the Small Bowel

1. Subcutaneous *c*alcinosis, *R*aynaud's phenomenon, *e*sophageal dysfunction, *s*clerodactyly, and *t*elangiectasia.

2. Esophagus.

3. Fibrosis and small vessel vasculitis.

4. Crowding of the valvulae and rigidity of the bowel.

Reference
Maglinte DDT, Kelvin FM, O'Connor K, et al: Current status of small bowel radiography, *Abdom Imaging* 21:247-253, 1996.

Cross-Reference
Gastrointestinal Radiology: THE REQUISITES, ed 2, p 115.

Comment
A number of connective tissue diseases can affect the small bowel. Scleroderma is caused by abnormal deposition of collagen in the skin, adjacent to blood vessels, and in various visceral organs. It may be isolated or may occur as part of the CREST syndrome, which includes other skin changes caused by calcinosis, sclerodactyly, Raynaud's disease, and telangiectasia, along with esophageal involvement. Mixed connective tissue disease (MCTD) is considered a distinct disease that has features of several connective tissue diseases, including systemic lupus erythematosus, scleroderma, polymyositis, and rheumatoid arthritis. In this condition, as well as scleroderma, the esophagus is the organ most often involved.

As mentioned, the major abnormality of scleroderma is the abnormal deposition of collagen into various tissues. Thus fibrosis is a major feature of this disease. However, there is also associated small vessel damage, particularly to the intestines, because much of this deposition produces vasculitis-type changes, with resultant long-term ischemia of the bowel. Malabsorption results because of stasis of the bowel contents, bacterial overgrowth, poor absorption of bile salts, and impaired lymphatic drainage. Diarrhea, weight loss, and bloating are all symptoms of this condition. Radiologically the changes of fibrosis, muscle atrophy, and vasculitis produce dilation of the small bowel, which is often termed *pseudoobstruction.* There is often dilation of the second portion of the duodenum as motility diminishes and it is compressed by the mesenteric vessels. Pneumatosis also can develop, but its underlying etiology is uncertain. A pathognomonic change seen in the bowel is crowding of the valvulae, or a "hidebound" appearance. The fibrosis of the bowel draws the valvulae closer together, producing more valvulae per inch (>5) than normal. The margins of the intestines also may be flattened. This flattening gives the bowel an accordion-pleated appearance.

Notes

CASE 110

Tumor Ingrowth in an Esophageal Stent

1. To maintain patency of the esophageal lumen in patients with esophageal carcinoma.

2. Granulation tissue or tumor overgrowth.

3. At the ends of the stent.

4. It's questionable, but MRI is not recommended within the first 6 weeks after stent placement.

Reference
Gollub MJ, Gerdes H, Baines MS: Radiographic appearances of esophageal stents, *Radiographics* 17:1169-1182, 1997.

Cross-Reference
Gastrointestinal Radiology: THE REQUISITES, ed 2, p 40.

Comment
The use of expandable esophageal stents has become more common for the treatment of severe esophageal problems. Currently the most common use of the stent is to maintain patency of the esophageal lumen in patients with esophageal carcinoma and less commonly in patients with tumors of the mediastinum, such as lymphoma. It also may be used in patients with benign conditions, such as tracheoesophageal fistulas, who have not responded to therapy. The stents are made of steel or titanium and expand after release from the device used to position them in the esophagus. The steel stents may be moved by the fields in an MR scanner, and it is usually recommended that they be in place for 6 weeks before scanning is performed. The radial force of the device holds them in place, but some have small wire struts at the ends to prevent migration. Some stents are also covered with nylon or another material to block fistula formation and prevent tumor ingrowth.

Complications may occur immediately after placement of the stent. These problems include migration and infolding of the device. Bleeding may occur at the ends as a result of the wire struts piercing the esophageal mucosa. Both bleeding and fistulas may develop at the ends of the stents because of the presence of the struts; thus not all makers use the struts. Late complications include migration, bleeding, and tumor ingrowth. If a mass or nodule appears at the end of the stent, it may be just granulation tissue or it may represent tumor overgrowth at the end of the device. Tumor ingrowth, as illustrated in this case, is uncommon because most stents have a covering of nylon or other material. However, on occasion, tumor grows through this material.

Notes

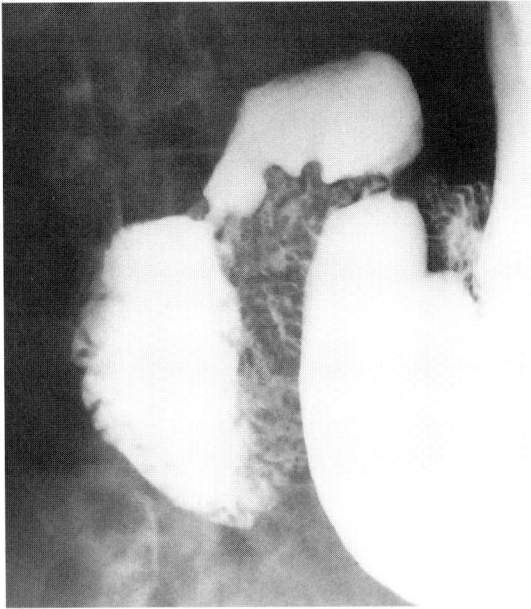

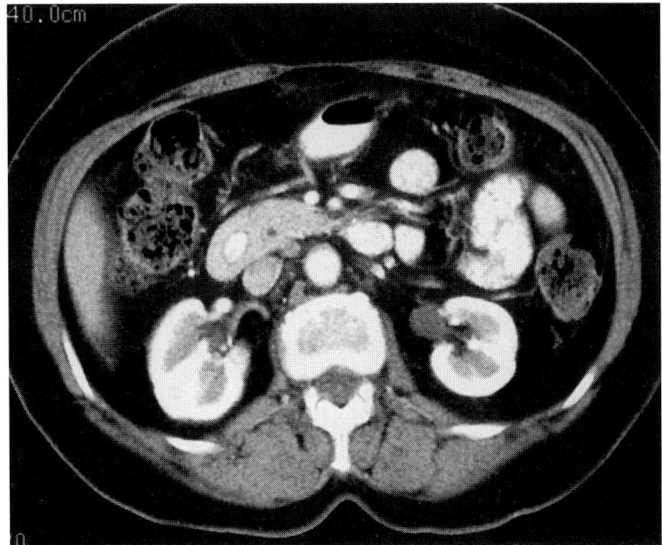

1. What anomaly is evident in this patient?
2. Embryologically, what portion of the pancreas becomes the head and uncinate?
3. Name a pancreatic complication of this condition.
4. In what age group does this condition present?

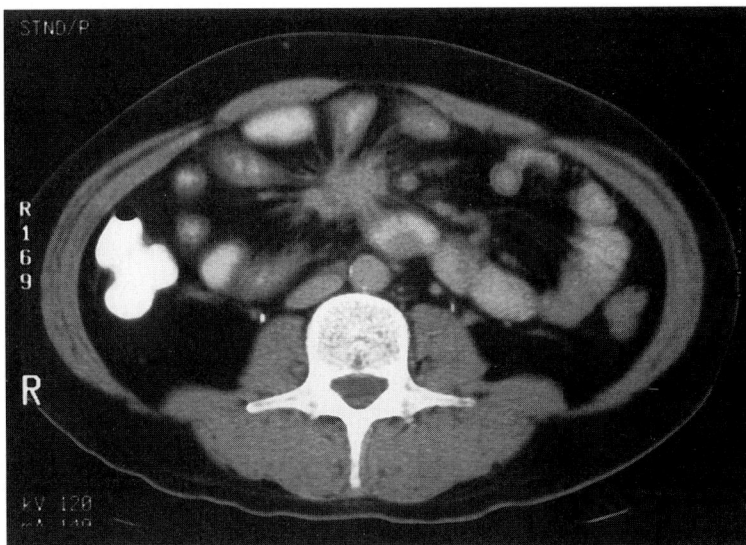

1. What is the most likely diagnosis?
2. In what site does this tumor most commonly occur?
3. What substance is excreted in the urine and confirms the diagnosis?
4. What is the major product secreted by this tumor?

Annular Pancreas

1. Annular pancreas.

2. Ventral pancreas.

3. Pancreatitis.

4. Half present in neonatal period, half in adulthood.

Reference

Rizzo RJ, Szucs RA, Turner MA: Congenital abnormalities of the pancreas and biliary tree in adults, *Radiographics* 15:49-68, 1995.

Cross-Reference

Gastrointestinal Radiology: THE REQUISITES, ed 2, p 138.

Comment

The embryologic development of the pancreas is complex and can lead to a variety of anomalies. Some are of no clinical significance, whereas others may present difficulties later in life. The pancreas forms as two distinct buds off of the biliary or hepatic bud, which comes from the duodenum. These buds are termed the *ventral* and *dorsal pancreatic buds.* The dorsal pancreatic bud is to the left of the midline and eventually forms the body and tail of the pancreas. The ventral bud develops to the right of the duodenum. It must rotate, along with the duodenum, to the left. This ventral bud later becomes the head and uncinate process of the pancreas.

Annular pancreas occurs when there is abnormal rotation of the ventral pancreas or the duodenum, both of which must rotate for proper pancreatic positioning. Some believe that the ventral bud adheres to the duodenum, so that as the structures rotate, the ventral pancreas develops and grows around the duodenum rather than in its normal position. The ventral duct continues to drain into the major papilla and joins with the biliary system, which is its normal embryologic anatomy.

The major pancreatic complication of annular pancreas is the development of acute or chronic pancreatitis. This condition affects as many as one quarter of patients with annular pancreas. Also, the annular pancreas produces duodenal narrowing or obstruction to varying degrees. About half of the cases of annular pancreas present in the neonatal period with duodenal symptoms. There may be other associated anomalies in the neonate as well. If the condition persists until adulthood, the annular pancreas may be discovered incidentally or when symptoms of pancreatitis or duodenal obstruction occur. These patients may become jaundiced as well. Surgery is necessary to correct the condition.

Notes

Carcinoid Tumor

1. Carcinoid tumor.

2. Appendix.

5. 5-HIAA.

4. Serotonin.

Reference

Picus D, Glazer HS, Levitt RG, et al: Computed tomography of abdominal arachnoid tumors, *Am J Roentgenol* 143:581-584, 1984.

Cross-Reference

Gastrointestinal Radiology: THE REQUISITES, ed 2, p 118.

Comment

Carcinoid tumors are unusual neoplasms that can arise in various structures of the intestinal tract and even the bronchi. The most common location in which carcinoids occur is the appendix. However, most symptomatic tumors arise in the small bowel, typically in the ileum. Rarely they are found in other parts of the intestinal tract, the abdominal cavity, and even the bronchi, which is an embryologic bud of the intestinal tract. Carcinoids are slow growing tumors that invade little by little. They are multiple in about 20% of the cases. All carcinoids are considered premalignant, but those of the small bowel are most likely to metastasize and those of the appendix rarely do so. These tumors belong to the group of lesions termed *APUD* (*a*mine *p*recursor *u*ptake and *d*ecarboxylation cell) *lesions.* They are hormonally active, and the major by-product they release is serotonin. Secretion of histamine, 5-hydroxytryptophan, and other hormones also has been described. Serotonin is converted in the liver and lungs to 5-hydroxyindoleacetic acid (5-HIAA), which is excreted in the urine and easily detected.

Carcinoid syndrome occurs when liver metastases (it rarely occurs without liver metastases) excrete hormonally active substances, which cannot be metabolized by the liver, directly into the venous circulation. This action produces vasomotor changes of flushing and vasodilation. Bronchospasm and wheezing may occur. Intestinal hypermotility, with diarrhea and cramping, is another symptom. With time, right-sided endocardial fibrosis and valve problems occur in the heart.

The primary tumor may appear as a polyp on conventional barium studies. However, the serotonin secreted by the tumor incites an intense desmoplastic response in the mesentery, producing the fibrotic response evident in this patient. There is marked fibrosis of the mesentery, with tethering and kinking of the small bowel loops. Bowel obstruction and even vascular obstruction are possible complications of this fibrosis.

Notes

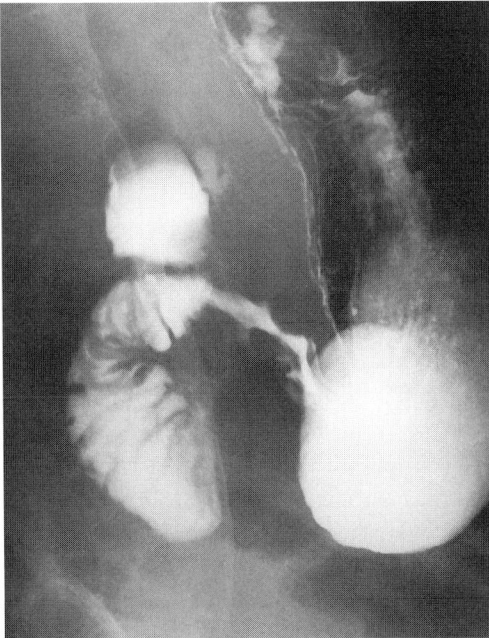

1. What is the most common cause of fistulas between the gallbladder and the duodenum?
2. What condition is associated with stone passage into the bowel?
3. What is the most likely cause of the fistula in this patient?
4. What other conditions also may produce this type of fistula?

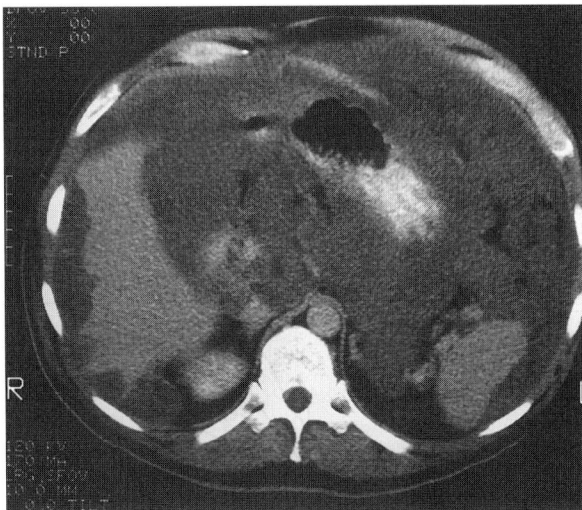

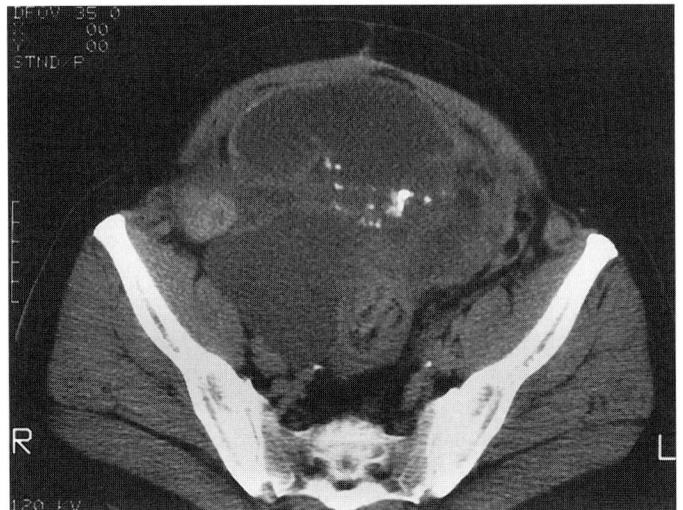

1. What gynecologic tumor may produce this condition?
2. What intestinal tumors cause this condition?
3. Do only malignant tumors produce this condition?
4. Name some other tumors associated with this condition.

Cholecystoduodenal Fistula Secondary to Crohn's Disease

1. Surgery.

2. Gallstone ileus.

3. Crohn's disease.

4. Cholecystitis, peptic ulcer disease, penetrating trauma, and neoplasms.

Reference

Levine MS: Crohn's disease of the upper gastrointestinal tract, *Radiol Clin North Am* 25:79-91, 1987.

Cross-Reference

Gastrointestinal Radiology: THE REQUISITES, ed 2, p 209.

Comment

The presence of a communication between the duodenum and the biliary system is quite common and typically is caused by a surgical connection between the bile ducts and the duodenum. However, the presence of a communication between the duodenum and the gallbladder is more unusual and often is associated with other conditions.

Most commonly a communication between the gallbladder and the duodenum is the result of a surgical procedure. This communication is common among patients with severe biliary disease or obstruction in whom the common bile duct must be surgically bypassed. This type of surgery is often reserved for patients with end-stage pancreatic disease, such as carcinoma, or patients who are medically unstable at the time of surgery. The next most likely condition to produce this finding is recurrent cholecystitis in which the adjacent duodenum is involved by the severe inflammatory process. With recurrent inflammation, a gallstone may erode through the gallbladder wall and into the adherent duodenum, producing a fistula. If the stone is large enough, it produces an obstruction, the so-called gallstone ileus condition. Other causes of fistula formation include peptic ulcer disease, with an ulcer eroding through the duodenum and into the gallbladder. Rarely a fistula may be the sequela of penetrating trauma. Neoplasms rarely produce fistulas.

In this individual the duodenum is rigid and featureless, which is typical of patients with Crohn's disease and less likely in patients with carcinoma or those undergoing radiation. Like other disorders of the gastrointestinal tract, Crohn's disease is known to produce fistulas. In this instance the gallbladder is not involved by Crohn's disease at the time of imaging and never becomes involved. However, the inflamed duodenum can still produce a fistula into adjacent structures, including the biliary system. Crohn's disease of the duodenum also can fistulize into the transverse colon and even the right renal pelvis.

Notes

Pseudomyxoma Peritonei

1. Mucinous cystadenocarcinoma of the ovary.

2. Mucinous appendiceal tumors.

3. No.

4. Mucinous tumors of the pancreas, stomach, or intestines.

Reference

Szucs RA, Turner MA: Gastrointestinal tract involvement by gynecologic diseases, *Radiographics* 16:1251-1271, 1996.

Cross-Reference

Gastrointestinal Radiology: THE REQUISITES, ed 2, p 125.

Comment

These CT images demonstrate low density material throughout the abdominal cavity, resembling ascites. However, in this instance the material appears loculated or cystic in the lower abdominal cavity. Scalloping of the liver edge also is present. Finally, areas of calcification are evident within the peritoneal cavity on some of the images. All these findings make this case atypical for conventional ascites and suggest the possibility of pseudomyxoma peritonei.

Pseudomyxoma peritonei is the presence of gelatinous or mucinous material in the peritoneal cavity. It is produced by the rupture of a mucin-producing neoplasm into the peritoneal cavity. It can be either a malignant process, such as a mucinous adenocarcinoma, or a benign process, such as a mucocele. Once the tumor ruptures, the cellular debris continues to produce mucin within the peritoneum, and the process tends to be progressive whether it is the result of a benign or a malignant cause.

In women by far the most common cause of pseudomyxoma peritonei is a mucinous neoplasm of the ovary, typically mucinous cystadenocarcinoma. In men the usual origin of the process is an appendiceal tumor, such as a mucocele of the appendix or a mucinous cystadenocarcinoma. Mucinous cystic tumors of the pancreas also may cause this condition. Mucinous tumors of the stomach, intestines, or bile ducts are even more rare. In this patient the scalloping of the liver and the calcification favor the diagnosis of a malignant mucinous process. Treatment is typically supportive because the material cannot be successfully removed surgically, and the remaining cells within the peritoneum will continue to produce the material.

Notes

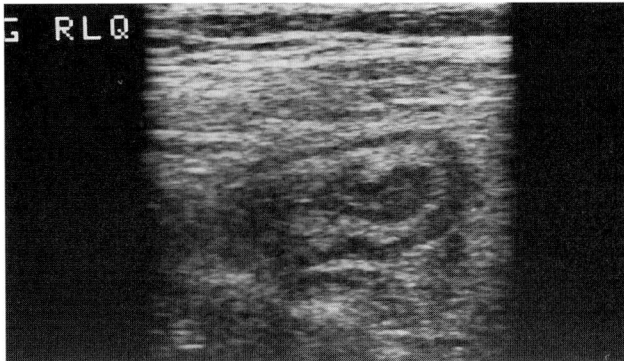

1. How large is a normal appendix as measured by ultrasound?
2. What is the most likely cause of this abnormality?
3. What other conditions may cause this abnormality?
4. What part of the appendiceal wall is brightly echogenic?

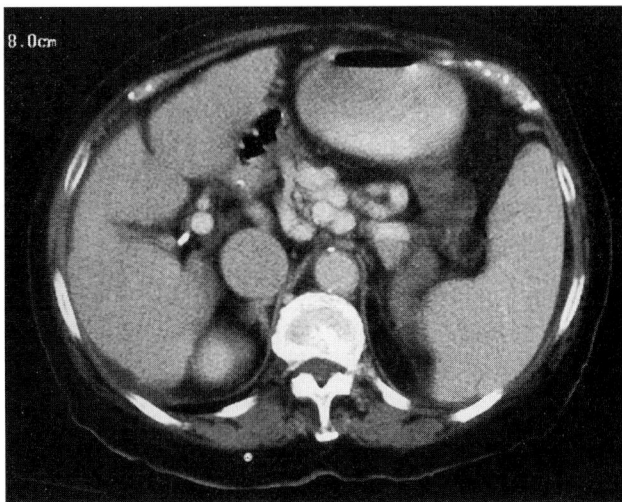

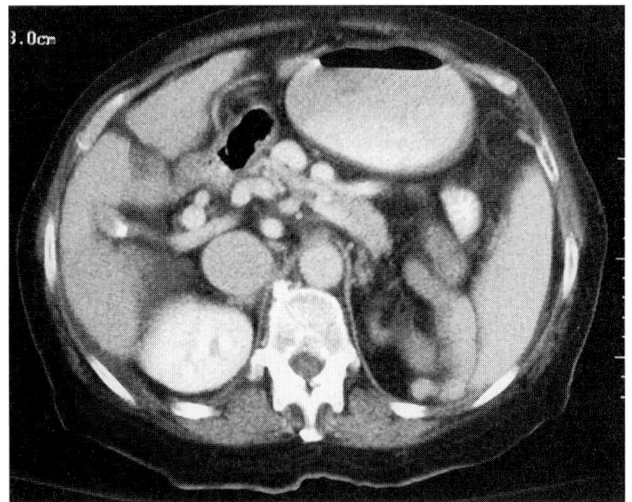

1. What underlying condition is present in this patient?
2. Name some neoplastic causes of this condition.
3. What is the most common cause of this condition?
4. What is the most common parasitic cause of this condition?

Crohn's Disease of the Appendix

1. 6 mm or less in diameter.

2. Appendicitis.

3. Inflammatory bowel disease (ulcerative colitis or Crohn's disease), other colonic inflammation, edema, ischemia, and adjacent inflammatory processes.

4. Submucosal layer.

Reference

Yacoe ME, Jeffrey RB: Sonography of appendicitis and diverti-culitis, *Radiol Clin North Am* 32:899-912, 1994.

Cross-Reference

Gastrointestinal Radiology: THE REQUISITES, ed 2, p 286.

Comment

Many consider sonography the modality of choice for the eval-uation of right lower quadrant symptoms, particularly in women. Identification of the appendix is a crucial part of the examination. However, successful diagnosis of appendicitis by ultrasound hinges on a well-performed examination and ad-herence to certain criteria. Both false positive and false negative diagnoses are possible when this modality is used.

The appendix is usually considered to be in a compressed state when it measures 6 mm or less in diameter. Compression must occur so that the true diameter can be determined. In-flamed appendices are typically not compressible. It may be im-possible to compress the appendix of an obese patient; thus the organ may appear somewhat larger, resulting in an incorrect di-agnosis of appendicitis if only the size criterion is used. The pres-ence of appendicoliths is strongly diagnostic of appendicitis. If there is discontinuity of the bright submucosal echogenic layer, it is often caused by necrosis and is indicative of appendicitis. Collections of fluid about the appendix often indicate abscess or peritoneal fluid, which also indicate appendicitis. The size crite-rion should not be the only factor used to make the diagnosis.

Many other conditions can produce changes in the appen-dix. Virtually any process that can affect the colon may also pro-duce changes in the appendix. Thus inflammatory bowel dis-ease, infectious colitis, bowel wall edema, and hemorrhage or ischemia also produce appendiceal wall thickening. Adjacent inflammation resulting from tuboovarian abscess or peritonitis also can produce appendiceal enlargement mimicking appen-dicitis. Crohn's disease of the appendix is an unusual entity. It may occur along with disease of the adjacent cecum and termi-nal ileum, or it may be an isolated finding, termed *granuloma-tous appendicitis.* This condition typically does not evolve into the extensive intestinal Crohn's disease that is commonly en-countered. Thus some consider this terminology inappropriate.

Notes

Portal Vein Thrombosis with Collateral Circulation

1. Obstruction of the portal vein.

2. Hepatocellular carcinoma, pancreatic carcinoma, and liver metastases.

3. Usually idiopathic. (There is no known cause in as many as half of all cases.)

4. Schistosomiasis.

Reference

Cho KC, Patel YD, Wachsberg RH, et al: Varices in portal hy-pertension: evaluation with CT, *Radiographics* 15:609-622, 1995.

Cross-Reference

Gastrointestinal Radiology: THE REQUISITES, ed 2, p 166.

Comment

These CT images demonstrate multiple venous collaterals oc-curring at the area where the portal vein should begin. This pre-sentation typically occurs when there is thrombosis of the por-tal vein and numerous collateral venous channels or varices must develop to carry the blood flow that normally courses through the portal vein. If this process occurs slowly, the devel-opment of these varices, which may eventually bleed or pro-duce symptoms, may be the only abnormality that occurs. If the thrombosis is severe, there may be serious venous conges-tion of the mesentery and intestines and possible ischemia of those structures. There also may be abnormalities in the en-hancement of the liver parenchyma on imaging studies caused by abnormalities in blood flow.

There are numerous causes for portal vein thrombosis, but in up to 50% of patients the exact cause is never found. Cir-rhosis is the most common intrahepatic cause for portal vein thrombosis because the stasis of blood flow in the portal veins predisposes the patient to thrombosis. Other vascular causes in-clude Budd-Chiari syndrome and venous congestion of the liver caused by congestive heart failure. Malignancies account for a high percentage of cases of portal vein thrombosis. The most common malignancy is hepatocellular carcinoma, which fre-quently invades the portal venous system with thrombosis. Pan-creatic carcinoma invades the portal system (superior mesen-teric or splenic vein) with thrombosis. A less likely cause is adenopathy in the portal hepatis with compression of the por-tal vein or intrahepatic metastases. Other conditions that in-crease a patient's tendency for thrombosis, such as polycythemia vera, can cause portal vein thrombosis. Inflammatory processes in the abdomen, such as abscesses, also have been known to cause portal venous thrombosis. Worldwide the most likely cause for this condition is schistosomiasis.

Notes

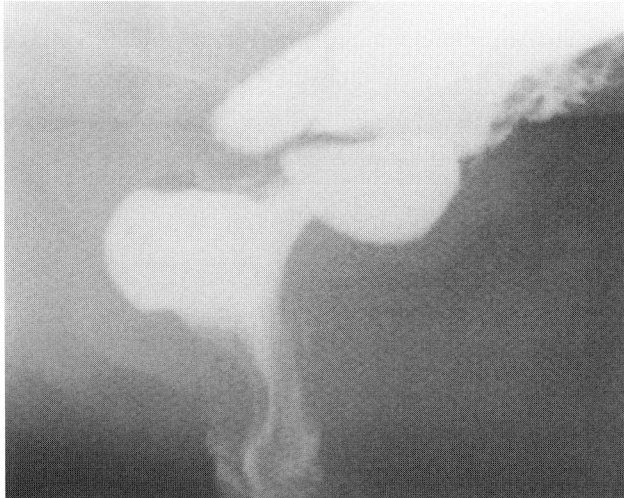

A

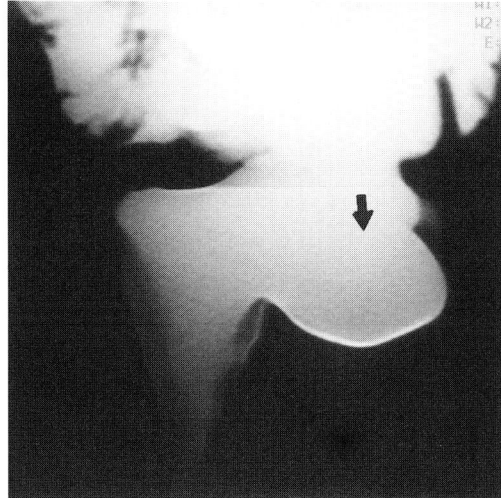

B

1. What constitutes a normal anorectal angle?
2. What muscle helps maintain the anorectal angle?
3. Between what two points is perineal descent measured?
4. What is the significance of a posterolateral rectal pouch?

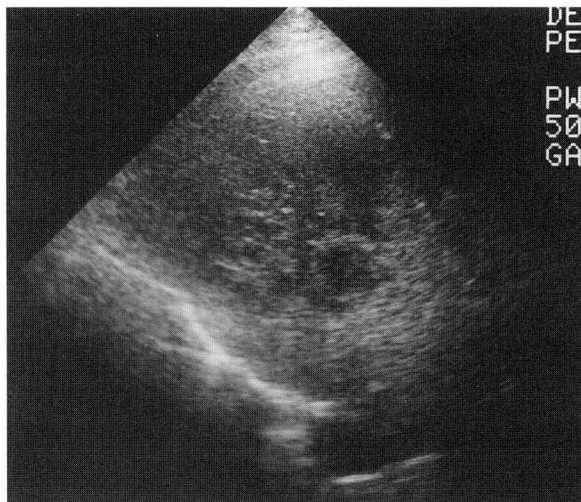

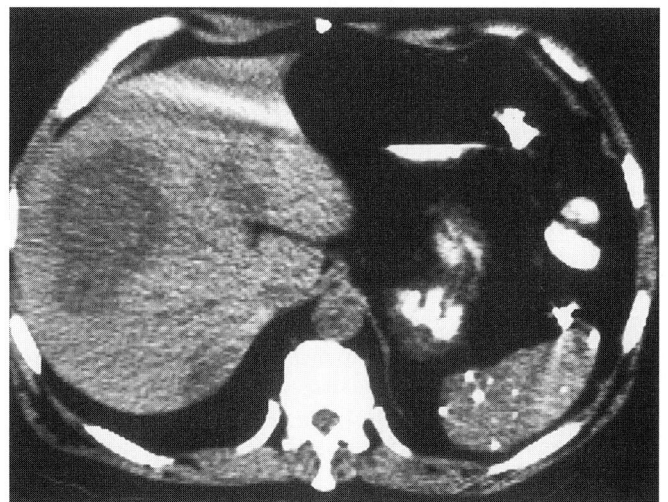

1. Name some possible differential diagnoses.
2. How often is air present in pyogenic liver abscesses?
3. Outside the intestines, amebiasis most commonly affects what site?
4. What is the treatment of choice for large liver abscesses (>5 cm in diameter)?

Rectocele (A) and Posterolateral Rectal Pouch (B)

1. Ranges from 70 to 130 degrees.

2. Puborectalis.

3. Anorectal junction and inferior aspect of the ischial tuberosities.

4. Usually found in patients who complain of severe straining during defecation.

Reference

Goei R, van Engelshoven J, Schouten H, et al: Anorectal function: defecographic measurement in asymptomatic subjects, *Radiology* 173:137-141, 1989.

Cross-Reference

Gastrointestinal Radiology: THE REQUISITES, ed 2, p 289.

Comment

Defecography has been used in the last two decades in an attempt to analyze the normal anorectal function during defecation. This procedure involves the introduction of a barium paste material into the rectum and then placement of the patient on a radiolucent commode in front of the fluoroscopic device, while defecation is recorded.

The analysis of a defecogram depends on the measurement of various structures, as well as their relationship to one another, which changes dynamically during defecation. The most common measurement is that of the anorectal angle, which is determined by drawing straight lines through the anus and posterior wall of the rectum and measuring their intersection. This angle approaches 90 degrees and helps maintain continence in the resting state. The puborectalis muscle, which produces this angle, must be contracted. However, during defecation, it must relax so that the anorectal angle becomes obtuse and approaches 180 degrees. Another important relationship exists between the anorectal junction and the ischial tuberosities, which help define the pelvic floor. These entities should be at the same level; if the anorectal junction descends too low during defecation, it indicates weakness of the musculature of the perineum.

Several abnormalities are discovered frequently during defecography. The most common is the rectocele, an anterior outpouching of the rectum that occurs during defecation. This anomaly is extremely common in women, and some regard a small rectocele as an insignificant finding. An enterocele is caused by loops of small bowel descending quite low into the pelvis during defecation, extending into the space between the rectum and vagina. Finally, a lateral rectal pouch is a herniation of the lateral wall of the rectum through the perineum and is often produced by chronic severe straining during defecation.

Notes

Pyogenic Liver Abscess

1. Metastasis, abscesses of various types, and necrotic tumor.

2. Less than 20% of the time.

3. Liver.

4. Percutaneous catheter drainage and antibiotic therapy.

Reference

Murphy BJ, Casillas J, Ros PR, et al: The CT appearance of cystic masses of the liver, *Radiographics* 9:307-322, 1989.

Cross-Reference

Gastrointestinal Radiology: THE REQUISITES, ed 2, p 179.

Comment

Abscesses of the liver are common among hospitalized patients. Abscesses may be the result of a pyogenic (bacterial) infection or may be caused by amebiasis or echinococcosis. This discussion pertains to pyogenic liver abscesses. Pyogenic hepatic abscesses can develop as a result of biliary obstruction with ascending cholangitis; portal vein phlebitis caused by abdominal inflammation (diverticulitis); hepatic artery septic emboli (endocarditis); direct extension from adjacent organs (penetrating ulcer); or trauma, usually penetrating or iatrogenic. Most often, hepatic abscesses are the result of biliary tract obstruction with cholangitis. Many years ago the most common cause was abdominal infection (e.g., appendicitis and diverticulitis with spread via the portal vein). Immunosuppression is another major factor contributing to the occurrence of liver abscess. Abscesses spread via embolic phenomena, yet the hepatic or portal systems are often solitary. If abscesses are caused by biliary tract obstruction, they are more likely to be multiple. Organisms that produce infection are often mixed; they may be aerobic or anaerobic. *Escherichia coli* is probably the most common causative organism, however.

Hepatic abscesses may be detected by either ultrasound or CT. On ultrasound, abscesses can have a variable appearance. Abscesses are often anechoic but may be isoechoic or even hyperechoic, as illustrated in this case. Debris and variable echogenicity are common findings. CT is the best method for demonstration of hepatic abscess. The masses are hypodense on both precontrast and postcontrast films. Their density overlaps with that of other liver lesions, such as hypodense tumors or cysts. Abscesses often have a peripheral rim of enhancement. Some may show a "cluster" sign in which small abscesses that are separated from one another by septa or liver tissue are clustered together to form one large lesion. Gas within the abscess is a specific sign but is present in less than 20% of cases. Treatment for small abscesses (<5 cm in diameter) is often just antibiotic therapy, but larger abscesses often require percutaneous catheter drainage.

Notes

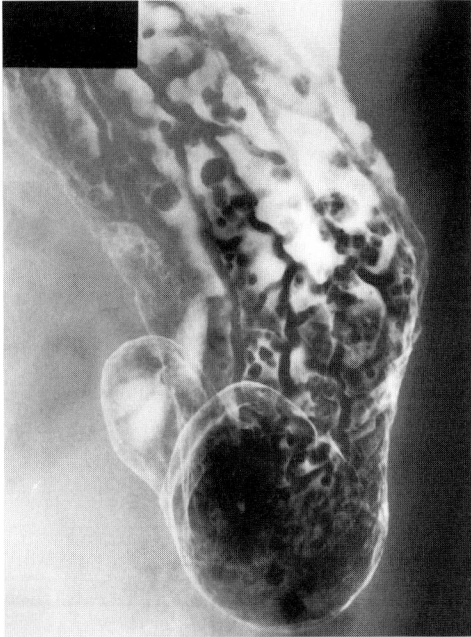

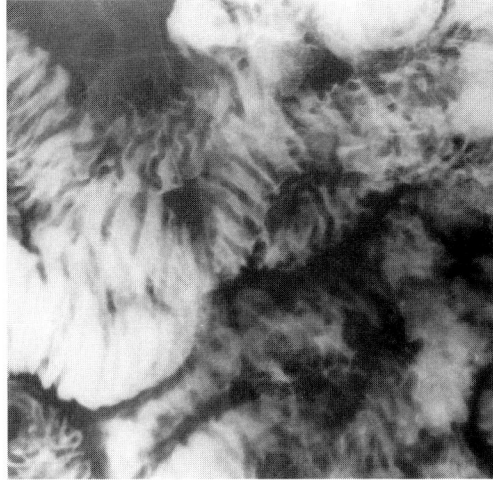

1. What intestinal diseases are associated with a peripheral eosinophilia?
2. What would help differentiate these possible entities radiologically?
3. What parts of the bowel wall are involved by eosinophilic gastroenteritis?
4. What is the relationship between eosinophilic granulomas and eosinophilic gastroenteritis?

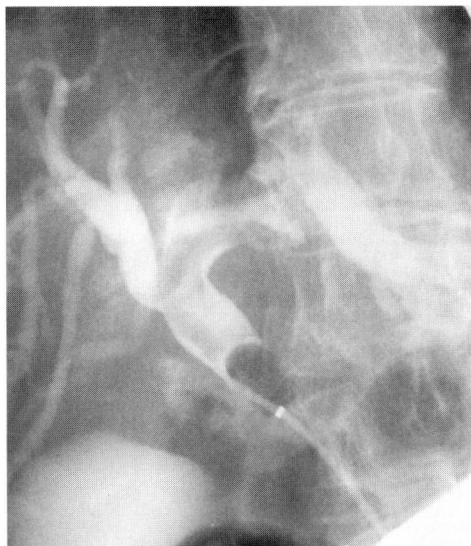

1. What is the most likely cause of this filling defect?
2. What parasitic infection often involves the biliary tract?
3. What is the most common cause of hemobilia?
4. What is the treatment of choice for hemobilia?

Eosinophilic Gastroenteritis

1. Parasitic infections and eosinophilic gastroenteritis.

2. Gastric involvement.

3. Most parts of the bowel, including the mucosa, muscularis, and serosa.

4. There is no relationship.

Reference

MacCarty RL, Talley NJ: Barium studies in diffuse eosinophilic gastroenteritis, *Gastrointest Radiol* 15:183-187, 1990.

Cross-Reference

Gastrointestinal Radiology: THE REQUISITES, ed 2, p 86.

Comment

Eosinophilic gastroenteritis is an unusual disease of the bowel. Its pathologic feature is an eosinophilic infiltration of the bowel wall. It produces symptoms of abdominal pain, nausea, vomiting, diarrhea, and rarely bleeding. Its major laboratory finding is a peripheral eosinophilia, which can be quite high. There is a relationship between this entity and food allergies, allergic conditions, asthma, and eczema. However, up to half of the patients have no known allergic condition. Clinically these patients respond well to steroids.

The eosinophilic infiltrate can involve any part of the bowel wall, resulting in different radiologic appearances. When it primarily involves the mucosa, the infiltrate will produce fold thickening and even slight nodularity or polyps. If the infiltration is in the muscularis, the lumen of the bowel is compromised and narrowed. The infiltration also may involve the serosa. Radiologic abnormalities include fold thickening, narrowing of the lumen, nodularity, and rarely ascites or adenopathy.

Both parasitic infections and eosinophilic granuloma can have peripheral eosinophilia, as well as small bowel fold thickening. However, eosinophilic gastroenteritis predominantly involves the stomach, whereas parasitic diseases rarely affect the stomach. Thus involvement of the stomach is an important differential point. Eosinophilic gastroenteritis also may involve the esophagus and colon. Eosinophilic granulomas are focal tumors composed of tissue with a heavy eosinophilic infiltrate, but they are typically isolated lesions. They are not related to eosinophilic gastroenteritis and do not have peripheral eosinophilia.

Notes

Blood Clot in the Biliary System

1. Blood clot.

2. Ascariasis.

3. Iatrogenic.

4. Superselective arterial embolization.

Reference

Okazaki M, Ono H, Higashihara H, et al: Angiographic management of massive hemobilia due to iatrogenic trauma, *Gastrointest Radiol* 16:205-209, 1991.

Cross-Reference

Gastrointestinal Radiology: THE REQUISITES, ed 2, p 199.

Comment

Filling defects within the bile ducts are most commonly caused by stones. However, these stones are round or faceted in configuration and usually easily identifiable as such. Tubular filling defects are less common. In most parts of the world the most common tubular filling defect is a parasitic worm, usually *Ascaris* species. However, in industrialized societies the most likely cause for a filling defect with this appearance is a blood clot. Sludge in the ducts is another possibility, but rarely is it visible in the bile ducts. Also, benign tumors could be another consideration.

Hemobilia can be difficult to diagnose. Often the endoscopist identifies bleeding or clots coming from the papilla, thus establishing the diagnosis. Many years ago, the most common cause for hemobilia was infection and mycotic aneurysm formation in the liver. Now, by far the most common cause for hemobilia is iatrogenic. The bleeding is often a sequela of liver biopsies, percutaneous biliary injections or drainages, and less commonly sphincterotomy. Penetrating injuries are another possible cause. Tumors rarely produce hemobilia, although both benign and malignant tumors can cause the condition. All of these events involve a penetrating wound to the liver. The trauma produces pseudoaneurysms of small hepatic arteries, which can fistulize into the biliary system, producing the bleeding. It is much less common for venous abnormalities to produce the bleeding. The best method of treatment for hemobilia is superselective hepatic artery catheterization with embolization of the arterial branch that is producing the bleeding.

Notes

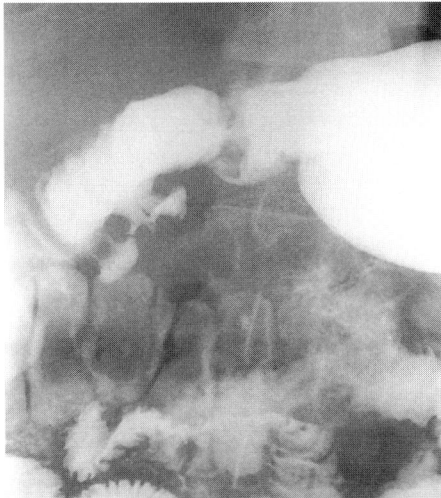

1. In patients with multiple endocrine neoplasia syndrome I, what organs are involved by tumors?
2. Give the location and incidence of extrapancreatic gastrinomas.
3. Approximately what portion of gastrinomas are malignant?
4. Besides ulcers, what is another common symptom of gastrinomas?

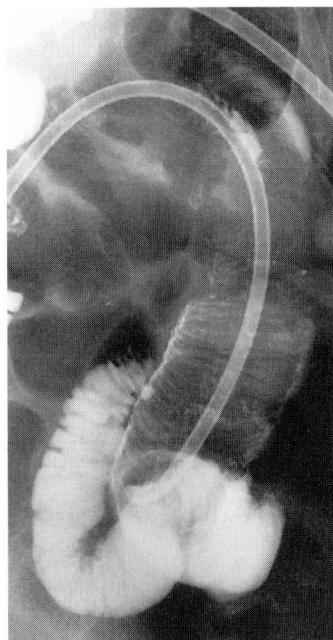

1. What is the most likely cause of the obstruction in this patient?
2. What mechanism produces this complication?
3. What unique complication may result when intestinal tubes with mercury bags are used?
4. What complication may result during the removal of an intestinal tube?

Duodenal Ulcers in Zollinger-Ellison Syndrome

1. Pancreas (gastrinoma), parathyroid, pituitary, and adrenal gland.

2. Duodenum (about 15%) and other organs (about 10%), such as paraaortic region, bladder, and ovaries.

3. Majority (approximately 60%).

4. Diarrhea.

Reference

Buetow P, Miller DL, Parrino TV, et al: Islet cell tumors of the pancreas: clinical, radiologic and pathologic correlation in diagnosis and localization, *Radiographics* 17:453, 1997.

Cross-Reference

Gastrointestinal Radiology: THE REQUISITES, ed 2, p 126.

Comment

Zollinger-Ellison (Z-E) syndrome is caused by gastrin secretion from non–islet cell tumors of the pancreas, so-called gastrinomas. The large majority (>75%) occur in the pancreas, but this tumor is also known to occur in ectopic locations. Approximately 15% of gastrinomas are found in the duodenum, and the remainder are in the paraaortic region, bladder, ovaries, and even liver. About one quarter are associated with multiple endocrine neoplasia syndrome I (MEN-I), which also causes tumors of the parathyroid, pituitary, and adrenal glands. The majority of gastrinomas are malignant and have a propensity for early metastases. Those tumors associated with the MEN-I syndrome have a lesser incidence of malignancy, however.

Clinically, patients develop peptic ulcer disease because of the acid hypersecretion related to the elevated gastrin levels. Most ulcers in patients with Z-E syndrome occur in the gastric antrum and duodenal bulb. Occasionally, ulcers occur in the distal duodenum. Although they are uncommon even in patients with Z-E syndrome, distal duodenal ulcers are so rare in healthy patients that they are considered a feature of the disease. Serum gastrin levels can be variable in patients with Z-E syndrome, although any level above 1000 units is indicative of the condition. Often a gastrin-provocative test using secretin is necessary to determine the presence of a gastrinoma. (This test produces a dramatic rise in serum gastrin levels in affected patients.)

The gastric acid hypersecretion may present as increased fluid in the stomach, along with thickened rugal folds. Many gastrinoma patients also complain of diarrhea. The increased acidity in the small bowel interferes with the function of the small bowel enzymes, resulting in diminished intestinal absorption. In severe cases a spruelike condition may ensue, with villous atrophy, malabsorption, and steatorrhea.

Notes

Intestinal Intussusception Along a Feeding Tube

1. Intussusception.

2. Peristalsis of the bowel causes telescoping of the intestines along the tube.

3. Gaseous distention of the mercury bag.

4. Retrograde intussusception.

Reference

Peskin SR, Langevin RE, Banks PA: Proximal jejunal intussusception associated with a long tube, *Dig Dis Sci* 31:657-660, 1986.

Cross-Reference

Gastrointestinal Radiology: THE REQUISITES, ed 2, p 103.

Comment

The use of enteric tubes for nutritional support is becoming increasingly common. The first tubes employed involved nasal access. These tubes could be quite long and have either a mercury bag attached or later a weighted tip so that peristalsis would carry them further into the intestine. Since the development of better interventional techniques, intestinal tubes are now often placed through the abdominal wall and into either the stomach or the proximal small bowel. These may be placed by the interventional radiologist or the gastroenterologist (via an endoscope), and sometimes they may be placed surgically. With the increasing use of nutritional support in the long-term care of chronically debilitated patients, these transabdominal catheters are becoming standard.

With the early transnasal catheters, bowel obstruction was a possible complication and typically was the result of intussusception, with the tip of the catheter serving as a lead point. However, when the tube was fixed to the nose, there could be telescoping of the bowel along the catheter. The peristaltic waves would cause the bowel to creep in a retrograde fashion along the catheter and telescope into itself. This telescoping is illustrated in this case. With the old mercury bag catheters, a rare complication was gaseous distention of the balloon tip.

The complication of obstruction is rarely detected, although it has been speculated that it may occur more frequently than previously thought. Many of these patients are extremely debilitated and may not complain of symptomatology. Also, the tip of the tube is not obstructed, and feedings could continue without difficulty, as they did in this case. Many episodes of silent intussusception caused by the placement of these tubes may go undetected. Besides obstruction, the other major complication possible is ischemia of the bowel, with resultant necrosis and perforation. In this patient the intussusception resolved spontaneously after withdrawal of the tube.

Notes

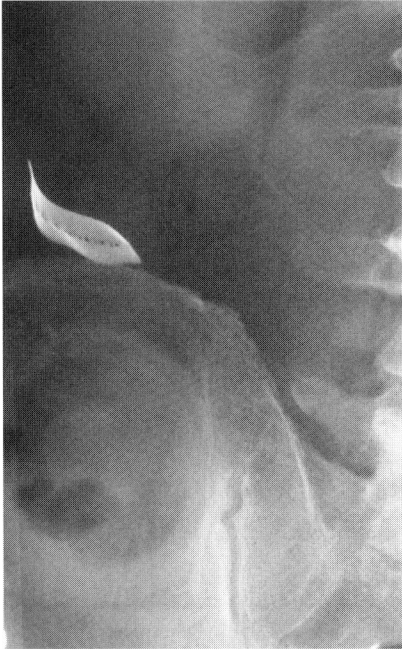

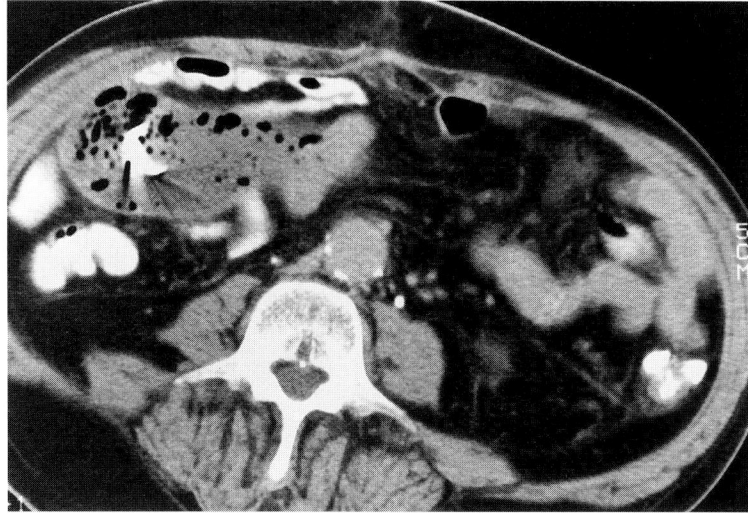

1. What abnormality is developing in the anterior abdomen?
2. What is the cause for the high density focus within this abnormality?
3. Why is it radiopaque?
4. What treatment may be performed by the radiologist?

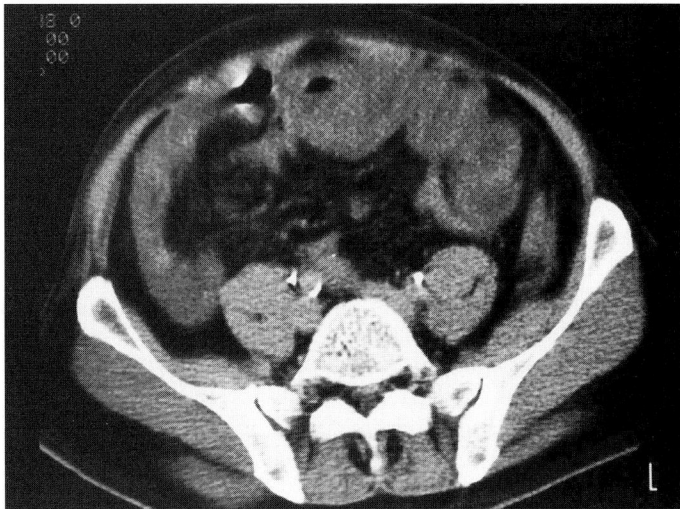

1. What diseases cause focal vasculitis of the intestines?
2. Which condition is the cause of most cases of ischemic bowel?
3. What pathologic change in the bowel occurs months after radiation therapy?
4. Multifocal ischemic changes often indicate what underlying condition?

CASE 127

Retained Surgical Sponge Within an Abscess

1. Abscess.

2. Retained surgical device (sponge).

3. Radiopaque material is embedded in a portion of it.

4. Percutaneous removal.

Reference

Kopka L, Fischer U, Gross A, et al: CT of retained surgical sponges (textilomas): pitfalls in detection and evaluation, *J Comput Assist Tomogr* 20:919-925, 1996.

Cross-Reference

Gastrointestinal Radiology: THE REQUISITES, ed 2, p 123.

Comment

This CT scan demonstrates an abnormal collection of fluid and air within the anterior abdomen consistent with an abscess. Of more importance, however, is the presence of a focus of high density within the abscess, which is indicative of some type of foreign object within the abdominal cavity. This finding could be the result of a penetrating trauma or perhaps something perforating the gastrointestinal tract. Another consideration is an iatrogenic cause (i.e., the introduction of some object into the peritoneal cavity during a medical procedure). This object could be a surgical sponge or towel or perhaps a surgical needle that was dropped into the peritoneal cavity. This complication is rare, considering the number of procedures performed daily.

Often it is difficult to diagnose a retained surgical sponge. All surgical sponges must have some radiopaque marker placed on them so that they can be identified on radiographs of the abdomen. Intraoperative radiographs are obtained if the sponge count taken during surgery is incorrect. This study usually detects most sponges that are lost within the abdominal cavity. However, often, because of incorrect counting, the surgeon may be unaware that a sponge has been lost within the abdominal cavity. Some of these objects produce no symptoms and are retained within the abdominal cavity until they are later discovered incidentally during a radiologic examination. Others may serve as a nidus for infection, leading to the development of an abscess, as in this patient. If the radiologist does not identify the high density structure within the abscess, the sponge may not be discovered. Surgical towels do not have radiopaque markers on them.

Surgery is the primary treatment when complications, such as abscess formation, occur as a result of a retained foreign object. However, the retained sponge can be removed percutaneously during drainage of the abscess.

Notes

CASE 128

Venous Occlusive Disease of the Intestines

1. Systemic lupus erythematosus, scleroderma, radiation therapy, and other collagen vascular diseases.

2. Hypotension or low flow states.

3. Thromboangiitis obliterans.

4. Embolic disease.

Reference

Scholz FJ: Ischemic bowel disease, *Radiol Clin North Am* 31:1197-1217, 1993.

Cross-Reference

Gastrointestinal Radiology: THE REQUISITES, ed 2, p 110.

Comment

The most common cause of ischemic changes in the intestines is hypotension or a low flow state brought on by shock, major surgery, or a cardiac abnormality. The next process to consider in ischemic disease of the intestines is arterial occlusion, which is either chronic (caused by atherosclerotic disease) or acute (as seen in embolic phenomena). The other part of the vascular system that must be considered in the patient with ischemia is the venous circulation.

Mesenteric venous occlusive disease accounts for 10% to 15% of cases of bowel ischemia. It can be produced by hypercoagulable states (polycythemia or disseminated intravascular coagulation), drugs (birth control pills), venous stasis (portal hypertension), malignancies (pancreatic and lung cancer), and mechanical obstructive processes of the portal system (tumors, fibrosis, or surgery). The thrombosis may occur in the portal vein and extend backward or occur primarily in the superior mesenteric vein. When the venous pressure increases in the portal system and mesenteric veins, there is often diminished blood flow to the intestines, resulting in arterial ischemia. Typically these patients have a gradual onset of symptoms, often including abdominal pain. However, the condition also has a fairly high mortality rate because, if it is not discovered early, progressive ischemia may ensue, with resultant necrosis of bowel.

Radiologically, visible changes include thickened bowel folds and thickening of the bowel wall. Many feel that ultrasound is helpful in evaluating the status of the blood flow in the mesenteric vessels. However, this examination can be difficult to perform because these patients often develop bowel distention, which hinders ultrasonography. CT is probably the modality of choice, particularly in patients with venous occlusion. It can demonstrate the ischemic changes in the intestines, evaluate for thrombus in vessels, and sometimes define the underlying etiology, such as tumor.

Notes

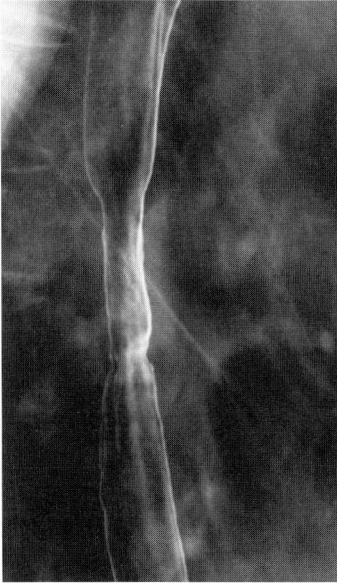

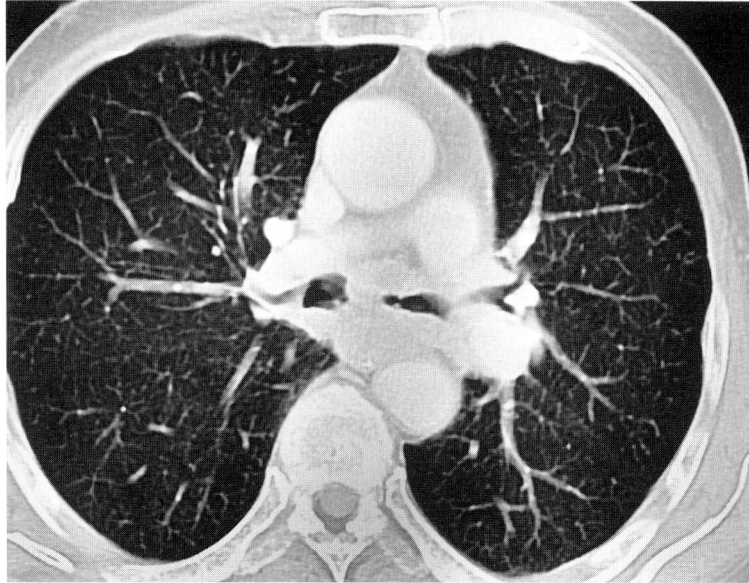

1. What is the most common cause of hematogenous metastases to the esophagus?
2. What tumor most frequently invades the esophagus through direct extension?
3. What hematologic neoplasms can involve the esophagus?
4. What is the most common site of secondary esophageal involvement by tumor?

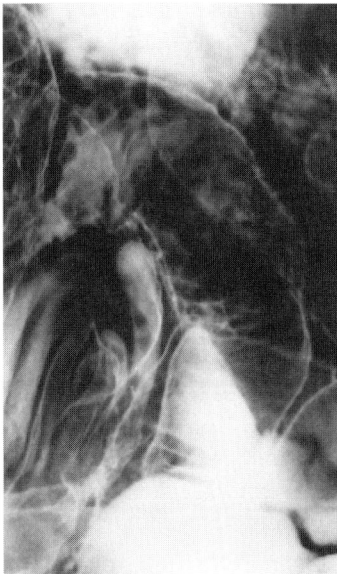

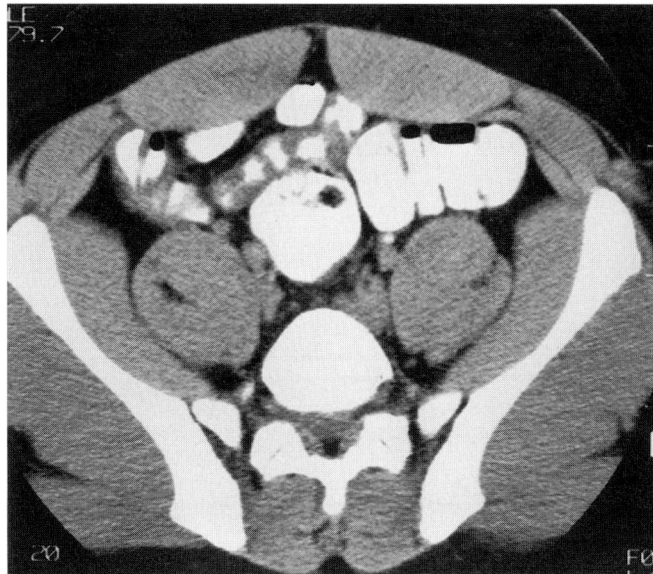

1. What infectious processes of the intestines are transmitted by the consumption of infected milk?
2. What self-limited infectious process often involves the terminal ileum?
3. What feature may distinguish *Yersinia* species infection from other inflammatory processes of the terminal ileum?
4. What fungal infection affects the distal small bowel?

Breast Metastases to the Esophagus

1. Breast cancer.

2. Gastric carcinoma.

3. Lymphoma and leukemia.

4. Middle of the esophagus, secondary to direct extension from lymph nodes.

Reference

Feczko PJ, Collins DD, Mezwa DG: Metastatic disease involving the gastrointestinal tract, *Radiol Clin North Am* 31:1359-1373, 1993.

Cross-Reference

Gastrointestinal Radiology: THE REQUISITES, ed 2, p 11.

Comment

Metastases to the esophagus are not uncommon findings on autopsy studies. However, it is somewhat more rare for them to be encountered in practice. The most common cause of secondary tumor involvement of the esophagus is direct invasion or extension of an adjacent neoplasm. The most common of these neoplasms is gastric carcinoma, which extends into the distal esophagus. Carcinoma of the lung also involves the esophagus either by direct extension or by secondary involvement of the mediastinal adenopathy. Breast cancer is the most likely distant tumor to secondarily involve the esophagus. It usually involves the esophagus by first spreading to mediastinal lymph nodes and then invading into the esophagus. However, it is also the most common cancer to have direct hematogenous metastases to the esophagus. Hematogenous metastases are quite rare. Although all tumors may metastasize to the esophagus, the hematogenous metastases are more commonly associated with breast cancer, Kaposi's sarcoma, melanoma, and hypernephroma.

Notes

Yersinia Species Infection of the Terminal Ileum

1. Tuberculosis and *Yersinia* organisms.

2. *Yersinia enterocolitica.*

3. Luminal narrowing is minimal.

4. Histoplasmosis.

Reference

Gardiner R, Smith C: Infective enterocolitides, *Radiol Clin North Am* 25:67-78, 1987.

Cross-Reference

Gastrointestinal Radiology: THE REQUISITES, ed 2, p 287.

Comment

The major inflammatory processes that affect the terminal ileum are Crohn's disease, tuberculosis, and *Yersinia* species infection. *Yersinia* organisms as pathologic agents have been recognized only over the past few decades, and little was known about them before that time. *Y. enterocolitica* is a gram-negative bacillus that can infect both animals and humans. It is seen predominantly in Scandinavia, Europe, and North America. Some believe it is transmitted by drinking infected cow's milk, although this is not the only method of infection. The infection occurs predominantly in the terminal ileum, and infection of other parts of the bowel is uncommon. It may occur in small epidemics. Clinically, patients complain of abdominal pain, fever, and sometimes diarrhea. There may be tenderness in the right lower quadrant, and the symptoms can mimic appendicitis quite easily.

Radiologically the abnormalities are usually confined to the terminal ileum. The disease process produces stages that can be apparent on serial studies. The initial phase produces nodular folds of the terminal ileum, with some bowel wall thickening and perhaps adenopathy. The infected bowel is often dilated or maintains its lumen when compared with bowel affected by other processes, such as Crohn's disease and tuberculosis. Lymphoid follicles may be prominent. In later phases, ulceration (mainly superficial aphthous ulceration) develops. Deep transmural ulceration is not a feature of this disease. After several (5 to 8) weeks, the inflammation may subside with no residual radiologic abnormalities evident. Antibiotics accelerate healing. During the active phase, some patients also complain of arthritis.

The main differential features that distinguish this entity from Crohn's disease include the lack of bowel lumen narrowing; the lack of deep ulceration; the short, self-limited clinical course; and healing without residual scarring.

Notes

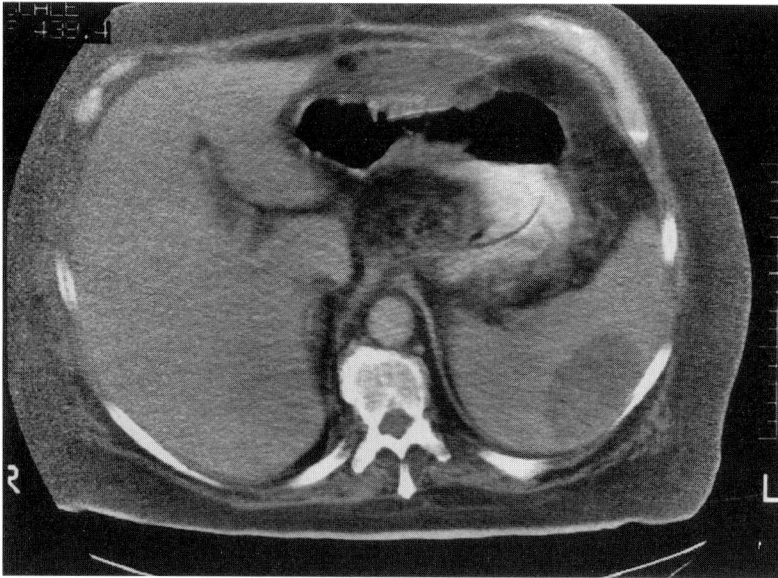

1. What is the most common benign splenic tumor?
2. Which benign splenic tumor may be isointense with the spleen on CT?
3. Which benign splenic tumor may calcify?
4. Which benign splenic tumor is associated with Klippel-Trenaunay-Weber syndrome?

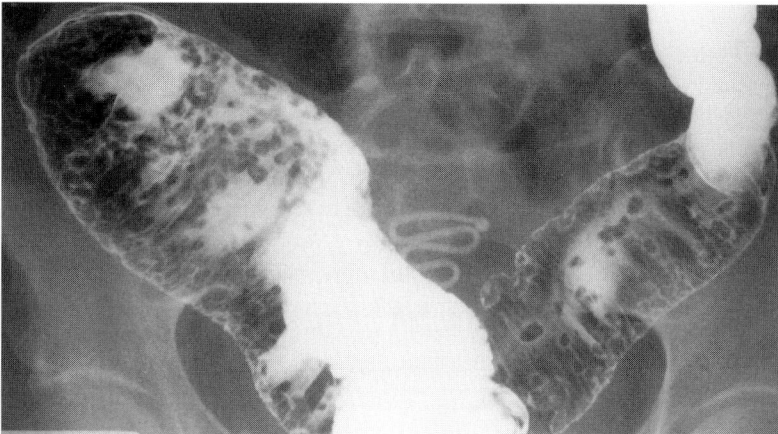

1. What diseases may produce these lesions?
2. To what finding does the term *pseudopolyp* refer?
3. What is "cobblestoning," and in what disease does it occur?
4. What histologic finding is associated with postinflammatory polyps?

Splenic Hemangioma

1. Hemangioma.

2. Hamartoma.

3. Hemangioma or lymphangioma.

4. Hemangioma.

Reference

Urrutia M, Mergo PJ, Ros LH, et al: Cystic masses of the spleen: radiologic-pathologic correlation, *Radiographics* 16:107-129, 1996.

Cross-Reference

Gastrointestinal Radiology: THE REQUISITES, ed 2, p 192.

Comment

The spleen is commonly affected by benign tumors. However, because most remain asymptomatic throughout life, splenic tumors are usually discovered incidentally at autopsy. The most common benign tumor of the spleen is the hemangioma, which occurs in up to 14% of the population. These tumors are typically asymptomatic but can produce symptoms of high output cardiac failure or thrombocytopenia if they become large enough. Hemangiomas may have internal calcifications and may be solitary or multiple lesions. Sometimes they can be part of a syndrome of generalized angiomatosis called *Klippel-Trenaunay-Weber syndrome.*

Hamartomas are solid masses that can grow quite large. A small percentage actually cause spontaneous splenic rupture. These tumors also can produce anemia or pancytopenia. Lymphangiomas may be capillary, cavernous, or cystic. They are typically subcapsular in location and may be either solitary or multiple. These tumors typically remain asymptomatic.

Hemangiomas and lymphangiomas are typically hypodense with the splenic tissue on CT examination. Hamartomas are isodense with the spleen on CT and may be difficult to distinguish from normal splenic tissue. Hemangiomas and lymphangiomas may contain calcification either peripherally or centrally, as phleboliths.

Notes

Postinflammatory Polyps

1. Almost any type of colitis.

2. Islands of normal or edematous mucosa surrounded by ulcerated or denuded mucosa.

3. Normal mucosa surrounded by linear ulceration; it occurs in Crohn's disease.

4. Regenerating normal mucosa.

Reference

Lichtenstein JE: Radiologic-pathologic correlation of inflammatory bowel disease, *Radiol Clin North Am* 25:3-24, 1987.

Cross-Reference

Gastrointestinal Radiology: THE REQUISITES, ed 2, p 255.

Comment

Several types of polypoid lesions occur in the colon during or after active colitis. Different terms have been used to describe these entities, and they are often interchanged, causing some confusion.

The term *pseudopolyp,* which many authors do not like to use, refers to islands of mucosa (either normal or edematous) that protrude into the lumen of the bowel. These growths are not adenomas, hamartomas, or hyperplastic polyps. Inflammatory pseudopolyps occur during active inflammation. Islands of intact but edematous mucosa protrude into the lumen because the surrounding mucosa has become sloughed or ulcerated as a result of severe inflammation. These islands are typically found in patients with ulcerative colitis and are less common among those with Crohn's disease. The term *cobblestoning* refers to another type of inflammatory pseudopolyp seen in patients with Crohn's disease. This appearance results when islands of normal mucosa become outlined by deep linear ulcers, which sometimes occur in patients with Crohn's disease. The aforementioned entities always coexist with active inflammation.

Postinflammatory polyps occur when the inflammatory process subsides or goes into remission. As the mucosa heals, there can be regenerative overgrowth of the mucosa, resulting in polyplike lesions. These lesions can occur in patients with any type of colitis, including ulcerative colitis, Crohn's disease, infectious colitis, and even ischemic colitis. Postinflammatory polyps may be large focal protuberances, small rounded nodules, or even branching growths. The branching growths are termed *filiform polyposis* because of their appearance. All these lesions represent colonic mucosa in some form, although it is regenerating or exophytic in its growth pattern. These lesions must be distinguished from the dysplastic lesions, which are premalignant, that occur in patients with ulcerative colitis.

Notes

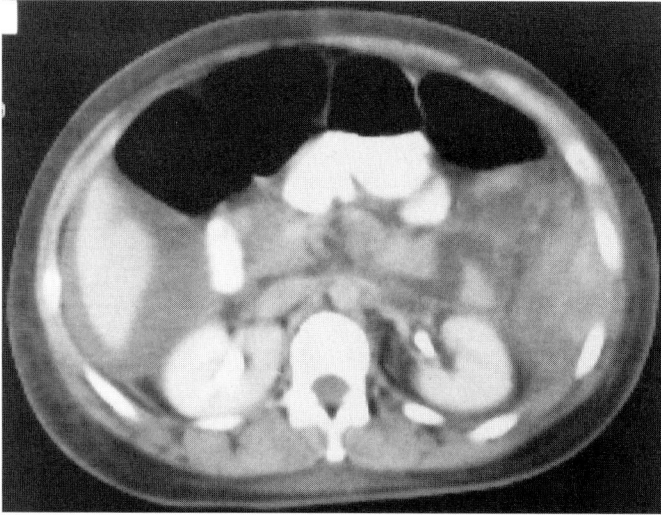

1. What is the most common cause of this abnormality in adults?
2. What is the most common cause of this injury in children?
3. What structure must be assessed to determine definitive treatment?
4. What is the most common treatment for this condition?

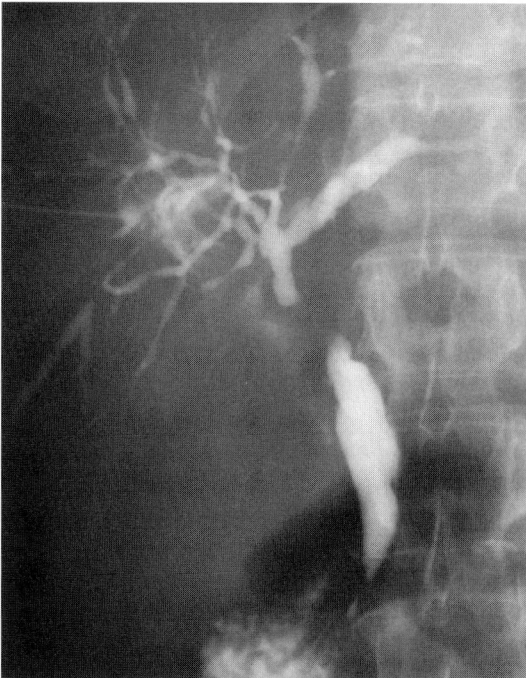

1. What is the diagnosis?
2. What underlying diseases are associated with this condition?
3. What infectious or parasitic conditions may produce this appearance?
4. Name an important complication that may occur in patients with this condition.

Pancreatic Laceration or Transection

1. Motor vehicle accident.

2. Child abuse or sports injury.

3. Integrity of the pancreatic duct.

4. Usually requires surgery.

Reference

Dodds WJ, Taylor AJ, Erickson SJ, et al: Traumatic fracture of the pancreas: CT characteristics, *J Comput Assist Tomogr* 14:375-378, 1990.

Cross-Reference

Gastrointestinal Radiology: THE REQUISITES, ed 2, p 157.

Comment

The pancreas is not often injured by blunt abdominal trauma. (It is injured in fewer than 12% of cases of blunt abdominal trauma.) The spleen and liver are much more commonly injured. However, the pancreas extends rather far anteriorly in the abdomen and crosses the spine, and both factors contribute to its risk of injury during blunt trauma. Motor vehicle accidents and deceleration injuries are the leading causes of pancreatic injury in adults, whereas child abuse or sports-related or bicycle injuries more typically produce the damage in children. Penetrating trauma is another frequent cause of pancreatic injury.

When pancreatic injury occurs, there is a high incidence of associated injuries to the bowel, spleen, liver, and blood vessels. The mortality for this injury approaches 20% because of both the pancreatic injury and all the other associated injuries. Patients with pancreatic injury have pain, leukocytosis, and elevated amylase levels. The injury may be just a contusion, a laceration, or a complete transection. The integrity of the pancreatic duct is important; if the duct is compromised or transected, surgical resection is required.

For this type of injury, CT is the imaging modality of choice. The appearance of the injury can be quite variable. Sometimes little or nothing can be seen. Changes related to pancreatitis, involving fluid, inflammation, or both, can be evident in the region. A contusion may produce a low density area in the parenchyma or an area of higher density if there is hemorrhage. The actual laceration or tear of the pancreatic tissue may be evident, particularly on high resolution scans through the pancreas. Surgery is frequently indicated for patients with this injury to at least drain the peripancreatic tissues of fluid that may accumulate. If the pancreatic duct is injured, the treatment usually requires surgical resection of the pancreas proximal to the injury. Ductal patency may have to be determined by endoscopic retrograde cholangiopancreatography.

Notes

Cholangiocarcinoma Complicating Sclerosing Cholangitis in Ulcerative Colitis

1. Sclerosing cholangitis of the biliary system.

2. Inflammatory bowel disease (usually ulcerative colitis), retroperitoneal fibrosis, ascending cholangitis (often after biliary tract surgery), acquired immunodeficiency syndrome (AIDS), and parasitic infections.

3. Recurrent bacterial infection, particularly after biliary-enteric bypasses; AIDS-related cholangitis caused by either cryptosporidiosis or cytomegalovirus; and parasites, including *Ascariasis lumbricoides* (roundworm) and *Clonorchis sinensis* (flatworm).

4. Cholangiocarcinoma.

Reference

Feczko PJ: Malignancy complicating inflammatory bowel disease, *Radiol Clin North Am* 25:157-174, 1987.

Cross-Reference

Gastrointestinal Radiology: THE REQUISITES, ed 2, p 205.

Comment

Primary sclerosing cholangitis typically occurs in young men. In some instances the disease is considered primary or idiopathic, with no known underlying etiology. The majority (70% or more) of cases are related to underlying inflammatory bowel disease, particularly ulcerative colitis. It is estimated that anywhere from 3% to 10% of patients with ulcerative colitis will develop sclerosing cholangitis. Pathologically the condition is caused by multifocal areas of periductal fibrosis, which produce the narrowing, with intervening normal areas developing ductal ectasia.

Similar radiologic changes are apparent in patients with recurrent biliary tract infections. The groups that typically develop this condition are postoperative patients with complications and the AIDS population. Worldwide the most likely cause is intestinal parasites, particularly *A. lumbricoides*. This roundworm migrates into the ducts from the small bowel and causes recurrent cholangitis.

The usual course of disease is one of secondary biliary cirrhosis, recurrent sepsis, and eventual hepatic failure. The time between the appearance of the initial symptoms and death is usually 5 to 10 years. Total colectomy may sometimes halt or diminish the course of the disease. Approximately 10% to 20% of patients with sclerosing cholangitis secondary to ulcerative colitis develop cholangiocarcinoma. Interestingly this condition does not develop in patients with Crohn's disease. Sometimes, total colectomy arrests the liver disease, but this effect is not predictable. If the disease progresses, the only treatment is liver transplantation.

Notes

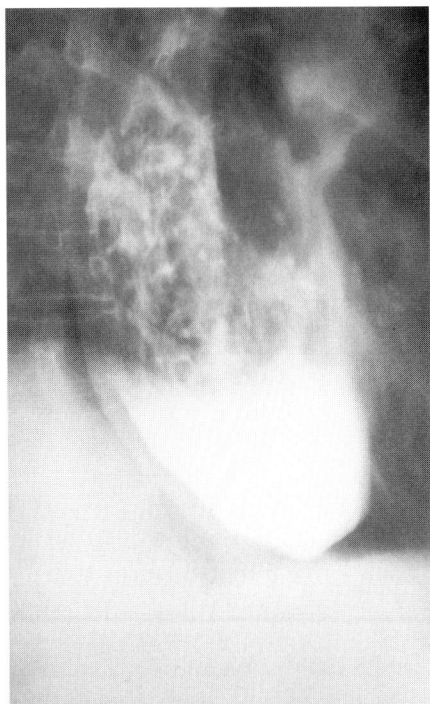

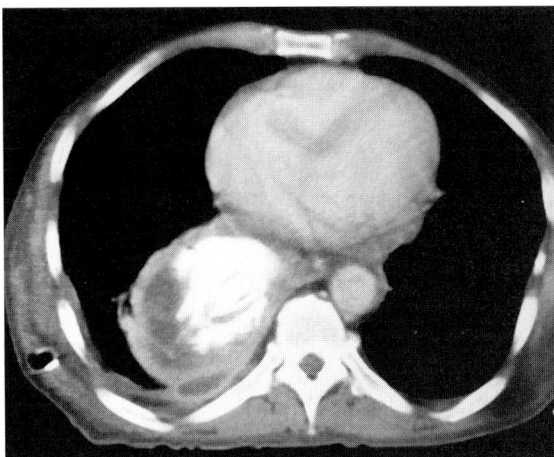

1. What is the underlying pathophysiologic defect in this patient?
2. What other disorders may mimic this condition?
3. What is an important complication of this disease?
4. Name other conditions that can result in esophageal carcinoma.

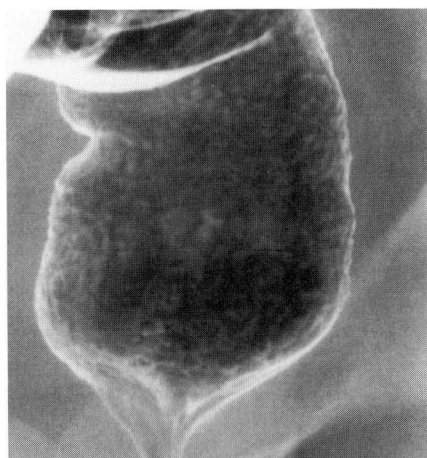

1. What is the most common form of bacteria-induced colitis?
2. What type of colitis does salmonella colitis mimic?
3. What type of colitis does tuberculous colitis mimic?
4. What may viral colitis mimic?

Esophageal Carcinoma Developing in Achalasia

1. Decreased number of ganglion cells in the esophagus.

2. Scleroderma, carcinoma of the gastroesophageal junction, and peptic stricture.

3. Esophageal carcinoma.

4. Lye strictures, celiac disease, radiation, head and neck tumors, and Plummer-Vinson syndrome.

Reference

Chuong JJH, DuBovik S, McCallum RW: Achalasia as a risk factor for esophageal carcinoma, *Dig Dis Sci* 29:1105-1108, 1984.

Cross-Reference

Gastrointestinal Radiology: THE REQUISITES, ed 2, p 21.

Comment

Achalasia is a fairly common but poorly understood disorder of esophageal motility, producing life-long dysfunction. It is a neurogenic disorder marked by a decreased number of ganglion cells in the esophagus. Abnormalities also have been found in the vagal trunks and nuclei. The underlying etiology for this loss of innervation is uncertain. The result is decreasing esophageal peristalsis and failure of the lower esophageal sphincter to relax. Achalasia occurs almost equally among men and women. Onset is typically in early adulthood, and later onset should raise suspicions of carcinoma, which may mimic the condition. With long-standing achalasia, the esophagus becomes markedly dilated and food is retained in the esophagus. Scleroderma, peptic strictures, and carcinoma at the gastroesophageal junction may produce a similar appearance.

One of the unusual complications of this condition is the development of esophageal carcinoma. This complication is said to affect approximately 5% of achalasia patients, although the classification of this condition as a complication is considered controversial because some feel its prevalence in those with achalasia is no higher than in the general population. The duration of the achalasia is usually 20 or more years before carcinoma is found. Typically, squamous cell carcinoma is present, but adenocarcinoma also has been noted. Other conditions that have a proven association with an increased incidence of esophageal squamous carcinoma include lye strictures, head and neck squamous tumors, celiac disease, Plummer-Vinson syndrome, and radiation exposure.

Notes

Campylobacter Colitis

1. Campylobacter colitis.

2. Ulcerative colitis

3. Crohn's colitis.

4. Either ulcerative colitis or Crohn's disease.

Reference

Brodey PA, Fertig S, Aron JM: Campylobacter enterocolitis: radiographic features, *Am J Roentgenol* 139:1199-1201, 1982.

Cross-Reference

Gastrointestinal Radiology: THE REQUISITES, ed 2, p 265.

Comment

Numerous infectious organisms produce colitis. The colon has only a few ways to respond to these infectious agents, and the resultant changes are similar to those seen in patients with idiopathic inflammatory bowel disease, ulcerative colitis, or Crohn's disease. The types of ulceration that occur may be seen in many conditions, but generally colitis caused by infectious agents mimics either ulcerative colitis or granulomatous colitis (Crohn's disease). Granular mucosa is produced by edema and hyperemia of the mucosa, as well as a decline in mucin production by the mucosa. Collar-button ulcers manifest a deeper ulceration that penetrates the muscularis mucosa into the submucosa and has branching at the margins of the ulcer. Aphthous ulcers are focal ulcers that are visible on a background of normal mucosa and are typically associated with Crohn's disease, although they can occur in other conditions.

Campylobacter colitis is the most common infectious colitis. It is produced by infection with *Campylobacter jejuni* and can affect both the colon and the small bowel. Interestingly this condition may produce diffuse granular inflammation, mimicking ulcerative colitis, but also has been known to produce focal aphthous ulcers, resembling Crohn's disease. Salmonella and shigella colitis are relatively common conditions. Several different species infect humans. Typically these infections produce diffuse ulceration, resembling ulcerative colitis. As the inflammation subsides, skip areas and other changes may become evident and may resemble the changes that occur in patients with Crohn's disease. Tuberculosis is an infection of the bowel that closely resembles Crohn's disease. Patients with tuberculous colitis have areas of severe inflammation with stricturing and intervening normal areas. They also have associated disease of the terminal ileum.

There has been an increase in the incidence of viral infections of the colon. Mild viral infections caused by herpesviruses or cytomegalovirus usually produce focal ulceration and resemble the aphthous ulcers of Crohn's disease. More severe infections result in the diffuse inflammation more typical of ulcerative colitis.

Notes

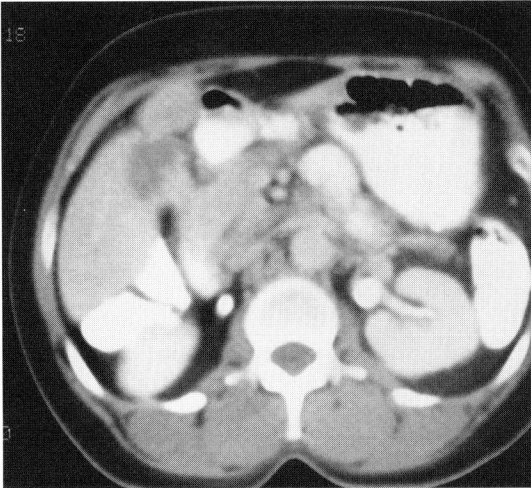

1. What is the most likely diagnosis?
2. What is the usual presentation of this entity?
3. In what group does this condition most commonly occur?
4. What other conditions may have a similar appearance?

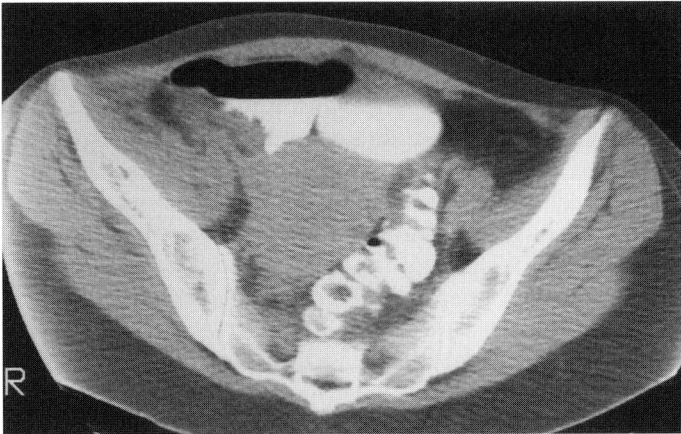

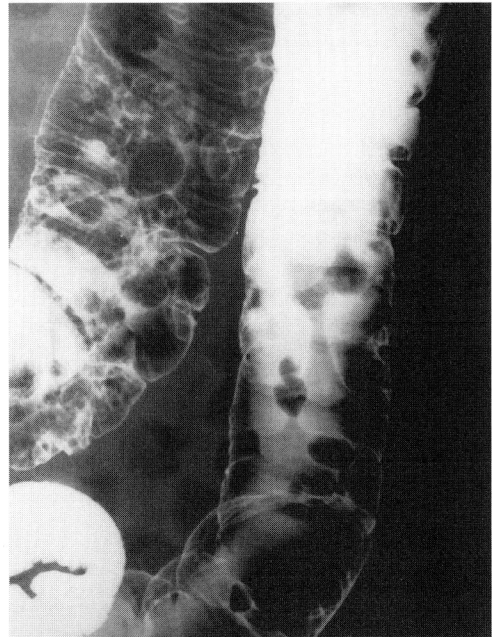

1. What are fibrotic changes of the mesentery termed?
2. With what polyposis syndrome is this finding associated?
3. What tumors may have this appearance?
4. When this occurs in a round shaped mass, what is it called?

Gallbladder Carcinoma

1. Gallbladder carcinoma.

2. Mass completely replacing the gallbladder.

3. Elderly women.

4. Gallbladder polyp or adenoma.

Reference
Lane J, Buck JL, Zeman RK: Primary carcinoma of the gallbladder: a pictorial essay, *Radiographics* 9:209-228, 1989.

Cross-Reference
Gastrointestinal Radiology: THE REQUISITES, ed 2, p 222.

Comment
Carcinoma of the gallbladder is one of the more common tumors of the gastrointestinal tract, ranking fifth, behind tumors of the colon, pancreas, stomach, and esophagus. However, the diagnosis can be difficult to make, despite the use of cross-sectional imaging modalities. Carcinoma of the gallbladder occurs most frequently among elderly women. This group also has a high incidence of cholecystitis. The presence of chronic inflammation and gallstones is considered a predisposing factor for the development of this tumor. Other predisposing factors include porcelain gallbladder (carcinoma is a complication in as many as 25% of these patients), inflammatory bowel disease, and familial adenomatous polyposis syndrome.

There are three different presentations or appearances of gallbladder carcinoma. The most common, occurring in more than half of patients, is that of a mass totally replacing the gallbladder. Cross-sectional imaging demonstrates a large subhepatic mass, and the gallbladder itself is not readily identifiable. This presentation can be confused with other types of liver tumors. The next most common appearance is diffuse thickening of the gallbladder wall, which may mimic chronic cholecystitis, particularly if gallstones are present. Sometimes the eccentric thickening of the wall helps to differentiate the tumor from inflammation. The least common presentation, as seen in this case, is that of an intraluminal polypoid mass. Gallbladder carcinoma with this appearance has the best prognosis, often because of its early detection, but it can be mistaken for a cholesterol polyp or a noncalcified stone.

Notes

Mesenteric Fibromatosis in Gardner's Syndrome

1. Retractile mesenteritis, mesenteric panniculitis or lipodystrophy, and mesenteric fibromatosis.

2. Gardner's syndrome (familial adenomatous polyposis syndrome [FAPS]).

3. Lymphoma, carcinoid tumors, and peritoneal carcinomatosis.

4. Desmoid.

Reference
Mata JM, Inaraja L, Martin J, et al: CT features of mesenteric panniculitis, *J Comput Assist Tomogr* 11:1021-1023, 1987.

Cross-Reference
Gastrointestinal Radiology: THE REQUISITES, ed 2, p 253.

Comment
Various fibrous conditions, which represent a combination of fibrosis, inflammation, and fatty replacement, can affect the mesentery. These conditions have been given several names, which are somewhat dependent on which component of the disease predominates. Terms used for this condition include *retractile mesenteritis, fibrosing mesenteritis, mesenteric panniculitis, mesenteric lipodystrophy*, and *desmoids*. Many use the broad category of fibrosing mesenteritis to describe this condition. Most often this condition occurs in patients without any predisposing factors. Patients with FAPS (the Gardner's type) are known to develop fibrotic lesions of the mesentery. The lesion may be an ill-defined fibrotic reaction, as in fibrosing mesenteritis, or it may be a more focal, rounded mass, which may be termed a *desmoid*.

The modality that allows the best visualization of these changes is CT. The tissue is denser than the mesenteric fat, although areas of fat may be seen within it. The fibrous tissue travels along the tissue planes and tends to surround structures, such as vessels or bowel, and may encase them to some degree. It also may be a more localized, ovoid mass that appears well defined, which is what some tend to refer to as a *desmoid*. This infiltrating fibrous reaction also mimics neoplastic processes, and it may be difficult to distinguish the two. Lymphoma, serosal spread of tumor, and even carcinoid tumors can resemble fibrosing mesenteritis. On barium studies of the bowel, the loops of bowel may be displaced or fixed in position.

Notes

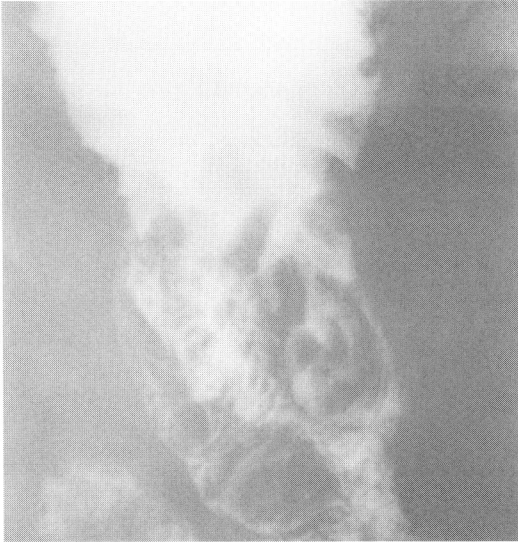
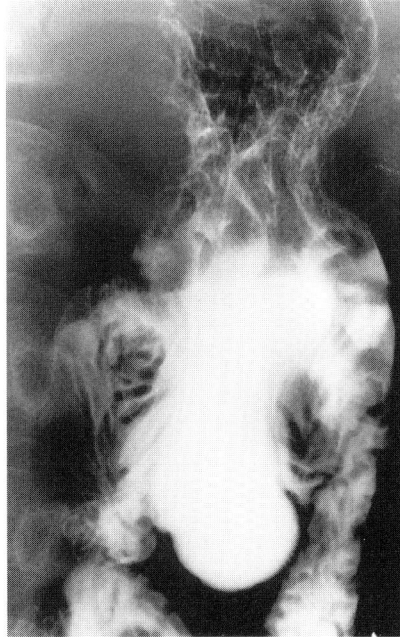

1. This patient has had a Billroth II gastrojejunostomy. What is the most likely cause of the mass in the gastric remnant?

2. Where are suture granulomas and surgical defects located?

3. What is the basis for bezoar formation in these patients?

4. What is the suggested interval for screening these patients for malignancy?

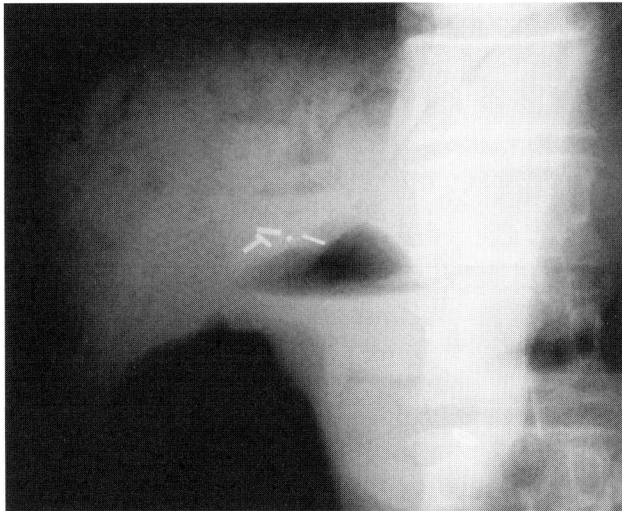
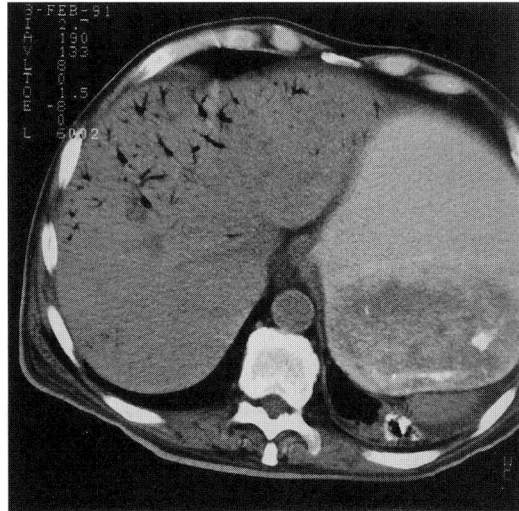

1. What is the most common cause of this abnormality?

2. What other conditions also may produce this abnormality?

3. What is the mortality associated with this entity?

4. What is the significance of this finding when it occurs in a liver transplant recipient?

Jejunogastric Intussusception After Billroth II Gastrojejunostomy

1. Jejunogastric intussusception.

2. Along the lesser curve between the cardia and the anastomosis.

3. Lack of acid secretion and diminished gastric motility lead to poor digestion of fibrous tissue.

4. Although controversial, most authors suggest screening for malignancy after 10 years.

Reference

Shaw PC, Op den Orth JO: Postoperative stomach and duodenum, *Radiol Clin North Am* 32:1275, 1994.

Cross-Reference

Gastrointestinal Radiology: THE REQUISITES, ed 2, p 80.

Comment

For many years, surgical resection of a portion of the stomach was used to treat peptic ulcer disease. Evaluation of these patients with a Billroth II gastrojejunostomy is difficult because of the distorted anatomy. However, these patients have a variety of problems that occur many years after the surgical procedure and often present for radiologic evaluation. The detection of a mass in the gastric remnant is an ominous finding. Although controversial, many believe that there is an increased incidence of gastric malignancy in these patients. This complication typically presents 10 years or more after the surgery. When a mass is encountered, the radiologist must be able to distinguish a neoplasm from other benign causes of intraluminal gastric masses.

Jejunogastric intussusception is an unusual complication of this operation. Several factors are believed to predispose a patient to this complication. First, the anastomosis may be too wide. Also, excessive mobility of the jejunum may contribute to small bowel peristalsis, pushing mucosa into the gastric remnant. The symptoms associated with this condition can vary. In long-standing, recurrent cases the patient may have a feeling of fullness, may vomit after eating, or may have severe pains that spontaneously disappear. If the intussusceptum becomes incarcerated, obstruction, necrosis, and bleeding may ensue. Radiologically, it can be diagnosed as a mass within the distal gastric remnant abutting the anastomosis. Careful fluoroscopic observation may reveal that the mass will spontaneously disappear. The size of the mass may vary throughout the examination.

Other common causes of masses include plication defects and granulomas resulting from surgery, which usually occur along the lesser curvature, where a row of sutures is placed. These patients are also at risk for developing bezoars because of the decrease in acid production and the diminished motility.

Notes

Portal Venous Gas

1. Infarcted bowel.

2. Ulcers, acute bowel dilation, endoscopic procedures, and necrotizing enterocolitis.

3. Although it has improved recently, it still approaches 50%.

4. It is often seen incidentally and may not be of any significance.

Reference

Cho KC, Baker SR: Extraluminal air: diagnosis and significance, *Radiol Clin North Am* 32:829-844, 1994.

Cross-Reference

Gastrointestinal Radiology: THE REQUISITES, ed 2, p 187.

Comment

Linear collections of air in the liver are usually one of two types of structures. The most common is air in the biliary system. This air is located centrally. Small branching collections of air in the periphery of the liver indicate air in the portal venous system. Rarely, air is central in the main portal vein, and this finding is identified only on CT examination. Portal venous gas carries a much more ominous connotation because bowel infarction or necrosis is the most common cause of this condition. This sign was once considered invariably fatal, but recent studies have shown that more than half of the patients can survive if treated aggressively, including treatment of the underlying cause. The portal venous gas itself typically does not produce any morbidity or mortality.

Other possible causes of portal venous gas include penetrating peptic ulceration. Sometimes acute gastric or intestinal dilation produces portal venous gas. It also has been reported in patients with inflammatory bowel disease, such as ulcerative colitis or Crohn's disease. Finally, portal venous gas may be iatrogenic in nature and has been described in patients who have had recent endoscopic procedures or air-contrast barium enemas. Often this finding resolves spontaneously and without sequelae, and the exact mechanism is uncertain because it is such a rare event. Occasionally portal venous gas is described in liver transplant recipients, but it does not appear to be related to either necrosis or rejection, and its significance is uncertain.

Notes

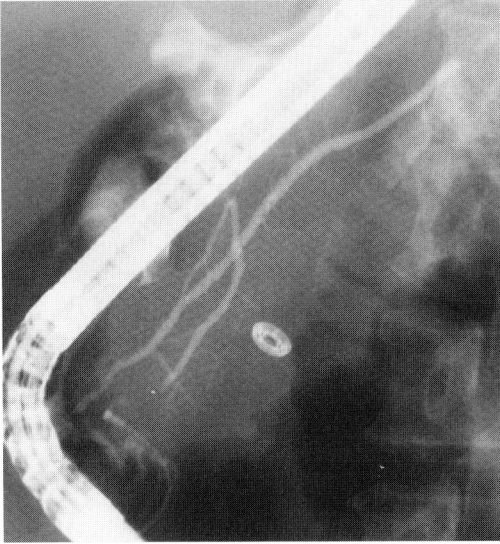

1. What is the most common congenital abnormality of the pancreatic ducts?
2. What complication is most often associated with pancreatic anomalies?
3. Which embryologic duct becomes the major duct of the pancreas?
4. Which duct drains the dorsal pancreas?

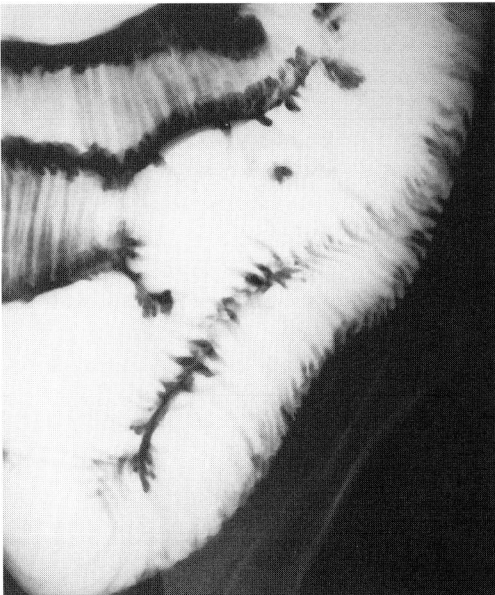

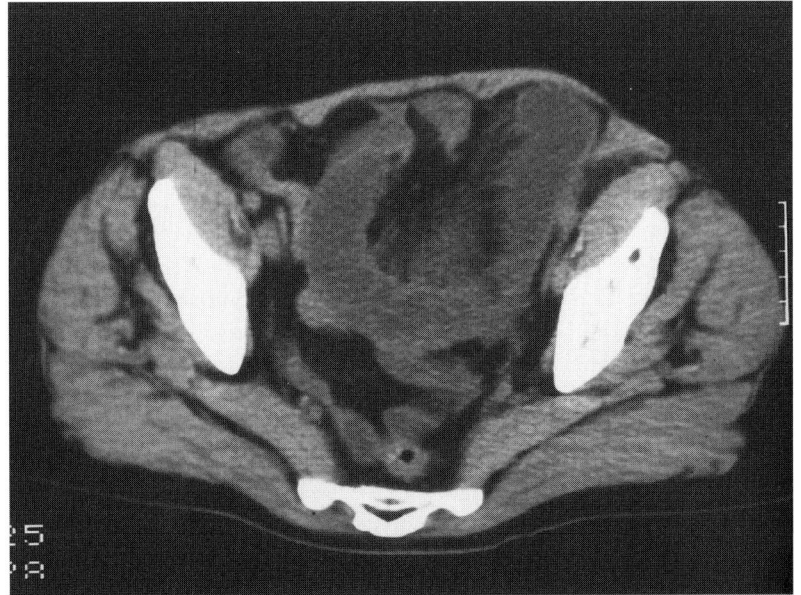

1. What is the underlying pathologic abnormality in patients with chronic radiation enteritis?
2. What is the radiologic feature of acute radiation enteritis?
3. What is the latent period for the development of chronic radiation enteritis?
4. What changes may be evident on CT?

Pancreas Divisum

1. Pancreas divisum.

2. Pancreatitis.

3. Duct of Wirsung.

4. Duct of Santorini.

Reference

Rizzo RJ, Szucs RA, Turner MA: Congenital abnormalities of the pancreas and biliary tree in adults, *Radiographics* 15:49-68, 1995.

Cross-Reference

Gastrointestinal Radiology: THE REQUISITES, ed 2, p 140.

Comment

The pancreas develops as two separate buds that fuse together during the first trimester of pregnancy to form a single pancreas. Not only do the two buds fuse their tissue, but the associated ductal structures must also join. Because of the complex nature of the ductal structures, anomalies affecting the drainage of the pancreatic ducts occur in a large percentage of individuals. Embryologically the ventral pancreas has the duct of Wirsung. As the ventral pancreas rotates, its duct (Wirsung) becomes the major duct in the head of the pancreas. It also is joined to the biliary system, and these ducts drain through the major papilla. The dorsal bud of the pancreas develops separately, and its duct is termed *Santorini.* Under normal circumstances the duct of Santorini fuses to the duct of Wirsung, and Santorini goes on to drain through Wirsung and into the major papilla. The portion of the Santorini duct that did drain into the duodenum usually involutes, and there is no separate papilla.

In pancreas divisum, of which there are several variations, the dorsal duct (Santorini) maintains its separate drainage into the duodenum via a minor papilla. The minor papilla may be located anywhere in the second or third portion of the duodenum. The dorsal duct may or may not join in some way to the ventral or main duct (Wirsung). The dorsal duct drains the body and tail, and the ventral duct drains the head and uncinate. In some instances, as in this case, there may be a tiny communicating branch between the two systems.

Most cases of pancreas divisum are discovered incidentally during endoscopic retrograde cholangiopancreatography. However, there is a higher than normal incidence of pancreatitis in these patients. Anytime pancreatitis occurs in a younger patient, the possibility of a pancreatic ductal anomaly should be considered.

Notes

Radiation Enteritis

1. Endarteritis obliterans.

2. Mild fold thickening, usually in a symmetric fashion.

3. Several months to many years (sometimes 10 years or more).

4. Bowel wall thickening and adjacent fibrotic changes.

Reference

Mendelson RM, Nolan DJ: The radiological features of radiation enteritis, *Clin Radiol* 36:141-148, 1985.

Cross-Reference

Gastrointestinal Radiology: THE REQUISITES, ed 2, p 110.

Comment

Radiation enteritis is a sequela of radiation therapy. (The treatment of a variety of conditions may consist of radiation involving the abdomen.) Acute radiation enteritis occurs during therapy and results from the loss of mucosal cells as the crypt cells of the mucosa become damaged by the radiation. There is edema and sometimes inflammatory change. Chronic radiation enteritis occurs several months to many years after the radiation therapy. This condition results from damage to the arterioles in the submucosa. The pathologic changes that ensue are related to ischemia and fibrosis. Patients with acute radiation enteritis complain of diarrhea, but chronic radiation enteritis causes diarrhea, bowel obstruction, and blood loss. There is little relationship between symptoms of acute radiation enteritis and the later development of chronic radiation enteritis.

In the acute phase of radiation enteritis the only changes apparent on small bowel examination are thickening of the valvulae and some bowel wall thickening. In the chronic phase a variety of abnormalities may be evident. The folds of the bowel may be thickened, and there is associated bowel wall thickening. In severe cases the folds may be completely effaced. In these instances rigidity or lack of peristalsis also may be evident in the bowel, perhaps with stenosis of the lumen. These latter changes are believed to be secondary to bowel wall fibrosis. The affected loops may be tethered and cannot be separated because of adhesions. Ulceration, which accounts for the blood loss, occurs but is usually not visible on radiographs. Small bowel obstruction is a common complication and may be related to the fibrotic stenoses or adhesions. The development of fistulas or sinus tracts is usually uncommon, unless there has been extensive surgical resection. CT is useful because features such as bowel wall thickening and fibrotic abnormalities are visible. It is often more helpful than the small bowel radiograph in evaluating the extent of disease.

Notes

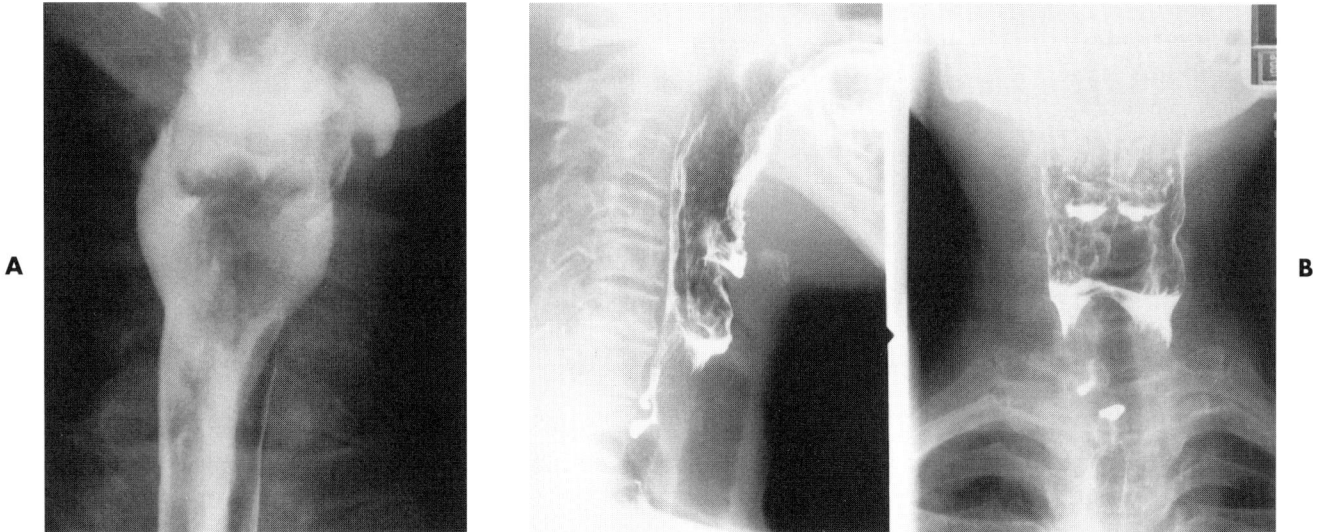

A

B

1. Through what does a Zenker's diverticulum protrude?
2. What are lateral diverticula of the pharyngoesophageal junction termed?
3. What possible etiologies produce hypopharyngeal outpouchings?
4. What embryologic source can produce pharyngeal diverticula?

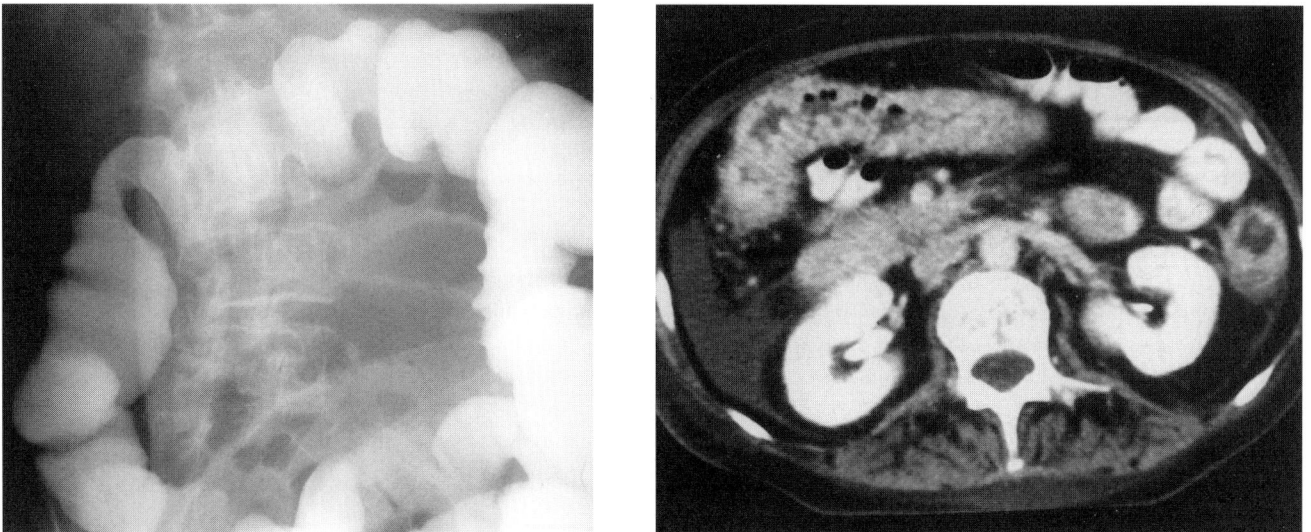

1. What is the most common cause of colon ischemia?
2. What modality is best for evaluating intestinal ischemia?
3. Where is the "watershed" region in the colon?
4. Small emboli to the colon may resemble what disease?

CASE 143

Lateral Hypopharyngeal Pouch (A) and Zenker's Diverticulum and Killian-Jamieson Diverticulum (B)

1. Killian's dehiscence.

2. Killian-Jamieson diverticula.

3. Muscular weakness or prolonged increases in pharyngeal pressures.

4. Branchial cleft remnants or anomalies.

Reference

Ekberg O, Nylander G: Lateral diverticula from the pharyngo-esophageal junction region, *Radiology* 146:117-122, 1983.

Cross-Reference

Gastrointestinal Radiology: THE REQUISITES, ed 2, p 30.

Comment

Numerous outpouchings have been identified in the hypopharynx and cervical esophageal region. The most common of these is the Zenker's diverticulum. These diverticula increase in frequency with age and can vary greatly in size. They develop in an area of relative muscular weakness termed *Killian's dehiscence,* which is a gap above the cricopharyngeus and between the inferior constrictor muscles. These diverticula typically occur in older patients and can produce symptoms related to the retention of swallowed food.

Killian-Jamieson, or lateral pharyngoesophageal, diverticula occur near the same level as the Zenker's diverticulum. Unlike Zenker's diverticula, which protrude posteriorly, these diverticula project laterally and may be either unilateral or bilateral. They develop below the transverse portion of the cricopharyngeus and probably protrude through a defect corresponding to where the inferior laryngeal nerve and vessels pass. They are typically small, with a narrow neck, usually only a few millimeters in diameter. They can occur in any age group. Symptoms can be quite vague, and many are found incidentally. Symptoms are more likely if the diverticula retain swallowed food debris.

Lateral hypopharyngeal outpouchings are large, wide-mouth bulges along the lateral contours of the hypopharynx. They may occur at the entrance site of the superior laryngeal vessels or above the hyoid bone near the tonsillar fossil. This abnormality is common among two groups. The first is elderly patients, in whom the etiology is probably progressive muscular weakness of the constrictor muscles. Young patients may develop these outpouchings as a result of prolonged increases in pharyngeal pressure, common among wind or brass instrument musicians. The outpouchings are usually transient bulges during the swallowing bolus and do not retain swallowed food debris. Rarely, diverticula in this region are the result of embryologic remnants of the branchial clefts, typically the second through fourth clefts.

Notes

CASE 144

Ischemia of the Colon

1. Low flow states.

2. CT.

3. Splenic flexure.

4. Carcinoma of the colon.

Reference

Scholz FJ: Ischemic bowel disease, *Radiol Clin North Am* 31: 1197-1218, 1993.

Cross-Reference

Gastrointestinal Radiology: THE REQUISITES, ed 2, p 266.

Comment

Ischemic bowel disease is a common clinical problem. Most often it is produced by low flow to the intestines, which occurs in patients who are in shock, those who are experiencing cardiac failure, and patients who have just had surgery, as well as in those with other conditions. Arterial obstruction is uncommon but can affect patients with atherosclerotic disease that obstructs mesenteric vessels or those with embolic disease who have cardiac abnormalities. Also, a small percentage of patients have ischemia caused by venous obstruction. Arteriography is not very useful in patients with ischemia because the demonstration of obstructed vessels is unlikely. CT is probably the best modality for defining the involved segments and identifying underlying pathologic conditions or complications.

Ischemic disease of the colon is often segmental in nature and rarely involves the entire colon. The different regions of the colon have separate blood supplies, although they are interconnected to some extent. The watershed regions are defined as the areas of transition between the superior and inferior mesenteric blood supplies. This term frequently refers to the splenic flexure, although sometimes it can refer to the rectosigmoid junction as well. The splenic flexure is a common location for ischemia in patients with low flow states because it is the farthest point of arterial flow to the colon. The right colon also is commonly involved because it is prone to ischemia resulting from distention. The right colon is the most distended segment of colon under most conditions.

Radiologically, ischemia first can be identified as thickening and edema of the bowel wall. Nodularity of the bowel wall could be the result of either edema or small areas of hemorrhage. The mucosa may become shaggy and begin to resemble inflammatory bowel disease. As ischemia heals, the colon may become fibrotic, with loss of haustral pattern and even pseudodiverticula formation. This fibrosis can be multifocal in nature.

Notes

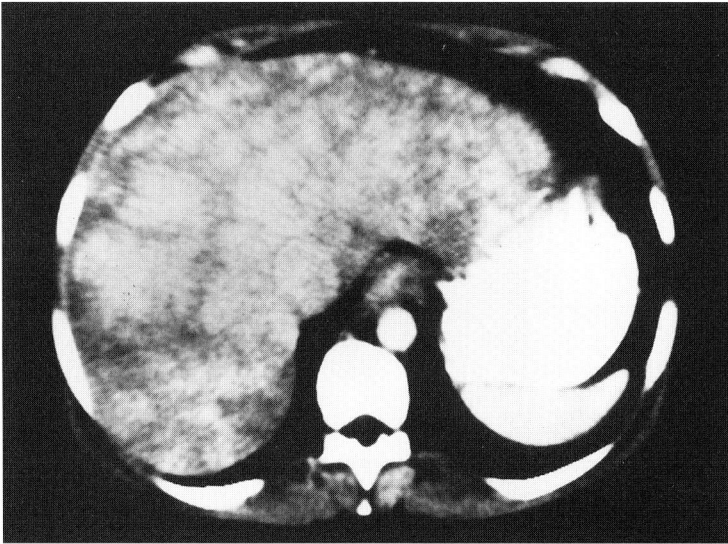

1. What is the most likely clinical condition in this patient?
2. Does liver dysfunction occur in patients with this condition?
3. Is there any long-term sequela?
4. What is the treatment?

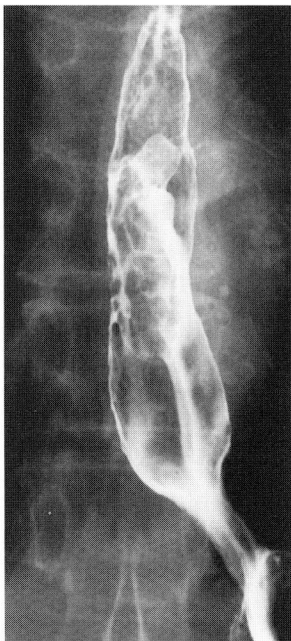

1. Name the primary esophageal neoplasms that may have this appearance.
2. Name the metastases known to produce intraluminal masses.
3. What "APUDoma" or endocrine tumor may occur in the esophagus?
4. What common skin tumor may occur as a primary esophageal neoplasm?

CASE 145

Passive Venous Congestion Caused by Congestive Heart Failure

1. Congestive heart failure.

2. Yes. It can be mild or severe.

3. Fibrosis (so-called cardiac cirrhosis).

4. Only the cardiac condition is treated.

Reference

Kawamoto S, Soyer PA, Fishman EK, et al: Nonneoplastic liver disease: evaluation with CT and MR imaging, *Radiographics* 18:827-848, 1998.

Cross-Reference

Gastrointestinal Radiology: THE REQUISITES, ed 2, p 166.

Comment

Elevated pressure in the right side of the heart can lead to passive venous congestion of the liver. The most common cause is congestive heart failure, which can be the result of ischemic heart disease, cardiomyopathy, constrictive pericarditis, or other diseases. Other conditions, such as pulmonary artery stenosis or right atrial myxoma, also can cause this problem. The chronically elevated venous pressure from the right side of the heart causes venous congestion that involves the hepatic veins. As the pressure in the hepatic veins elevates, the liver becomes swollen because of hepatic sinusoidal engorgement, and eventually edema develops. In patients with long-standing venous congestion there is a decrease in hepatic blood flow and a decrease in hepatic arterial oxygen, resulting in hepatic hypoxia. Depending on the severity and chronicity of the venous congestion, there can be associated abnormalities of liver function. In patients with long-standing disease, fibrotic tissue can develop between the lobules, eventually leading to what is termed *cardiac cirrhosis*. Microscopically there may be evidence of necrosis of hepatocytes or at least some atrophy. On occasion the liver failure may predominate clinically over the cardiac failure.

The relevant imaging findings may be apparent on ultrasound or CT. Diminished flow is evident on Doppler ultrasound examination. The appearance of the liver on CT is the so-called nutmeg liver produced by enhancing lobules of hepatocytes, which are still functioning, and areas of edema that do not enhance. Similar findings may be noted in patients in the early stages of Budd-Chiari syndrome.

Notes

CASE 146

Spindle-Cell Tumor of the Esophagus

1. Squamous carcinoma, leiomyosarcoma, spindle-cell carcinoma, and fibrovascular polyp.

2. Kaposi's sarcoma and melanoma.

3. Oat-cell tumor of the esophagus may be a primary lesion.

4. Melanomas may arise directly from the esophageal mucosa.

Reference

Agha FP, Keren DF: Spindle-cell squamous carcinoma of the esophagus, *Am J Roentgenol* 145:541-545, 1985.

Cross-Reference

Gastrointestinal Radiology: THE REQUISITES, ed 2, p 4.

Comment

Large, bulky intraluminal tumors of the esophagus are rare. However, their appearance is distinctive, and a certain group of lesions is known to produce this appearance. First, normal squamous carcinoma of the esophagus may grow as a bulky intraluminal mass. Other esophageal neoplasms that have this appearance are leiomyosarcoma, spindle-cell carcinoma, and fibrovascular polyp. Extraordinarily rare tumors of the esophagus include primary esophageal melanoma, oat-cell carcinoma of the esophagus, and adenocystic carcinoma. Hematogenous metastases from Kaposi's sarcoma, melanoma, or hypernephroma also have been given this description.

Spindle-cell carcinoma of the esophagus has a bi-phasic composition and even clinical nature. It is composed of both carcinomatous and sarcomatous elements. There is also a nonneoplastic component of the stroma, producing further confusion. These tumors were initially described as carcinosarcomas, indicating their dual histologic appearance. These tumors also were termed *pseudosarcomas* because the sarcomatous component did not seem to metastasize readily. However, it is now common practice to lump all of these descriptive terms under the category of spindle-cell carcinoma, recognizing that there is a variability in the histologic appearance and clinical course.

These tumors are quite aggressive and metastasize early in their course. The prognosis is quite poor, probably no better than that of ordinary esophageal carcinoma. Because of their bulky appearance, spindle-cell tumors present clinically with dysphagia. Although these growths may be easily removed with surgery, their propensity for distant metastases makes these tumors difficult to manage.

Notes

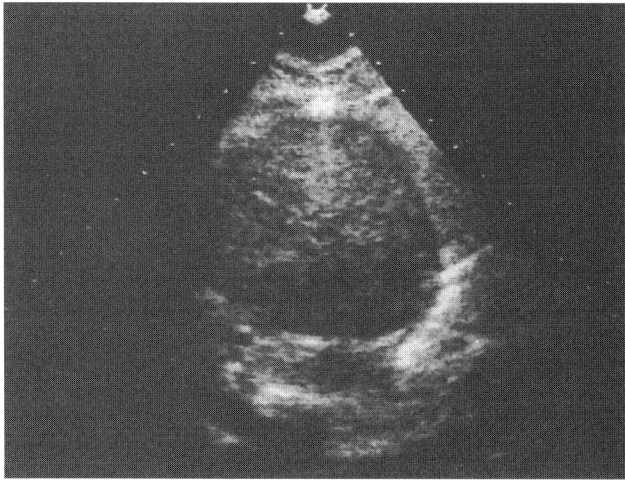

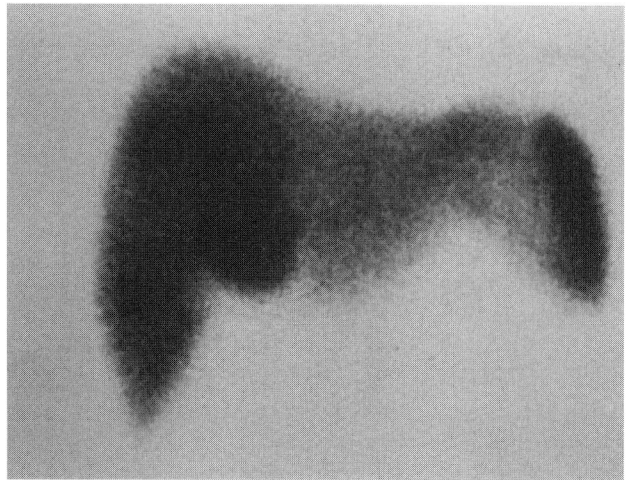

1. Why is this lesion "hot" on the sulfur colloid scan?
2. In what demographic group does this tumor occur?
3. Is this tumor associated with the consumption of any type of drugs?
4. Where is the vascular supply usually located in this lesion?

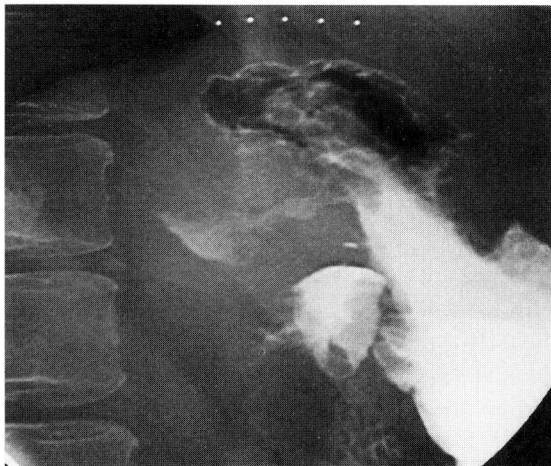

1. What contrast material should be used to evaluate fistulas?
2. If this is a postoperative fistula, what was the underlying condition?
3. What stomach tumor could have this appearance?
4. Do pseudocysts spontaneously communicate with the intestinal tract?

Focal Nodular Hyperplasia

1. Contains Kupffer cells.

2. Young women, same as adenomas.

3. No.

4. Centrally.

Reference

Buetow PC, Pantongrag-Brown L, Buck JL, et al: Focal nodular hyperplasia of the liver: radiologic-pathologic correlation, *Radiographics* 16:369-388, 1996.

Cross-Reference

Gastrointestinal Radiology: THE REQUISITES, ed 2, p 178.

Comment

Focal nodular hyperplasia (FNH) of the liver is the second most common benign tumor of the liver after hemangiomas. The tumor is a hyperplasia of normal, nonneoplastic liver tissue that has an abnormal arrangement and is similar to a hamartomatous type of lesion. It is believed to develop as some type of response to a congenital vascular abnormality in the region, and there is a slight association between hemangiomas and FNH. Histologically the liver tissue is arranged in small nodules, with septa in between. Arterial vessels feed the nodules from a centrally located artery that is often within a central scar or septum. They do not have a portal venous supply. FNH contains Kupffer cells in most instances.

Adenomas and FNH are similar in that they both occur in young women, although FNH also occurs in children and older patients. Unlike adenomas, FNH is not associated with oral contraceptive use. This tumor is rarely found in men. FNH must be differentiated from other hepatic tumors, such as adenomas, fibrolamellar hepatomas, and giant cavernous hemangiomas. All these tumors are large vascular tumors that affect young women and often have a central scar.

Focal nodular hyperplasia is easily detected on ultrasound as a well-defined lesion with echogenicity different from that of the normal liver. A large central vessel may be detectable on Doppler scanning. On CT scanning the lesion may be of similar density as the liver and difficult to distinguish from the normal liver parenchyma. A central scar or low density area may be visible. Because of the functional reticuloendothelial cells, FNH is usually detectable on sulfur colloid scanning. FNH is often isointense with the liver parenchyma and in some circumstances (as in this case) appears as an area of increased uptake. However, it is now recognized that a substantial portion of FNH is evident as a cold defect on liver scans. On MRI, FNH is slightly hyperintense on T2W images, but the central scar is often markedly hyperintense.

Notes

Pancreatic Pseudocyst Communicating with the Stomach

1. Barium.

2. Pseudocyst of the pancreas.

3. Ulcerating stromal cell tumor (leiomyosarcoma).

4. Yes.

Reference

Safait HD, Rice RP: Gastrointestinal complications of pancreatitis, *Radiol Clin North Am* 27:73-79, 1989.

Cross-Reference

Gastrointestinal Radiology: THE REQUISITES, ed 2, p 150.

Comment

This case demonstrates contrast tracking out of the posterior wall of the stomach into a collection located posteriorly in the region of the pancreas or lesser sac. At first glance, it appears to be a large ulcer, extending far beyond the wall of the stomach, but if it were an ulcer, it would have to be a penetrating ulcer with a walled-off cavity or abscess, which could be a diagnostic consideration. Another possibility is some type of cavitating tumor with ulceration or communication with the stomach. A likely consideration is a tumor, such as a leiomyosarcoma, that is known to ulcerate and communicate with the gastric lumen. The tumor often grows exophytically in relation to the gastric lumen. The final consideration is that this track communicates with a pancreatic process, most likely a pseudocyst or abscess.

Pancreatic pseudocysts are thin walled collections of fluid that develop in the weeks after an episode of acute pancreatitis. They are more common than once realized. Many small pseudocysts resolve spontaneously with time, and others remain stable. Larger pseudocysts (greater than 4 or 5 cm in diameter) often do not resolve and put the patient at risk of developing complications, such as rupture, bleeding, and infection. The treatment of these larger pseudocysts may be external drainage or internal drainage into the intestinal tract. In this case the pseudocyst was drained into the posterior wall of the stomach, which could be done surgically or endoscopically. Also, pseudocysts may drain spontaneously into the intestinal tract, and this drainage has reportedly occurred in the duodenum, stomach, and sometimes even the colon. CT remains the primary method of evaluation of this problem. Either dilute barium or water-soluble contrast may be used to demonstrate the communication, although barium is often better at demonstrating small leaks or fistulas.

Notes

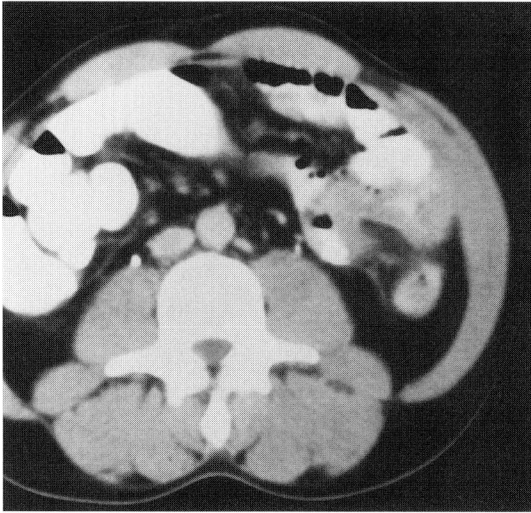

1. What type of process is involving the small bowel?
2. What small bowel disease may have this appearance?
3. What type of trauma could produce this appearance?
4. What should be the next study for further evaluation?

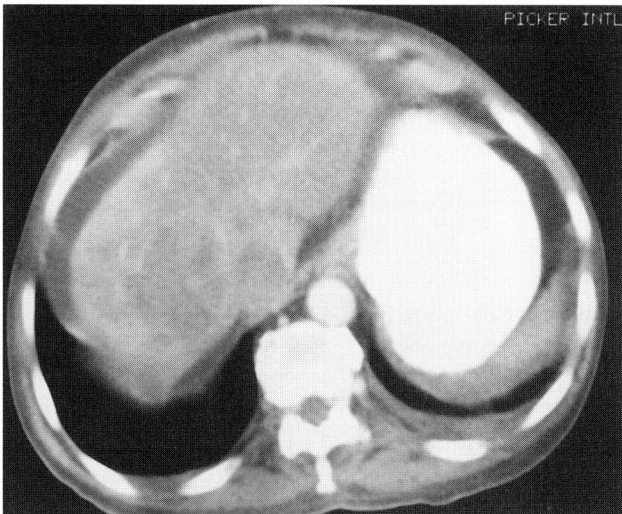

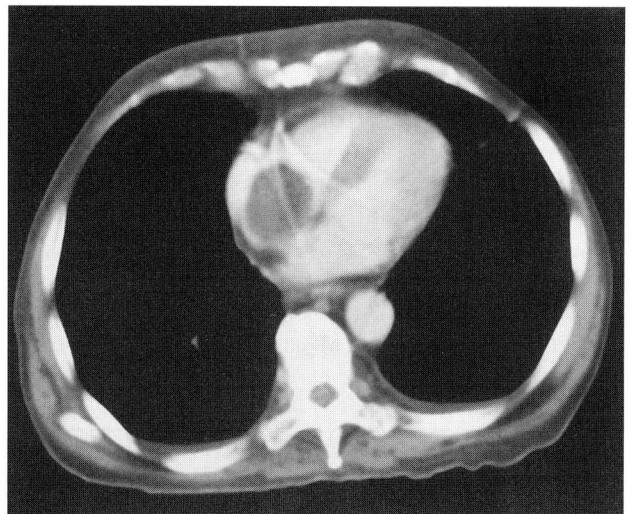

1. What liver tumors have an elevated serum alpha-fetoprotein level?
2. What infection predisposes an individual to this tumor?
3. The presence of what parasite increases the likelihood of this tumor's development?
4. What is the most common predisposing condition for this tumor in North America?

Small Bowel Perforation Secondary to Swallowed Foreign Body

1. Inflammatory.

2. Crohn's disease.

3. Direct blow or seat belt injury.

4. Small bowel enteroscopy.

Reference

Raptopoulos V: Abdominal trauma: emphasis on computed tomography, *Radiol Clin North Am* 32:969-987, 1994.

Cross-Reference

Gastrointestinal Radiology: THE REQUISITES, ed 2, p 127.

Comment

The CT image shows a short segment of small bowel, likely jejunum, that is thickened and some fluid collections around it. There may be some tracking of contrast into the soft tissues around the small bowel. These findings are consistent with some type of inflammatory process involving the proximal small bowel. The most likely cause is Crohn's disease. Crohn's disease can affect any portion of the intestinal tract. It produces bowel wall thickening evident on cross-sectional imaging and results in the development of fistulas and other inflammatory changes around them. Trauma to the small bowel also may produce some bowel wall thickening and adjacent inflammatory changes. Possibilities include penetrating injury to the area or direct blunt trauma. Possible seat belt injury should be considered as well. This patient eventually underwent surgery, and the culprit was a swallowed foreign body (chicken bone) that had lodged in the intestines and caused perforation.

As far as detecting the site of the abnormality and providing a clue as to the nature of the problem, CT is fairly sensitive. However, it is not that specific in determining the exact cause. Some people advocate small bowel enteroclysis for investigation of a known small bowel abnormality, but it may have been inappropriate in this instance because small bowel perforation was suspected. If the cause had been Crohn's disease, enteroclysis would have been safe, but given the final diagnosis, there was a risk of further perforation and intraperitoneal spillage. Small bowel enteroscopy with a 2-meter small caliber scope is now being used to evaluate small bowel pathologic findings detected on other studies, and sometimes it is used to evaluate the small bowel in the absence of known disease. This method is somewhat more specific than enteroclysis, and use of the device allows the clinician to obtain tissue biopsy.

Notes

Hepatocellular Carcinoma with Tumor Thrombus

1. Hepatocellular carcinoma and hepatoblastoma in children.

2. Hepatitis.

3. Liver flukes.

4. Cirrhosis, usually alcoholic.

Reference

Ito K, Honjo K, Fujita T, et al: Liver neoplasms: diagnostic pitfalls in cross-sectional imaging, *Radiographics* 16:273-293, 1996.

Cross-Reference

Gastrointestinal Radiology: THE REQUISITES, ed 2, p 175.

Comment

Hepatocellular carcinoma, or hepatoma, is the primary malignant tumor of the liver. It is a relatively slow-growing tumor, but it has a strong tendency to invade adjacent structures and extend along vascular channels, making resection at the time of discovery difficult. There is a strong propensity for the tumor to extend into the hepatic veins, producing thrombosis (Budd-Chiari syndrome), or to involve the portal vein with thrombosis, resulting in varices. Symptoms are minimal, and the tumors often do not become clinically apparent until they are advanced, with local invasion. The tumor can be detected on a blood test by an elevated alpha-fetoprotein level.

Hepatoma is more common in the Orient. Predisposing factors include hepatitis B or C infection, which is quite common in the region. Also, parasitic infections of the liver, such as liver flukes, increase the possibility of hepatoma. The tumor is less common in North America but has a slightly increased incidence in men because the major predisposing factor in the United States is alcoholic cirrhosis. Other conditions that increase the incidence of this tumor are the use of anabolic steroids; exposure to hepatocarcinogens, such as aflatoxins; and certain storage diseases, such as hemochromatosis.

Hepatocellular carcinoma has a wide range of appearances and can mimic both benign tumors and metastatic disease. The most common pattern is that of a large, solitary mass. Another form is that of multifocal, distinct masses, which can resemble metastatic disease. Finally, the tumor can be diffuse and extensive, infiltrating throughout the liver without distinct lesions or borders. Sometimes the tumor is identified as a hepatoma only because of the vascular invasion that is so common in these tumors.

Notes

Challenge Cases

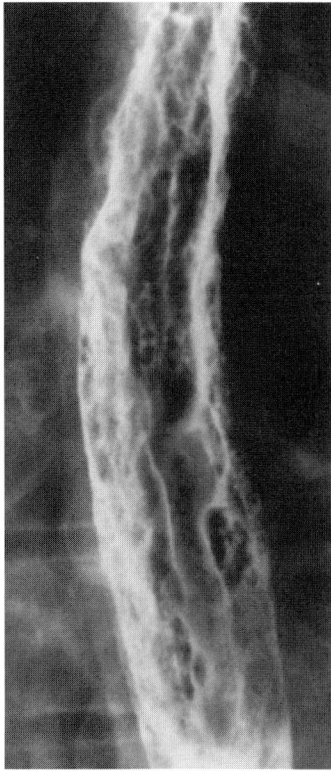

1. What type of primary esophageal neoplasm may have this appearance?
2. What hematologic neoplasms can involve the esophagus?
3. What infectious process could have this appearance?
4. What common benign condition also should be considered?

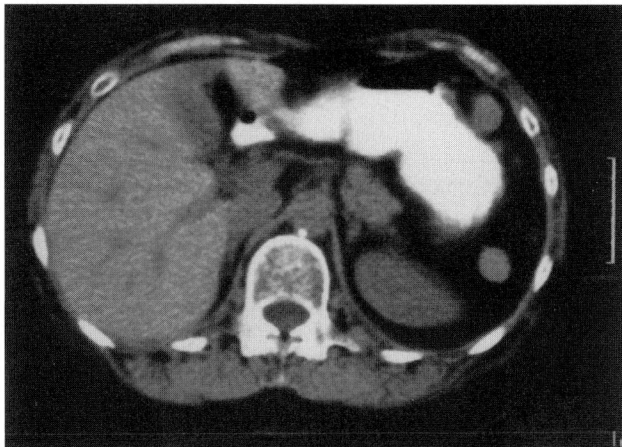

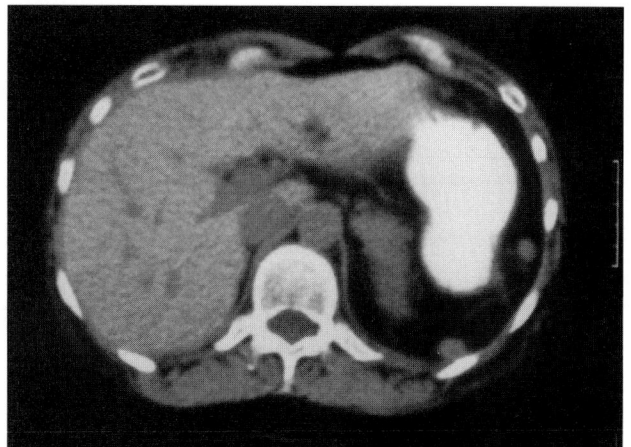

1. What is this condition called?
2. Of what is it the sequela?
3. How common is this condition?
4. Does it produce any clinical problems?

Leukemia of the Esophagus

1. Verrucous or varicoid esophageal carcinoma.

2. Both lymphoma and leukemia.

3. Candidiasis.

4. Varices.

Reference

Buck JL, Pantongrag-Brown L: Tumors of the esophagus, *Semin Roentgenol* 29:351, 1994.

Cross-Reference

Gastrointestinal Radiology: THE REQUISITES, ed 2, p 11.

Comment

Both lymphoma and leukemia can occur in the esophagus when the disease is diffuse and extensive but rarely occur when it is a primary process. Both lymphoma and leukemia of the esophagus typically produce multifocal lesions. These lesions may appear as diffuse fold thickening and irregularity or as multiple nodules, usually submucosal in location. Thus their radiologic appearance may mimic that of other diffuse esophageal malignancies or hematogenous metastatic processes to the esophagus. These lesions usually regress readily with treatment of the primary tumor but have been known to produce symptoms of dysphagia.

Other causes of multiple filling defects in the esophagus include unusual appearances of squamous esophageal carcinoma, such as varicoid carcinoma or verrucous squamous carcinoma. Squamous papillomas of the esophagus, which is a benign condition, could present as multiple filling defects as well. Probably the most common infectious condition that could have this appearance is candidiasis of the esophagus. Other infectious diseases are less likely. Varices of the esophagus present as multiple submucosal filling defects and have an appearance similar to that shown in this case. Glycogen acanthoses, which produce mucosal nodules in the older population, never become this large.

Notes

Splenosis

1. Splenosis.

2. Trauma to the spleen.

3. Between 20% and 50% of patients with splenic trauma are affected.

4. Rarely.

Reference

Gentry LR, Brown JM, Lindgren RD: Splenosis: CT demonstration of heterotopic autotransplantation of splenic tissue, *J Comput Assist Tomogr* 6:1184-1187, 1982.

Cross-Reference

Gastrointestinal Radiology: THE REQUISITES, ed 2, p 188.

Comment

The CT scan demonstrates multiple rounded masses in the left upper quadrant. These masses enhance and are solid and homogeneous in density. In the patient with a history of splenic trauma or splenectomy the most likely diagnosis is splenosis. Other considerations include adenopathy, peritoneal metastatic implants from ovarian or other abdominal tumors, endometriosis, and multiple accessory spleens. The absence of the spleen suggests that it has been removed for some reason.

In patients with splenosis, splenic tissue becomes implanted within the abdominal cavity, and these implants begin to grow and function like normal splenic tissue. Trauma is by far the leading cause of splenosis, although surgery may sometimes produce this condition. The implants can be located anywhere in the abdominal cavity and even within the hemithorax if there has been penetrating trauma. The splenic tissue obtains its vascular supply from the serosal and mesenteric surfaces. Clinically these small splenic growths produce few symptoms. Sometimes they are the source of abdominal pain. Probably of more concern is their potential misdiagnosis as some type of neoplastic process. Nuclear scanning is the definitive method for demonstrating that this tissue is splenic in origin.

Notes

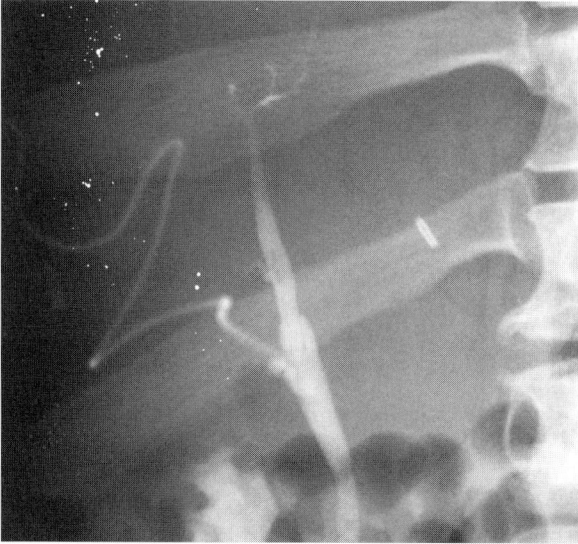

1. This patient has had a liver transplant. What is the most common cause of an anastomotic stricture?

2. What causes intrahepatic strictures?

3. If transplantation was performed to treat sclerosing cholangitis, does the condition ever recur?

4. The patency of what other structure must be evaluated in liver transplant patients?

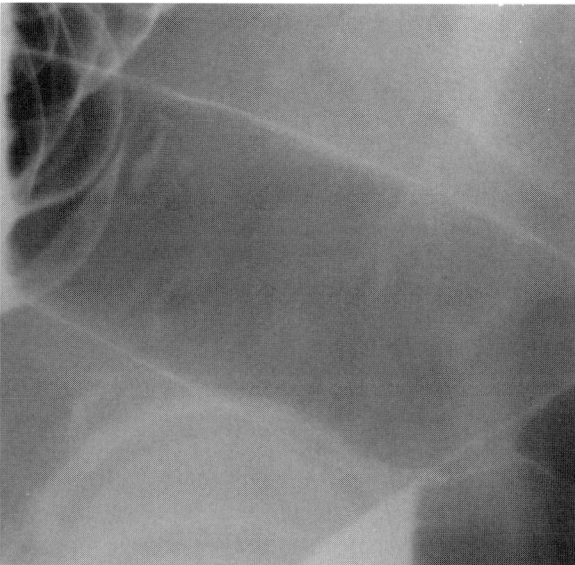

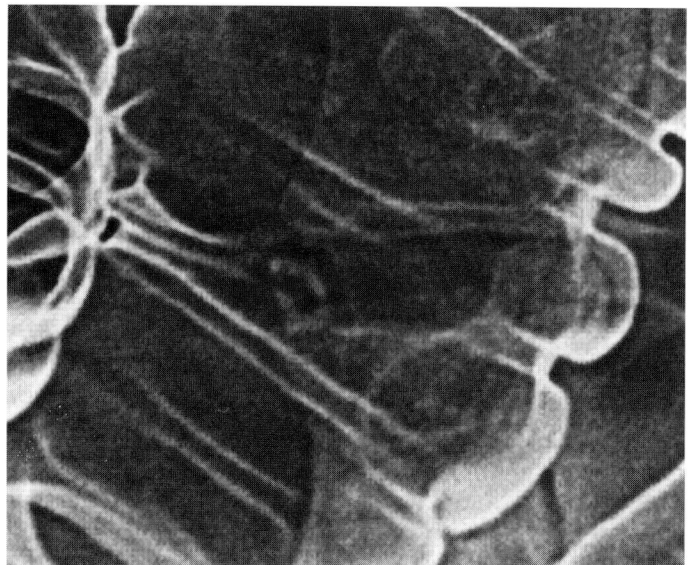

1. Both patients shown have the same history, and both have only this abnormality. What could produce this abnormality?

2. What type of ulcer does this resemble?

3. How long does this condition last?

4. Is there any need for treatment?

CASE 153

Chronic Rejection After Liver Transplantation

1. Scarring and fibrosis resulting from surgery.

2. Ischemia and chronic rejection.

3. Rarely (but this subject is controversial).

4. Hepatic artery.

Reference

Sheng R, Zajko AB, Campbell WL, et al: Biliary strictures in hepatic transplants: prevalence and types in patients with primary sclerosing cholangitis vs those with other liver diseases, *Am J Roentgenol* 161:297-300, 1993.

Cross-Reference

Gastrointestinal Radiology: THE REQUISITES, ed 2, p 204.

Comment

Liver transplantation is becoming increasingly common. Also, transplant patients are surviving much longer, and it is fairly common for them to undergo multiple studies of the biliary system after transplantation. One of the major complications involving the biliary system in these patients is the development of strictures. There are two major areas of stricturing—at the anastomosis and in the intrahepatic ducts.

Strictures at the anastomosis occur in up to 20% of patients receiving care at major institutions. Many of the anastomotic strictures are a postsurgical complication caused by a combination of scarring, fibrosis, and retraction related to the surgery. The theory is that these strictures usually occur within the first year after transplantation. Prolonged cooling of the transplant seems to result in a higher incidence of stricturing. Ischemia caused by arterial occlusion is believed to play only a minor role in the development of anastomotic strictures.

Intrahepatic strictures also occur in between 20% and 30% of transplant patients. Intrahepatic strictures may occur in conjunction with anastomotic strictures, but the two are not related. Intrahepatic strictures occur from several months to years after transplantation and can be the result of a combination of ischemia, chronic rejection, and infection. After transplantation, the hepatic artery is the sole blood supply to the intrahepatic bile ducts, and occlusion of the hepatic artery is a fairly common complication. Many intrahepatic strictures are believed to be ischemic in nature. There is some controversy regarding whether a patient with sclerosing cholangitis (PSC) who develops strictures can have recurrence of disease after transplantation. Strictures are no more common in PSC patients than in non-PSC patients. There are a few reports of possible PSC recurrence, but the pathologic findings often do not support this diagnosis, and the actual recurrence of PSC after transplantation is currently considered rare.

Notes

CASE 154

Biopsy Ulcer or Scar

1. Ulcer or scar at biopsy or polypectomy site in the colon.

2. Aphthous ulcer.

3. Several weeks to months.

4. No.

Reference

Ott DJ, Chen MYM: Specific acute colonic disorders, *Radiol Clin North Am* 32:871-885, 1994.

Cross-Reference

Gastrointestinal Radiology: THE REQUISITES, ed 2, p 268.

Comment

Radiologists commonly perform colon examinations on patients who have had recent endoscopy, usually because the initial examination was incomplete or because some pathology was encountered and further evaluation of the colon is recommended. Sometimes this examination can be done the same day as the endoscopic procedure, although it is generally advisable to wait several days to a week if a biopsy has been performed. Both of the patients in this case had double-contrast colon examinations within several weeks of colonoscopy. Both patients had polyps removed at the abnormal sites shown. This procedure has been described only recently, and it was not until the advent of double-contrast colon examination, with the finer mucosal detail, that these lesions were finally recognized.

The major differential point is that these lesions are not mistaken for aphthous ulcers. The abnormality itself can be considered an ulcer, which it technically represents. However, it is iatrogenic in nature and does not indicate any other processes. Without obtaining a proper history, the radiologist could erroneously suspect that the patient is developing focal ulcers, as seen in Crohn's disease or perhaps an infectious colitis. There is an entity of nonspecific ulcer of the colon, typically encountered in the cecum, that could have this appearance.

Both of the lesions shown were encountered within several weeks after colonoscopy and biopsy. These abnormalities may be present for up to several months after the procedure, until the scarring subsides and they are no longer visible radiologically. If the biopsy site scars substantially, some changes may persist permanently.

Notes

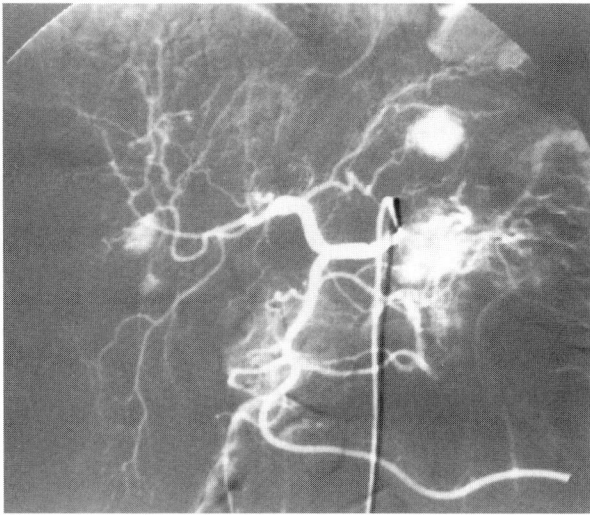

1. What pancreatic tumors are the most vascular?
2. Which pancreatic tumor is associated with multiple endocrine neoplasia syndrome I (MEN-I)?
3. Which pancreatic tumors occur in patients with von Hippel-Lindau disease?
4. What is the most common islet cell tumor?

A 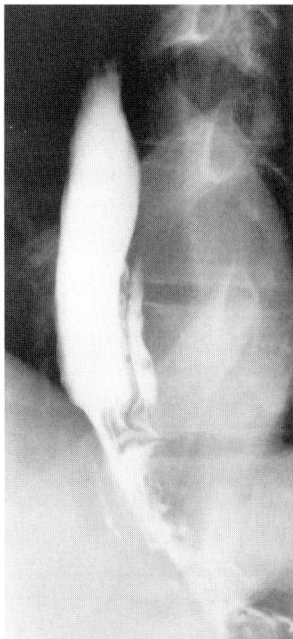 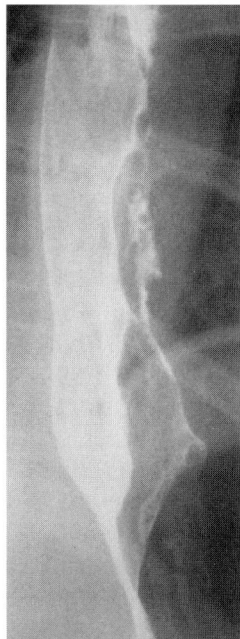 B

1. What is the most common cause of esophageal perforation?
2. What conditions produce a Mallory-Weiss tear of the esophagus?
3. In what location do Mallory-Weiss tears most frequently occur?
4. What other conditions may produce intramural tracking of barium in the esophagus?

Islet Cell Tumor of the Pancreas with Liver Metastases

1. Islet cell tumors.

2. Any islet cell tumor but usually gastrinoma.

3. Islet cell tumors.

4. Insulinoma.

Reference

Buetow PC, Parrino TV, Buck JL, et al: Islet cell tumors of the pancreas, *Am J Roentgenol* 165:1175-1179, 1995.

Cross-Reference

Gastrointestinal Radiology: THE REQUISITES, ed 2, p 147.

Comment

Islet cell tumors of the pancreas are a group of tumors that arise from the islets of Langerhans. They also are termed *APUDomas* because they have certain chemical properties indicating that they arise from what are termed *APUD* cells, a type of neuroendocrine tissue. APUD cells migrate from the neural crest embryologically. Although this tissue is found most often in the pancreas, these tumors also can arise in nonpancreatic locations, usually in the paraspinal tissues. Islet cell tumors are classified according to the active hormone they excrete, although not all are functioning. In order of their frequency, these tumors are insulinoma, gastrinoma, nonfunctioning islet cell, glucagonoma, vipoma, and somatostatinoma. Islet cell tumors, most often gastrinomas, are associated with multiple endocrine neoplasia syndrome (MEN-I). They also present as a complication of von Hippel-Lindau disease. Most are not associated with any syndrome, however.

Islet cell tumors are quite different from the more common pancreatic adenocarcinoma. Islet cell tumors are usually hypervascular on angiography, whereas adenocarcinoma is hypovascular. On arteriograms, adenocarcinoma is shown to encase and narrow blood vessels. Islet cell tumors, however, are very vascular (>80%) and show evidence of neovascularity. Also, their metastases can be quite vascular, as illustrated in this case. The tumor can be identified with angiography. Sometimes the tumors are quite small, but their hormone activity is significant. These tumors may be identified by venous sampling of the splenic vein and portal system, which helps to better localize them. It is uncertain whether MRI can play a significant role in their detection, although they are bright on T2W images.

Notes

Intramural Tracking of Barium After Endoscopy with Sclerotherapy of Varices (A) and Crohn's Disease (B)

1. Endoscopy.

2. Although vomiting is the most common cause, coughing, straining, seizures, and blunt trauma also are causes.

3. Usually at the cardia of the stomach, and less commonly in the distal esophagus.

4. Endoscopy; perforation caused by nasogastric tube passage, balloon dilation, or other therapeutic maneuver; Crohn's disease; and surgery.

Reference

Phillips LG, et al: Esophageal perforation, *Radiol Clin North Am* 22:607-613, 1984.

Cross-Reference

Gastrointestinal Radiology: THE REQUISITES, ed 2, p 19.

Comment

Tracking of contrast material in the wall of the esophagus is an ominous sign, yet it is not unusual in large hospitals where numerous procedures are performed daily. Patients in whom contrast runs parallel to the lumen (but does not leak into the mediastinum) have what is often termed a *double-barrel esophagus.* Despite the fact that this finding signifies a breach in the integrity of the mucosa of the esophagus, the majority of these abnormalities heal spontaneously and often require no further intervention on the part of the physician because the full thickness of the esophageal wall is not breached.

The majority of mucosal tears of the esophagus are related to instrumentation use during a procedure, typically fiberoptic endoscopy. Although tears may occur in a healthy esophagus, often an underlying pathologic condition, such as a web or other type of stricture, in the area contributes to the tear. This type of intramural dissection of contrast is common among patients who have had esophageal dilation performed immediately before the imaging study. In those hospitals in which endoscopists routinely request postdilation esophagrams, this finding may be encountered frequently. The patient in one of the cases illustrated has had repeated injection sclerotherapy of varices, and it is probably a varix that is filling with the contrast.

A Mallory-Weiss tear is a mucosal tear usually associated with vomiting or retching but it can result from other causes of increased intraabdominal pressure. The most serious complication is bleeding, although it often stops spontaneously. Typically the tear occurs on the gastric side of the gastroesophageal junction, in the cardia. However, it can be encountered in the distal esophagus as well. Radiologic diagnosis is rare because endoscopy is usually performed on these patients. Crohn's disease also can produce tracts through the wall of esophagus, similar to those it produces in other parts of the gastrointestinal tract.

Notes

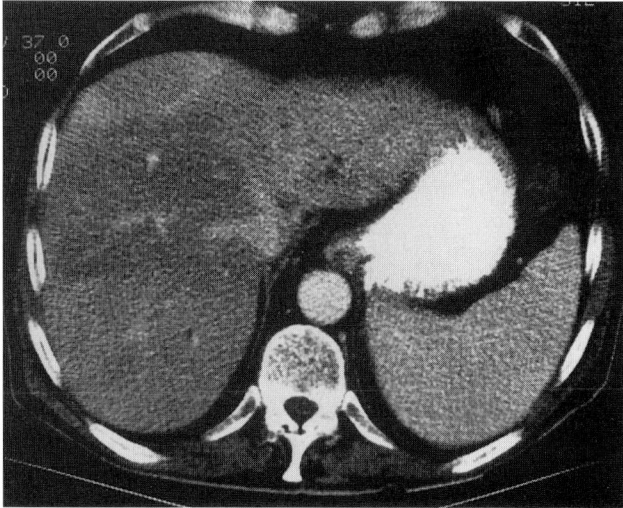

1. Name the possible causes for this appearance.
2. If the liver has received radiation, what condition produces this change?
3. What results from diffuse liver radiation therapy?
4. What are the long-term sequelae of liver radiation therapy?

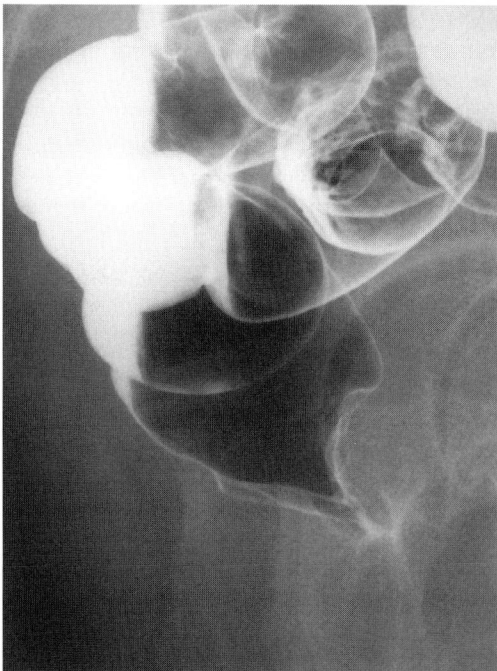

1. What is a predisposing factor for anal canal tumors?
2. What tumor is known to arise from embryonic tissues in this location?
3. Which tumor in this location has the worst prognosis?
4. What gender is most frequently involved by these tumors?

CASE 157

Radiation-Induced Liver Defect

1. Focal fatty infiltration and radiation defect.

2. Edema.

3. Hepatomegaly, ascites, and liver dysfunction.

4. Atrophy and fatty infiltration.

Reference

Unger EC, Lee JKT, Weyman PJ: CT and MR imaging of radiation hepatitis, *J Comput Assist Tomogr* 11:264-268, 1987.

Cross-Reference

Gastrointestinal Radiology: THE REQUISITES, ed 2, p 168.

Comment

Radiation to the liver is usually incidental and occurs when the liver is included in the port for radiation of an adjacent structure. In this instance the patient had gallbladder cancer and required radiation to shrink the tumor before surgery. Treatment of esophageal, gastric, or pancreatic tumors and lymphoma can result in liver damage. Damage to the liver can occur with a single 1200-rad dose or can be the result of a cumulative effect when a series of doses exceeds 4000 rad. The hepatocytes are actually more radiosensitive than the Kupffer cells. Patients who have a large portion of liver in the field can develop substantial liver dysfunction.

Radiation to the liver produces focal radiation hepatitis. This condition is caused by lobar congestion, hyperemia, and hemorrhage. There is damage to the central veins, resulting in local passive congestion. This venous stasis produces immediate congestion. In the long term there is loss of hepatocytes, fibrosis, and atrophy, with loss of the central veins. In the early phase, CT demonstrates an area of low attenuation that is sharply demarcated by the treatment port. This area does not follow an anatomic distribution. With time, the border of the field becomes less distinct. Ultrasound reveals an hypoechoic area. Nuclear sulfur-colloid scans are fairly normal because the Kupffer cells tend to survive the radiation. However, nuclear hepatobiliary scans are abnormal because of the loss of hepatocytes in the radiated area.

Notes

CASE 158

Cloacogenic Carcinoma

1. Viral infection.

2. Cloacogenic carcinoma.

3. Cloacogenic carcinoma.

4. Women.

Reference

Sink JD, Kramer SA, Copeland DD, et al: Cloacogenic carcinoma, *Ann Surg* 188:53-59, 1978.

Cross-Reference

Gastrointestinal Radiology: THE REQUISITES, ed 2, p 247.

Comment

Tumors occurring at the anal canal can be squamous cell carcinoma, adenocarcinoma, or the rare cloacogenic carcinoma. Adenocarcinomas typically arise from the lower rectal mucosa and extend into the anal canal. They have a tendency to produce metastases to the local lymph nodes. Squamous carcinomas of the anus arise from the mucosa of the anal canal. Their damage is produced by local invasion and later spread to the regional lymph nodes.

Cloacogenic carcinoma arises from the embryologic cloacogenic zone, which basically is the transition region between the anus and distal rectum. The glands in this location can give rise to what is termed a *cloacogenic tumor.* Histologically the tumor can consist of a mix of several cell types, including transitional, squamous, and cylindrical cells. There are two general groups of cloacogenic tumors—poorly differentiated small cell tumors and large cell tumors of either squamous or transitional origin. The small cell tumor has a poor prognosis, with involvement of regional lymph nodes and distal metastases. Both types have a worse prognosis than either squamous carcinoma or adenocarcinoma.

On barium enema the tumors are difficult to distinguish from one another. However, cloacogenic carcinoma tends to have its center of growth near the anorectal junction. It also has extensive growth outside the lumen of the rectum, with a large extraluminal component compared with adenocarcinoma.

Notes

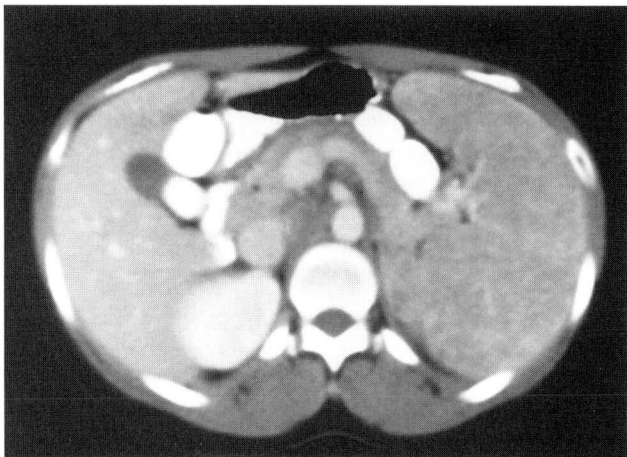

1. What is the most common cause of splenomegaly?
2. What pulmonary disease produces splenomegaly?
3. Name some neoplasms that may enlarge the spleen.
4. Name some storage diseases associated with splenomegaly.

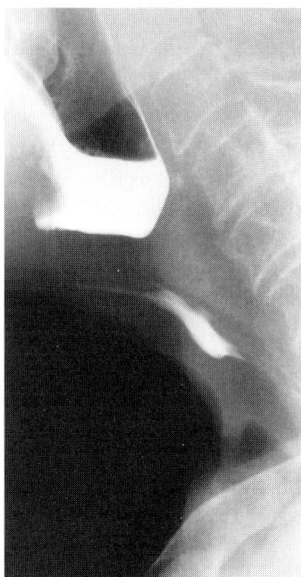

A

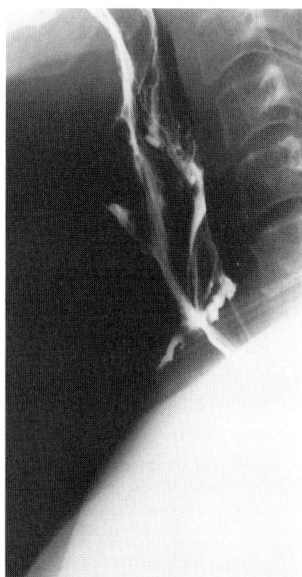

B

1. What is the significance of the mass posterior to the hypopharynx in this patient who just underwent laryngectomy to treat carcinoma?
2. What is the significance of a postoperative tracheoesophageal fistula?
3. What other complications may occur after laryngectomy?
4. What is the cause of a "hairy" or "hirsute" esophagus?

Splenomegaly in Gaucher's Disease

1. Infection.

2. Sarcoidosis.

3. Lymphoma, chronic lymphocytic leukemia, metastases, and primary splenic tumor.

4. Gaucher's disease, amyloidosis, hemochromatosis, and Niemann-Pick disease.

Reference

Lanir A, Hader H, Cohen I, et al: Gaucher disease: assessment with MR imaging, *Radiology* 161:239-244, 1986.

Cross-Reference

Gastrointestinal Radiology: THE REQUISITES, ed 2, p 190.

Comment

Numerous diseases produce enlargement of the spleen. The most common are usually infectious processes with secondary splenomegaly resulting from the reaction of the reticuloendothelial system to the infection. Direct infection of the spleen by abscess is less common. An extremely common cause in certain populations is vascular congestion caused by cirrhosis, portal hypertension, or both. Congestive heart failure and splenic vein occlusion are other vascular causes. Patients with anemia often have splenomegaly, which may be related to the filtering of the damaged red blood cells by the spleen. It also may be the result of extramedullary hematopoiesis, which can occur in the spleen. Neoplastic conditions always must be considered, and the most common are lymphoma and certain types of leukemia. Metastases and primary tumors of the spleen are rare. Other conditions to consider are space-occupying lesions, such as hematomas or cysts. Sarcoidosis occasionally produces splenomegaly, as do some collagen vascular diseases.

Storage disorders may cause deposition of material in the spleen. These diseases include Gaucher's disease, hemochromatosis, and amyloidosis. In Gaucher's disease there is a metabolic disorder causing deposition of glucocerebrosides in the spleen and reticuloendothelial system. The disease produces hepatosplenomegaly. Splenectomy may be necessary as the spleen becomes massively enlarged and compresses adjacent structures. CT reveals an enlarged homogeneous spleen. Sometimes it is low in attenuation because of the nature of the material deposited. MRI also can be used to assess this disease.

Notes

Pseudotumor After Laryngectomy (A) and Surgical Tracheoesophageal Fistula for Phonation (B)

1. Indicates pseudotumor from the inferior constrictor and cricopharyngeus muscles.

2. Normal finding created to aid in phonation.

3. Aspiration, bezoars, recurrent tumor, and benign strictures.

4. If a skin flap is used for reconstruction of the hypopharynx, the hair on the skin may continue to grow.

Reference

Balfe DM, Koehler RE, Setzen J, et al: Barium examination of the esophagus after total laryngectomy, *Radiology* 143:501-508, 1982.

Cross-Reference

Gastrointestinal Radiology: THE REQUISITES, ed 2, Chapter 1.

Comment

Radical surgical resection of the neck is still a common approach to the treatment of tumors of the larynx and hypopharynx. Invariably these tumors are squamous in origin, and surgery remains the best approach for confinement of the tumor. However, the extensive surgical resection that ensues produces marked changes that make interpretation of the postlaryngectomy esophagram difficult. Virtually all of these patients have some type of swallowing difficulties and often present to the radiologist for evaluation of these problems.

During surgery, muscle groups may be removed, or the attachments of these muscle groups (i.e., the cartilages) are removed. A common finding on esophagrams is a large soft tissue mass posterior to the hypopharynx that is displacing it forward. This mass should not be mistaken for recurrent tumor; it represents normal muscle groups (inferior constrictor and hypopharynx). As a result of the surgery, these muscles have lost their attachments and bunch together posteriorly, as well as hypertrophy in some instances. Other problems that may produce dysphagia include strictures (as a result of either surgery or radiation). Bezoars have been known to develop in the hypopharynx.

Fistulas sometimes develop between the upper trachea and either the cervical esophagus or the hypopharynx. The majority of these are surgically created so that the patient can continue to phonate. By covering up the tracheostomy hole, the patient can exhale out of the mouth via this fistula. He or she can then form words and communicate, despite loss of the vocal cords. However, this fistula can lead to complications of aspiration if it is too large, and not all surgeons perform this procedure.

Notes

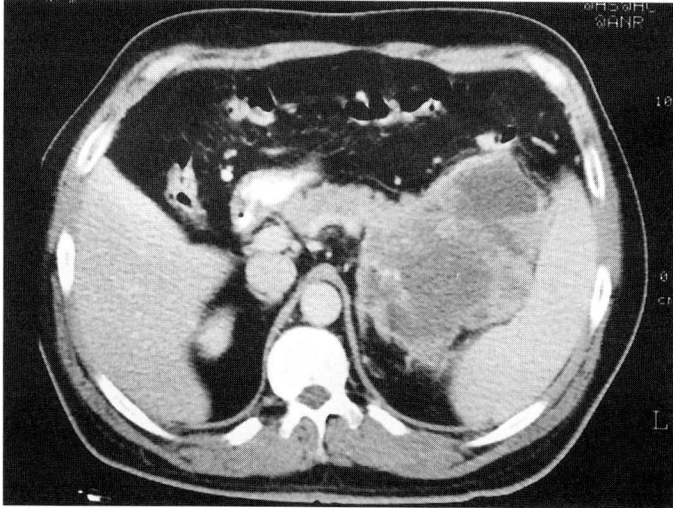

1. Name possible cystic tumors of the pancreas.
2. How do cysts appear in microcystic adenoma?
3. What are the cysts like in mucinous neoplasm?
4. What is the malignant potential of mucinous cystic tumors of the pancreas?

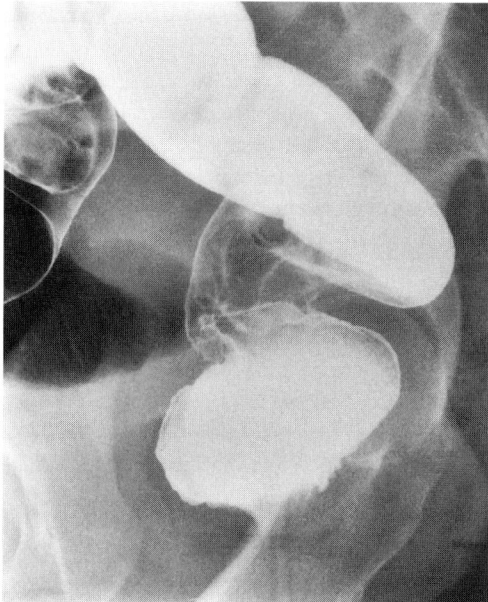

1. What sexually transmitted disease may cause rectal ulceration and stricturing?
2. What problem do patients with spastic pelvic floor syndrome experience?
3. Name the rectal inflammation that results from internal prolapse.
4. Name another sequela of repeated internal prolapse and ulceration.

CASE 161

Mucinous Cystic Tumor of the Pancreas

1. Microcystic adenoma, mucinous cystic neoplasms, papillary epithelial neoplasm, rarely islet cell tumors, and cystic teratoma.

2. Multiple small cysts of varying size.

3. Large, either single or just a few septated cysts.

4. All are potentially malignant.

Reference

Ros PR, Hamrick-Turner JE, Chiechi MV, et al: Cystic masses of the pancreas, *Radiographics* 12:673-686, 1992.

Cross-Reference

Gastrointestinal Radiology: THE REQUISITES, ed 2, p 152.

Comment

Several neoplasms of the pancreas present as cystic lesions, although all are fairly rare compared with ductal adenocarcinoma, which almost never has cysts. One of the most common cystic tumors is microcystic adenoma, which has multiple small cysts of varying size. If the cysts are too numerous to count, the diagnosis should be considered microcystic adenoma. This condition occurs in older women. This tumor is associated with von Hippel-Lindau disease. It is a hypervascular tumor that develops central necrosis and scarring, often with calcification.

The term *mucinous cystic neoplasms* describes what has been termed *mucinous cystadenoma* and *mucinous cystadenocarcinoma.* These tumors are difficult to distinguish, and because cystadenomas have malignant potential, they are now classified together, and all are considered malignant or potentially malignant. The cysts in patients with these tumors are large. Often the cyst is unilocular, resembling a pseudocyst, or large, with multiple distinct septations. These tumors are hypovascular, and if they calcify, they do so in a peripheral location.

Another tumor that may resemble a mucinous cystic neoplasm is a cystic teratoma, although this tumor is rare. This tumor also has multiple large cysts and dystrophic calcification. Papillary epithelial neoplasms can be cystic. The cyst is usually thick walled, with mural tumor projections. This tumor occurs in young women and is considered a low grade malignancy. Also, islet cell tumors that undergo necrosis may show cystic changes.

Notes

CASE 162

Solitary Rectal Ulcer Syndrome

1. Lymphogranuloma venereum.

2. Failure of the pelvic floor to relax during defecation.

3. Solitary rectal ulcer syndrome.

4. Colitis cystica profunda.

Reference

Goei R, Baeten C, Janevski B, et al: The solitary rectal ulcer syndrome: diagnosis with defecography, *Am J Roentgenol* 149:933-936, 1987.

Cross-Reference

Gastrointestinal Radiology: THE REQUISITES, ed 2, p 268.

Comment

Several pathologic conditions may occur in the rectum of the patient with a defecation disorder. One of these is termed *solitary rectal ulcer syndrome.* This terminology is used to describe patients with chronic straining and defecation problems who develop ulceration in the rectum. However, the term *solitary* is incorrect in that many of these patients have multiple but focal ulcers in the rectum.

The etiology of solitary rectal ulcer syndrome is believed to be related to excessive straining during defecation. Patients who strain often produce internal intussusception or prolapse of the rectal mucosa. The middle to upper portion of the rectum is more mobile, and during excessive straining throughout defecation, the proximal rectal mucosa may be pushed into the lumen and may intussuscept into the distal rectum or even externally through the anal canal. This invagination of the rectal mucosa results in stretching of the submucosal vessels and focal ischemia. Also, there may be direct trauma to the mucosa as it is pushed against or through the anal canal. Both of these etiologies are believed to be the basis for the development of the ulceration. The ulcers typically occur along the anterior rectum because it is most mobile but can be seen laterally or posteriorly as well. The condition causes a distinctive pathologic change, with replacement of the lamina propria with fibroblasts and thickening of the muscularis mucosa. Patients with spastic pelvic floor syndrome (i.e., failure of relaxation of the puborectalis during defecation) also develop solitary rectal ulcer syndrome because the rectal mucosa is traumatized by its contact with the fixed puborectalis muscle.

Defecography is important in the diagnosis of this condition. It can demonstrate the presence of intussusception during defecation or the failure of the puborectalis to relax during defecation. Findings on barium enema are variable, but sometimes small ulcers or thickening of the valves of Houston are evident. Sometimes stricturing or polypoid lesions (colitis cystica profunda) are visible. Solitary rectal ulcer syndrome must be differentiated from other causes of proctitis.

Notes

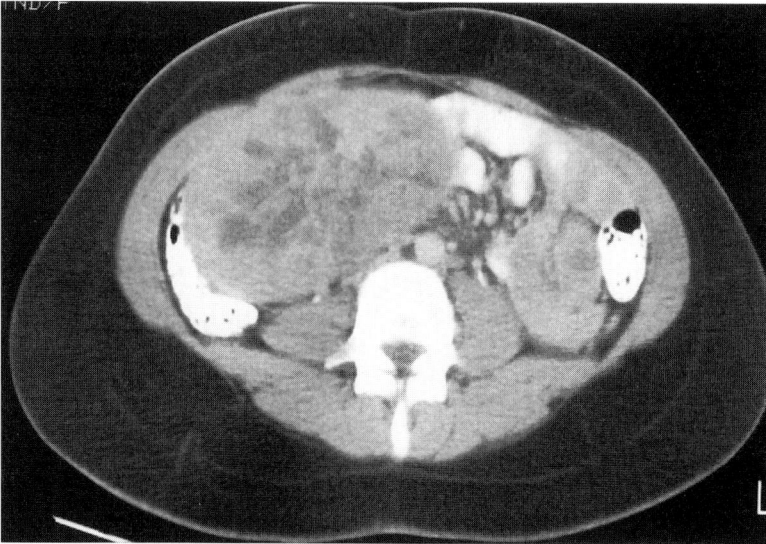

1. In this young patient, what are the diagnostic possibilities?
2. What malignancies of the liver may calcify?
3. What type of hepatoma occurs in young patients?
4. What conditions predispose an individual to develop this lesion?

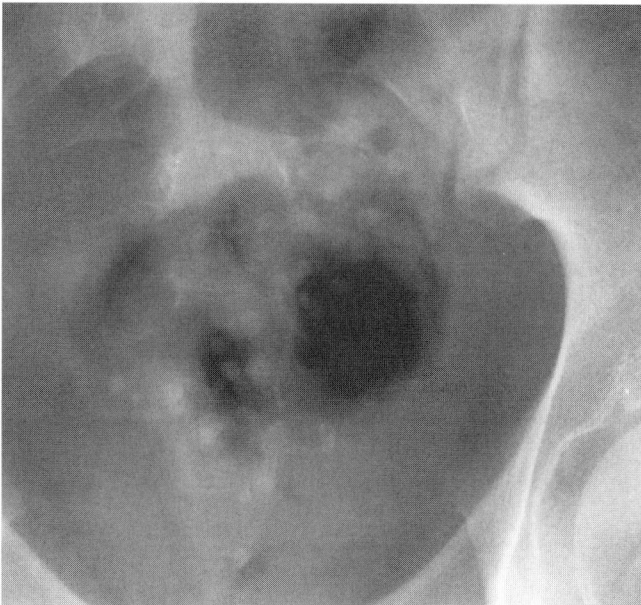

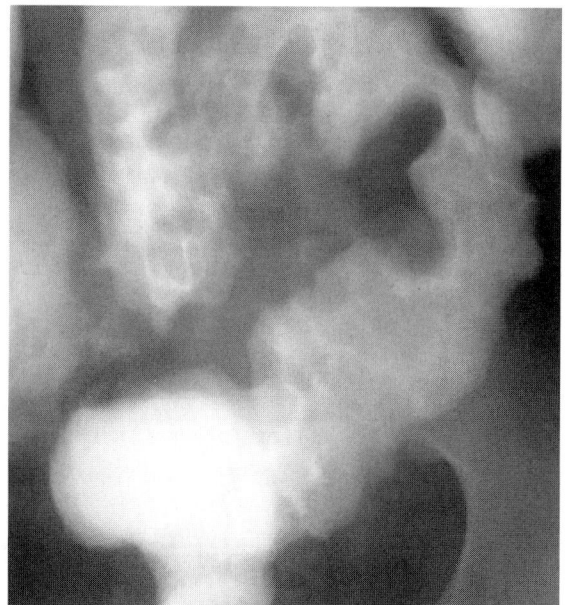

1. Name some diagnostic possibilities for this radiologic appearance.
2. What age group does this lesion affect?
3. What vascular tumors may involve the colon?
4. How does the appearance of cavernous hemangiomas differ from the appearance of capillary hemangiomas?

Fibrolamellar Hepatoma

1. Focal nodular hyperplasia, hepatic adenoma, and fibrolamellar hepatoma.

2. Fibrolamellar hepatoma, hepatoblastoma, intrahepatic cholangiocarcinoma, and metastases.

3. Fibrolamellar hepatoma.

4. None.

Reference

McLarney JK, Rucker PT, Bender GN, et al: Fibrolamellar carcinoma of the liver: radiologic-pathologic correlation, *Radiographics* 19:453-471, 1999.

Cross-Reference

Gastrointestinal Radiology: THE REQUISITES, ed 2, p 176.

Comment

Neoplasms of the liver in young patients can be caused by several different cell types. The most commonly encountered are focal nodular hyperplasia (FNH) and hepatic adenoma. Hemangiomas and metastases also must be considered. The appearance of this tumor in conjunction with a central scar or low density areas is suggestive of FNH but also can occur in other conditions.

Fibrolamellar carcinoma is an unusual variant of conventional hepatocellular carcinoma (HCC). The demographic population affected by fibrolamellar carcinoma is quite different from that affected by HCC; fibrolamellar carcinoma occurs in a much younger population, even in children. Also, the usual predisposing factors associated with HCC, such as cirrhosis or long-standing hepatitis, are not associated with fibrolamellar carcinoma. There is not believed to be any associated risk factor for the development of fibrolamellar hepatoma, but this possibility must be a strong consideration when liver masses are encountered in a young adult. The radiologic diagnosis can be difficult to make because the lesion may resemble other liver tumors. It typically has a central "scar" or area of fibrous or necrotic tissue that can resemble FNH in its appearance. Fibrolamellar hepatoma does calcify and has been described in up to 50% of patients. On CT scans the tumor is initially hypodense, particularly its central scar. However, delayed images show increasing homogeneity of the lesion with the surrounding liver, simulating a hemangioma. A poorly performed CT scan may underestimate the size of the lesion. Nuclear scanning may help differentiate the mass from FNH because fibrolamellar hepatoma does not have Kupffer cells.

The prognosis for patients with fibrolamellar hepatoma is much better than that for patients with HCC, and the lesion is potentially curable with surgery. Vascular invasion and other abnormalities of HCC are much less common in fibrolamellar hepatoma. This lesion also responds well to chemotherapy.

Notes

Hemangioma of the Colon

1. Ischemia, inflammatory bowel disease, hemorrhage, lymphoma, and hemangioma.

2. Typically a younger age group.

3. Hemangiomas and lymphangiomas.

4. Cavernous hemangiomas are more diffuse; capillary hemangiomas are localized.

Reference

Dachman AH, Ros PR, Shekitka KM, et al: Colorectal hemangioma: radiologic findings, *Radiology* 167:31-34, 1988.

Cross-Reference

Gastrointestinal Radiology: THE REQUISITES, ed 2, p 248.

Comment

Hemangiomas of the colon, as well as the rest of the gastrointestinal tract, are rare lesions. Clinically, patients with hemangiomas experience recurrent bleeding, which can be massive at times. High mortality is associated with this condition because patients may exsanguinate before the diagnosis is made and proper treatment is initiated. Proper diagnosis is necessary because an endoscopic biopsy or other simple procedure could prove to be disastrous. This lesion occurs in a much younger age group and can affect even pediatric patients. It is a much different lesion from the vascular ectasias that occur in the elderly. Most of these hemangiomas are located in the rectosigmoid region, although they have been reported in all parts of the colon.

Histologically there are two different types of hemangiomas to consider. Also, there are often lymphangiomatous components to these tumors, and some are considered a mixed variety of tumors. Cavernous hemangiomas are by far the most common. These develop in the submucosa and extend for varying lengths. They may be quite large and resemble neoplasm, ischemia, or inflammatory bowel disease.

Approximately one half of patients with cavernous hemangiomas have phleboliths visible on plain radiographs. This finding is crucial because it is pathognomonic of the condition. Also, phleboliths are much less common in younger patients who are diagnosed with this condition. Capillary hemangiomas are less common and are encapsulated. They occur as focal lesions and do not have phleboliths. Preoperative diagnosis of focal lesions is difficult because they cannot be differentiated from polyps or tumors.

These lesions are usually diagnosed by barium enema initially. Angiography may be performed, but the vascularity can range from hypervascular (typical hemangioma) to hypovascular, thus making the diagnosis more difficult. CT may help determine the extent of bowel involvement, but endoluminal ultrasound may be more beneficial in this regard because it could detect subtle vascular abnormalities in the submucosa.

Notes

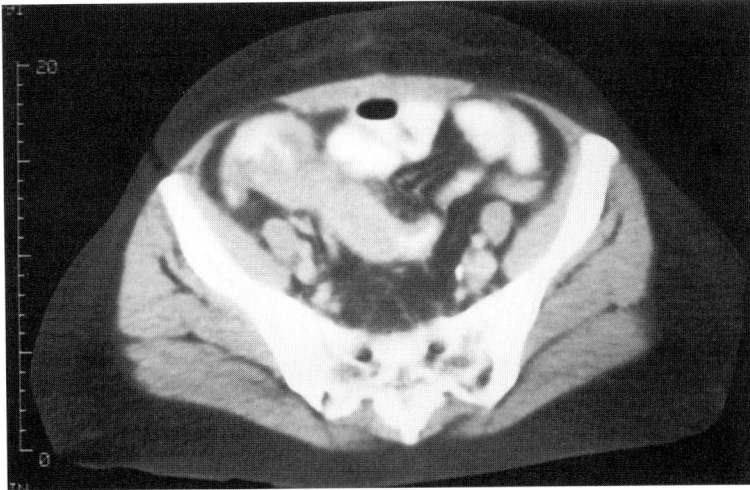

1. What may produce palpable right lower quadrant masses in children?
2. What abdominal masses occur in patients with Gardner's syndrome?
3. What is the most common location of Burkitt's lymphoma?
4. What virus can be associated with lymphoma?

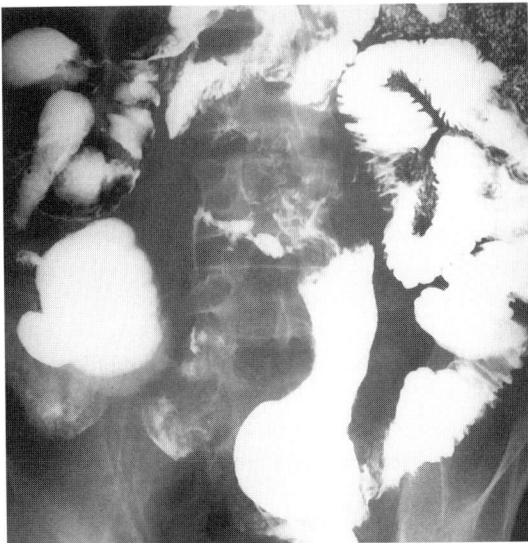

1. What is the most common primary malignancy of the small bowel?
2. Where is lymphoma most frequently found in the small bowel?
3. Where is adenocarcinoma most frequently found?
4. Name some conditions that predispose an individual to small bowel carcinoma.

Burkitt's Lymphoma of the Small Bowel

1. Crohn's disease, appendicitis, and lymphoma.

2. Desmoid tumors.

3. Distal ileum.

4. Epstein-Barr virus.

Reference

Laufer L, Barki Y, Schulman H, et al: Calcification in an un-treated case of Burkitt's lymphoma: radiographic, ultrasound and CT diagnosis, *Pediatr Radiol* 24:180-184, 1994.

Cross-Reference

Gastrointestinal Radiology: THE REQUISITES, ed 2, p 250.

Comment

This patient had a palpable abdominal mass in the right lower quadrant. In the pediatric age group, this mass most likely is the result of an inflammatory process, usually appendicitis. A more long-standing inflammatory process is Crohn's disease. Intussusception is another cause of palpable masses in children. Unusual processes that occur in children include duplication cysts and malpositioned kidneys. Malignant possibilities include lymphoma and perhaps some unusual sarcomas.

Burkitt's lymphoma is an unusual neoplasm predominantly affecting children. The type found in North America usually presents in the distal ileum and can be felt or seen as a mass in the right lower quadrant. It is extremely typical of Burkitt's lymphoma to involve this area, and the diagnosis should be strongly considered in any child who has a palpable mass in the region. Other areas are rarely involved. In the type of Burkitt's lymphoma common in Africa, the jaw and retroperitoneal lymph nodes are frequently involved, but this is not typical of the type of Burkitt's lymphoma common in North America. The tumor is associated with the Epstein-Barr virus, as are some other lymphomas. A feature of this lymphoma is its rapid doubling time. It grows in an extremely aggressive fashion, involving and displacing bowel loops in the region. It also responds fairly dramatically to chemotherapy.

Notes

Adenocarcinoma of the Small Bowel in Crohn's Disease

1. Adenocarcinoma.

2. Ileum.

3. Proximal small bowel, duodenum, and jejunum.

4. Sprue, Crohn's disease, and Peutz-Jeghers syndrome.

Reference

Feczko PJ: Malignancy complicating inflammatory bowel disease, *Radiol Clin North Am* 25:157-174, 1987.

Cross-Reference

Gastrointestinal Radiology: THE REQUISITES, ed 2, p 106.

Comment

Considering all malignancies of the small bowel beginning at the duodenal bulb, adenocarcinoma is the most common primary malignancy. Despite this fact, adenocarcinoma is a relatively rare tumor. It is found more frequently in the duodenum and proximal jejunum. (Lymphoma predominates in the distal small bowel.) The rarity of small bowel malignances is believed to be a result of a combination of the sterility of small bowel contents, rapid transit of material, and the immune function of the small bowel.

Several conditions are believed to lead to the development of adenocarcinoma of the small bowel. First, adenomatous polyps, particularly of the villous type, have a strong malignant potential. Both adenomas and adenocarcinomas are found more frequently in the proximal jejunum. Patients with celiac disease (sprue) also have a known predilection for the development of carcinoma. Sprue can lead to small bowel lymphoma, small bowel carcinoma, and esophageal carcinoma. Maintaining a gluten-free diet may diminish the likelihood of malignancy, probably because of a resulting decrease in the immune status of the small bowel. Crohn's disease is also associated with an increased incidence of malignancy. Typically, malignancy occurs in patients with long-standing Crohn's involvement of the small bowel. Bypassed loops of bowel were once considered particularly vulnerable, but this surgery is no longer performed. Unlike conventional carcinoma of the small bowel, which forms annular masses, Crohn's carcinoma is a subtle, infiltrating type of tumor. It spreads through tissue planes and is difficult to detect preoperatively because the strictures it forms resemble Crohn's disease. Many Crohn's carcinomas are found incidentally after small bowel resection. Adenocarcinoma should be considered any time a patient with long-standing Crohn's disease has a significant worsening of his or her symptoms.

Notes

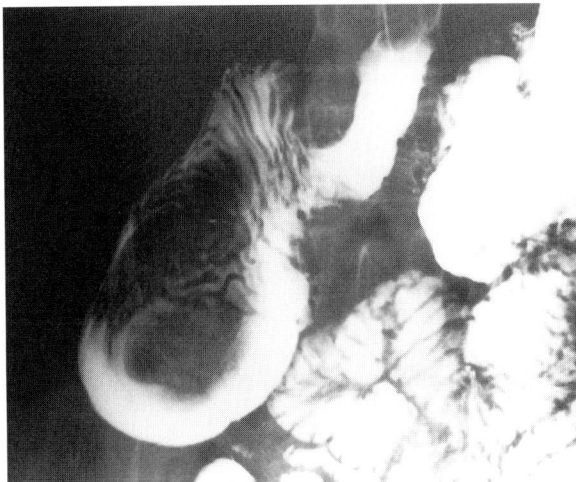

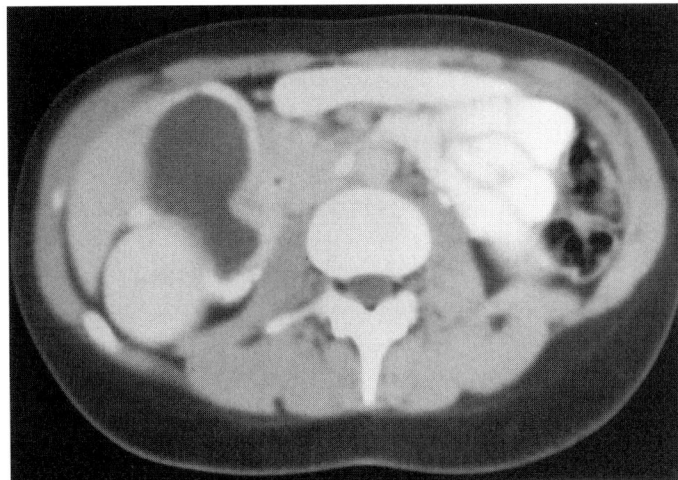

1. Name some possible causes for this abnormality.
2. If this patient has congenital anomalies, what is a likely diagnosis?
3. What modality may be helpful for further evaluation?
4. How often do duplication cysts communicate with the bowel lumen?

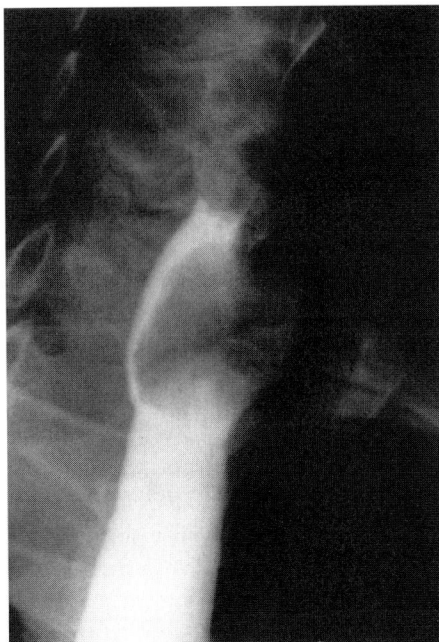

1. This patient vomited a mass into his mouth. What is the most likely diagnosis?
2. Where are these tumors most commonly located?
3. What age group and gender typically develop these tumors?
4. What other types of tumors may have this appearance?

Duodenal Duplication Cyst

1. Pancreatic pseudocyst, intraluminal duodenal diverticulum, choledochocele, and duplication cyst.

2. Duplication cyst.

3. Endoscopic ultrasound.

4. Rarely. Most do not communicate.

Reference

Guibaud L, Fouque P, Genin G, et al: CT and ultrasound of gastric and duodenal duplications, *J Comput Assist Tomogr* 20:382-386, 1996.

Cross-Reference

Gastrointestinal Radiology: THE REQUISITES, ed 2, p 120.

Comment

Cystic lesions about the duodenal sweep can be caused by a variety of conditions. The most common cause is some type of pancreatic pseudocyst arising from the head of the pancreas. Also, a choledochocele may produce a cystic lesion, although probably not as large as the one shown in this case. The rare intraluminal duodenal diverticulum may fill with secretions and no longer communicate with the lumen, producing this appearance as well.

Duplication cysts are epithelium-lined structures that attach to portions of the intestinal tract. They tend to occur on the mesenteric side of the bowel, sharing a portion of the wall of the bowel, usually the serosal or muscular coat. Most duplications do not communicate with the lumen of the bowel, although communication rarely occurs. Most are spherical or ovoid. These cysts fill with fluid, are epithelium lined, and may increase in size. The most common site of an intestinal duplication is the ileum. The duodenum is an uncommon site, accounting for very few duplications. Duplications of the duodenum often are associated with other anomalies (e.g., malrotation, atresias, anal anomalies) and, as in this patient, are an incidental finding. Endoscopic ultrasound to determine the involvement of the bowel wall may be helpful in further diagnosis and treatment planning. Surgery is the only treatment but may be difficult in the duodenum because of the possible involvement of ductal structures.

Notes

Fibrovascular Polyp of the Esophagus

1. Fibrovascular polyp or tumor.

2. Cervical or upper thoracic esophagus.

3. Older men.

4. Spindle-cell tumors (carcinosarcoma), leiomyosarcoma, adenocarcinoma, and even foreign bodies.

Reference

Levine MS, Buck JL, Pantongrag-Brown L, et al: Fibrovascular polyps of the esophagus: clinical, radiographic and pathologic findings in 16 patients, *Am J Roentgenol* 166:781-786, 1996.

Cross-Reference

Gastrointestinal Radiology: THE REQUISITES, ed 2, p 10.

Comment

Fibrovascular polyps of the esophagus, which are composed of a mix of fibrovascular tissue and adipose tissue, are rare. These tumors are sometimes termed *angiolipomas, fibrolipomas,* or *hamartomas.* Because of the presence of fatty tissue, fibrovascular polyps appear low density on CT examination, which is a hallmark feature. They have a propensity to develop in the upper portion of the esophagus, particularly in the cervical region, which is the opposite of most esophageal tumors, typically seen in the middle to distal esophagus. These polyps occur more commonly in the elderly but are seen in middle-aged individuals and are more frequent in men.

Because of their soft nature, these tumors can grow quite large before producing symptoms. The cervical location exposes the polyps to repeated peristalsis and dragging by ingested materials that cause the tumors to become pedunculated or mobile. Thus the most dramatic clinical finding is when the patient states that he or she has regurgitated a mass into the oropharynx and then swallowed it. Beyond this bizarre presentation, fibrovascular polyps can obstruct the esophagus or even the airway, with fatal results. Most of these tumors grow quite large before producing symptoms of dysphagia. As they grow, the polyps conform to the lumen of the esophagus, eventually growing large enough to distend the esophagus and produce an esophageal appearance mimicking achalasia. Small tumors can be removed endoscopically, but larger lesions require surgery. These tumors may cause bleeding, but malignant transformation is rare.

A piece of food retained in the esophagus closely mimics the appearance of this tumor. A tumor with a similar radiologic appearance is the spindle-cell tumor. Rarely, adenocarcinomas or leiomyosarcomas may appear as large intraluminal masses.

Notes

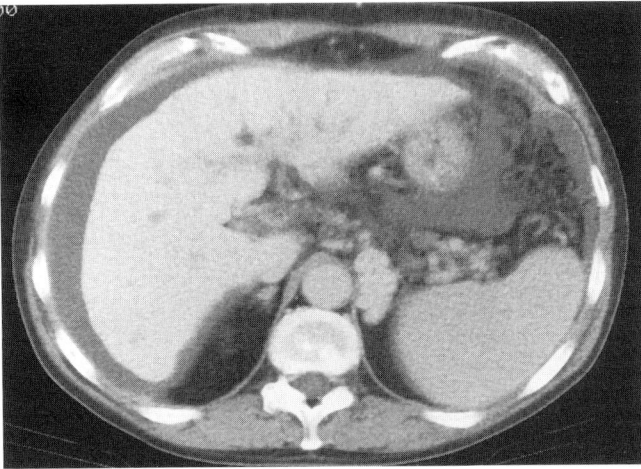

1. What storage diseases may result in increased liver density?

2. What drugs increase liver density?

3. What is the cause of primary hemochromatosis?

4. What is the long-term complication of this condition?

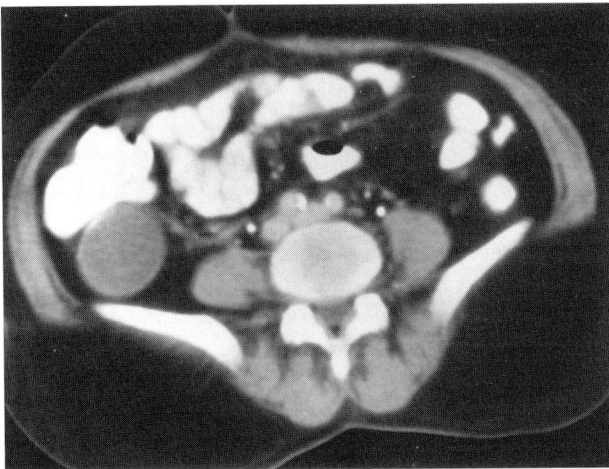 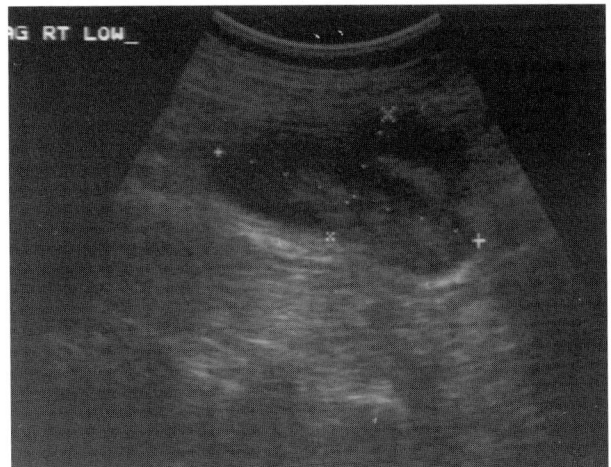

1. What abnormality often produces this condition?

2. What neoplastic processes may have this appearance?

3. If this mass ruptures, what condition may result?

4. What is meant by the term *myxoglobulosis?*

Hemochromatosis

1. Hemosiderosis, hemochromatosis, and glycogen storage disease.

2. Amiodarone and gold therapy.

3. Genetics (inherited disorder).

4. Hepatocellular carcinoma.

Reference

Stark DD: Hepatic iron overload: paramagnetic pathology, *Radiology* 179:333-335, 1989.

Cross-Reference

Gastrointestinal Radiology: THE REQUISITES, ed 2, p 185.

Comment

The CT scan shows a diffuse increase in the density of the liver in relation to the spleen. Only a few conditions produce an overall increase in density of the liver. Usually, this finding is the result of hemosiderosis or hemochromatosis. Glycogen storage diseases may increase liver density, but they also cause fatty infiltration of the liver, so the density is more often normal to hypodense in patients with those conditions. Amiodarone is a drug that contains large amounts of iodine. During long-term amiodarone therapy, iodine is deposited in the liver, resulting in an increase in density. Gold therapy in patients with rheumatoid arthritis also leads to an increase in liver density. Patients who have endured long-term arsenic poisoning as a result of drinking contaminated water also develop this appearance of the liver on CT.

Hemosiderosis is iron deposition in organs that does not produce organ damage. Hemochromatosis is iron overload that eventually damages the liver and other organs. Primary hemochromatosis is an inherited disorder of abnormal iron deposition. Secondary hemochromatosis is caused by the excessive liberation of iron from red blood cells, which occurs in conditions such as hemolytic anemias. Also, excessive blood transfusions (dialysis patients) or excessive iron intake can produce hemochromatosis. Hemochromatosis also results in cirrhosis, diabetes mellitus, and hyperpigmentation.

The liver is the organ most severely affected by hemochromatosis. Other organs affected include the spleen, kidneys, heart, endocrine glands, and gastrointestinal tract. Cirrhosis of the liver occurs and may be irreversible even if the iron levels can be effectively lowered. Hepatocellular carcinoma is a common late complication of hemochromatosis.

Notes

Mucocele of the Appendix

1. Obstruction of the appendiceal lumen.

2. Cystadenoma or cystadenocarcinoma.

3. Pseudomyxoma peritonei.

4. Type of mucocele with numerous small globules of mucin in the lumen.

Reference

Madwell D, Mindelzun R, Jeffrey RB: Mucocele of the appendix: imaging findings, *Am J Roentgenol* 159:69-72, 1992.

Cross-Reference

Gastrointestinal Radiology: THE REQUISITES, ed 2, p 286.

Comment

The term *mucocele of the appendix* describes a condition in which the appendiceal lumen is dilated by thick mucinous secretions. Sometimes this dilation leads to marked enlargement of the lumen until it becomes cystic or masslike. Mucoceles are usually the result of some type of process obstructing the lumen of the appendix. These processes include scarring, a fecalith, a tumor, or a cecal lesion. Tumors that produce this condition are cystadenomas and cystadenocarcinomas. Benign causes greatly exceed malignant causes of this process by a wide margin. Patients tend to complain of a dull pain in the right lower quadrant. Sometimes a mass may be clinically palpable.

Radiologically, on plain films there may be rimlike calcification about the mucocele. A mass effect may be evident on plain films or on barium enema, but this finding is indistinguishable from an inflammatory mass or abscess. On ultrasound the lumen of the appendix is visibly anechoic, although there may be some echoes or debris at the dependent portion of the lumen. Through transmission also is increased. CT examination shows that the appendiceal lumen is dilated and filled with a low density material. It may be soft tissue density, or the density may approach that of water. CT is also good for identifying rimlike calcifications.

Myxoglobulosis is a variant of a mucocele in which the lumen is filled with multiple small globules of mucin. When a mucocele ruptures, it may produce a condition known as *pseudomyxoma peritonei.* This condition can occur as a result of either benign or malignant causes of mucocele.

Notes

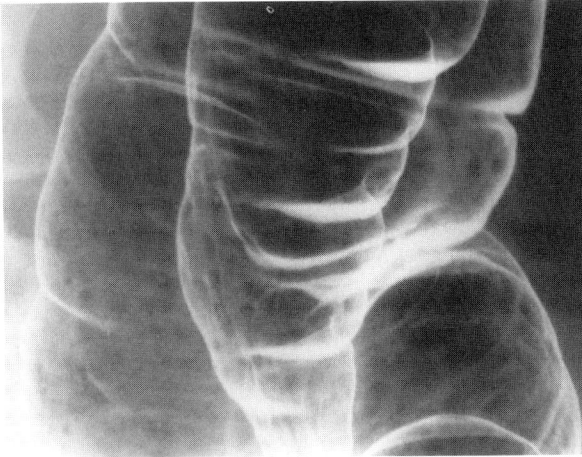

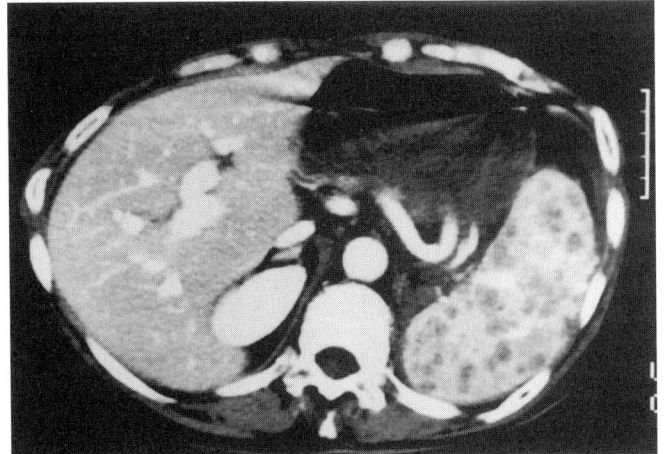

1. What is the incidence of lymphoid follicles among healthy adults?
2. Name some pathologic processes that cause prominent lymphoid follicles.
3. Patients with a compromised body system may have numerous lymphoid follicles. Name the body system.
4. What pulmonary condition presents as small nodules in the gastrointestinal tract?

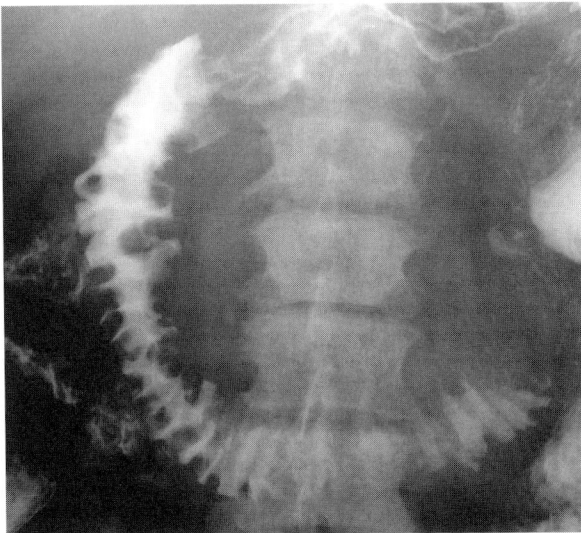

1. What conditions may produce elevated serum gastrin levels?
2. What are the major symptoms of elevated gastrin levels?
3. What structures in the body contain histamine?
4. What organs are involved in systemic mastocytosis?

C A S E   1 7 1

Sarcoidosis of the Colon

1. Approximately 10%.

2. Intestinal infections and parasites, Crohn's disease, dysgammaglobulinemia, ulcerative colitis, leukemia, and lymphoma.

3. Immune system (particularly patients with immunoglobulin deficiencies).

4. Sarcoidosis.

Reference

Kenney PJ, Koehler RE, Shackelford GD: The clinical significance of large lymphoid follicles of the colon, *Radiology* 142:41-46, 1982.

Cross-Reference

Gastrointestinal Radiology: THE REQUISITES, ed 2, p 256.

Comment

The intestinal tract represents one of the largest components of the human immune system. Thus any process that leads to a response from the immune system can manifest itself in the gastrointestinal tract, often in the form of lymphoid follicles in the bowel wall. Lymphoid follicles are common in children and less common in adults, although they are present in up to 10% of healthy adults. Normal lymphoid follicles range up to 5 mm in diameter, although they may be larger. Size is not a crucial point in differentiating normal and abnormal lymphoid follicular responses. Any inflammatory condition of the gut, such as inflammatory bowel disease, infections, or parasites, may produce a diffuse response of the immunologic tissue of the bowel. Also, systemic processes, such as leukemia and lymphoma, are known to infiltrate the lymph tissue of the gut. Finally, when there is a dysfunction of the immune system, enlarged lymphoid follicles may develop. This process is particularly evident in patients with immunoglobulin deficiencies.

Perhaps the rarest cause of enlarged lymphoid follicles of the colon is sarcoidosis. Sarcoidosis is a systemic granulomatous disease of unknown etiology that is manifested pathologically by noncaseating granulomas containing multinucleated giant cells. Although commonly the chest and adjacent lymph nodes are involved, other organs, such as the spleen and even the liver, may be involved. Also, sarcoidosis can affect the eye, skin, heart, muscles, and even nervous system. There are several reports of sarcoidosis of the gastrointestinal tract found incidentally at biopsy. The condition typically manifests itself as small nodules or bumps along the wall of the bowel. Rarely, sarcoidosis causes a fibrotic narrowing. The intestinal organ most commonly involved is the stomach, and then the colon. In the colon the condition manifests itself as prominent lymphoid follicles. Sarcoidosis should be considered in any patient with known sarcoidosis and nodules of the bowel wall. Treatment is steroids, and response is usually rapid.

Notes

C A S E   1 7 2

Systemic Mastocytosis (Urticaria Pigmentosa)

1. Gastrinoma, histamine release, achlorhydria, pernicious anemia, and G-cell hyperplasia.

2. Abdominal pain secondary to peptic ulcer disease and diarrhea caused by malabsorption.

3. Mast cells.

4. Skin, gastrointestinal tract, bone, liver, and spleen.

Reference

Avila NA, Ling A, Worobec AS, et al: Systemic mastocytosis: CT and US features of abdominal manifestations, *Radiology* 202:367-371, 1997.

Cross-Reference

Gastrointestinal Radiology: THE REQUISITES, ed 2, p 113.

Comment

A number of clinical conditions produce elevated serum gastrin levels. The most well known cause is Zollinger-Ellison (Z-E) syndrome, resulting from a gastrin-producing tumor. Another condition associated with elevated gastrin is mastocytosis. Mastocytosis is an accumulation of mast cells in the skin and various other organs. Mast cells are responsible for storage and release of histamine. Histamine increases gastrin levels, although not to the extent seen in patients with Z-E syndrome (often in excess of 1000 pg/ml).

Mastocytosis typically involves the skin. When the mast cells are disturbed and release histamine, they produce raised elevations, accounting for the disease description *urticaria pigmentosa.* It is less commonly known that other organs may be involved with a mast cell infiltrate; this occurrence is termed *systemic mastocytosis.* The gastrointestinal tract (small bowel) is the second most commonly involved organ after the skin; the bone, liver, and spleen also can be involved. There can be both local and systemic release of histamine. Clinically, patients complain of bouts of diarrhea, flushing, and tachycardia. Alcohol consumption may precipitate the symptoms, and the condition is treated with histamine receptor antagonists.

Radiologically, small bowel examination shows thickened folds and sometimes bowel wall thickening. Elevated mucosal lesions and "bull's eye" lesions have been described. Because of the increased gastrin levels, there is a high incidence of peptic ulcer disease, as well as increased fluid in the small bowel. All of these abnormalities may be present in the individual with Z-E syndrome. However, mastocytosis can involve the bone marrow, producing diffuse sclerotic changes. In this case the lumbar vertebra are quite dense. This change, along with the fold abnormalities, suggests the diagnosis of mastocytosis.

Notes

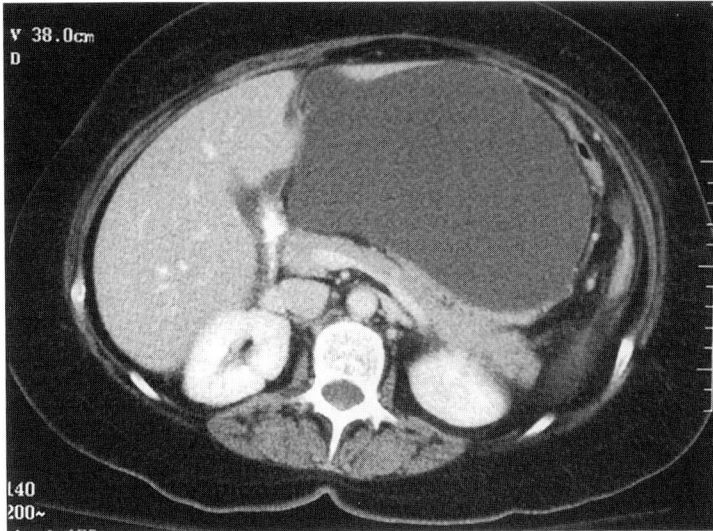

1. If this patient had cholecystectomy 2 weeks ago, what is the most likely diagnosis?
2. Name some causes for this condition.
3. What effect does bile have on the peritoneal cavity?
4. What is the best method for evaluation of this complication?

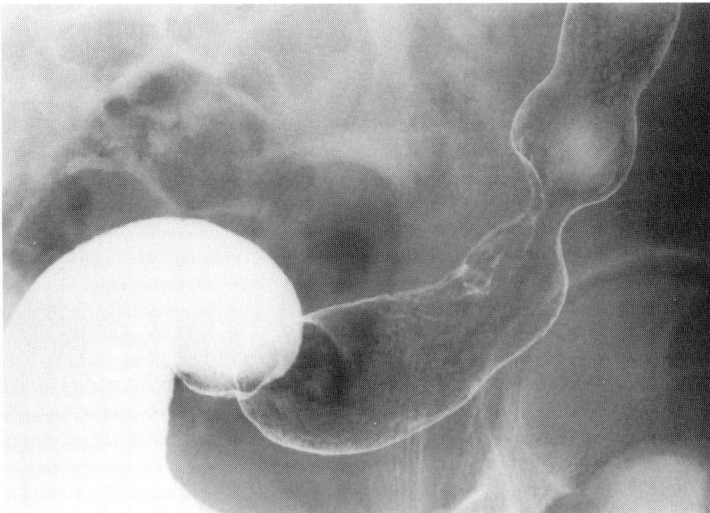

1. What is the significance of strictures in the patient with ulcerative colitis?
2. What is the premalignant change in ulcerative colitis termed?
3. What colitic patients have an increased incidence of malignancy?
4. What is the approximate risk associated with this condition?

CASE 173

Biloma

1. Leakage from the bile ducts with biloma.

2. Inadvertent laceration of a duct, poor suturing of a duct, and slippage of a catheter.

3. Mild peritonitis.

4. Direct injection of the ducts.

Reference

Ghahremani GG, Crampton AR, Bernstein JR, et al: Iatrogenic biliary tract complications: radiologic features and clinical significance, *Radiographics* 11:441-456, 1991.

Cross-Reference

Gastrointestinal Radiology: THE REQUISITES, ed 2, p 214.

Comment

This case illustrates the development of a large fluid collection in the upper abdomen after cholecystectomy. Cholecystectomy is one of the most frequently performed surgical procedures, and a laparoscopic approach is being used in an increasing number of these procedures. Despite its frequency, cholecystectomy is fraught with complications. Fluid collections visible on CT examination after surgery could be caused by abscess, hemorrhage with hematoma, or a collection of bile (biloma).

Bilomas are collections of bile and are usually visible in the upper abdomen. They are an infrequent but serious complication that can occur after any type of manipulation or trauma to the biliary tract, and they are often iatrogenic in nature. Bile leakage into the peritoneal cavity is a serious complication in that bile induces a peritonitis, and patients have fever and peritoneal signs, mimicking an abscess or infection. Bilomas may result from cutting or perforating one of the bile ducts, usually inadvertently. Often, anomalous ducts either draining into the gallbladder or near the cystic duct are cut during cholecystectomy, unbeknownst to the surgeon. Another cause of biloma is inadequate suturing or slippage of a suture or clip off of a ligated duct, resulting in leakage. Sometimes the T tube slips out of the extrahepatic ducts, and bile drains into the peritoneal cavity because of this malpositioned tube, which is what occurred in this patient.

Usually, direct injection of the bile ducts is necessary to identify with certainty the exact site of leakage. This identification is important because surgical repair of the leaking duct is often necessary. Of course, the leakage is worse if there is postoperative obstruction of the ducts caused by a retained common bile duct stone. Although catheter drainage can be performed, ligation of the leaking duct is still necessary for adequate treatment.

Notes

CASE 174

Dysplasia and Carcinoma in Ulcerative Colitis

1. Strictures can be benign or malignant.

2. Dysplasia.

3. Typically those with pancolitis; it is less common among those with left-sided colitis.

4. 10% chance of malignancy after 10 years, with a slight increase with age.

Reference

Feczko PJ: Malignancy complicating inflammatory bowel disease, *Radiol Clin North Am* 25:157-174, 1987.

Cross-Reference

Gastrointestinal Radiology: THE REQUISITES, ed 2, p 242.

Comment

It has been known for several decades that patients with ulcerative colitis are at increased risk for developing colorectal carcinoma. This incidence increases with age, and those who develop ulcerative colitis in childhood are at the greatest risk. Patients with pancolitis have the greatest risk, whereas those with colitis confined to the left side have a lesser risk. Inflammation of the rectum (i.e., proctitis) does not appear to be associated with increased risk. Patients with recurrent inflammation seem to have a higher incidence of cancer, but even one episode of severe colitis may lead to cancer at a later date. The overall incidence of cancer is believed to be around 10%.

Carcinoma in patients with long-term ulcerative colitis is different than in the ordinary population. There is a much higher incidence of synchronous malignancies (25% or greater). These tumors tend to have a higher incidence of poor differentiation and are often mucinous in nature. Also, the growth of the malignancies can be unusual, including plaquelike lesions and scirrhous tumors.

For the past two decades, there has been an emphasis on screening these patients for neoplastic and preneoplastic changes. The term *dysplasia* refers to a mucosal change that is believed to be a marker lesion for malignancy. It can be found at and near sites of malignancy in patients with ulcerative colitis. Often, dysplasia is multifocal in nature. Some consider it a premalignant condition because of its strong association with later carcinomatous change. Colonoscopy has been used to randomly biopsy the mucosa and detect areas of dysplastic mucosa. Occasionally the dysplasia is visible radiologically. It has several features. Sometimes it has a plaquelike or "mosaic tile" appearance. Other times it has the appearance of an ordinary polyp. When dysplasia is detected, proctocolectomy is often considered because of the condition's strong relationship to malignancy.

Notes

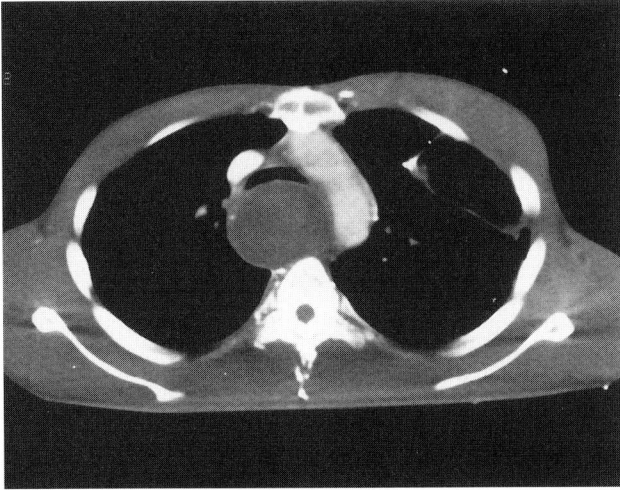

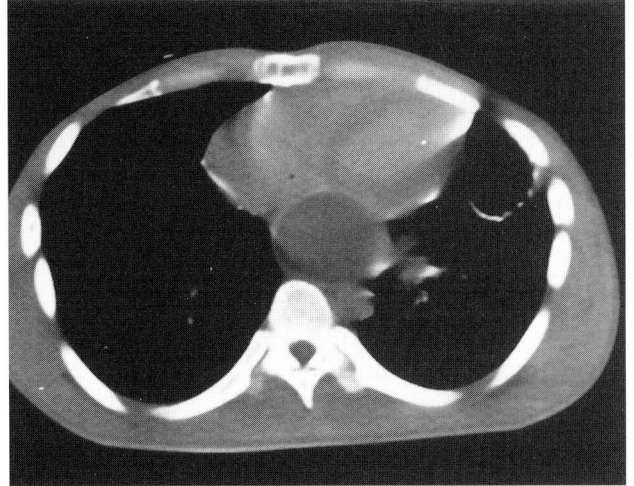

1. What are the indications for colonic interposition to treat esophageal disease?
2. Name a few of the complications associated with this condition.
3. Does malignancy ever develop within the colonic interposition?
4. What occurs in the bypassed esophagus?

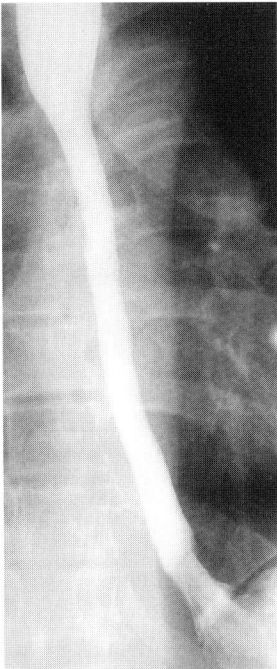

1. What iatrogenic condition may produce these changes?
2. Name two skin conditions that affect the esophagus as depicted in this case.
3. Name a diffuse intestinal condition that may stricture the esophagus.
4. What long-term complication may occur with diffuse stricturing?

Mucocele of the Esophagus After Colonic Interposition

1. Typically, benign disease, such as severe strictures, perforation, and failed surgical procedures, and rarely malignancy.

2. Leakage at an anastomosis is the most common; fistulas, strictures, ischemia, aspiration, food retention, and mucocele of the bypassed esophagus also can occur.

3. Rarely, but colonic malignancy has been reported in the colonic interposition.

4. A mucocele may develop within several months of the surgery.

Reference
Glickstein MF, et al: Esophageal mucocele after surgical isolation of the esophagus, *Am J Roentgenol* 149:729-730, 1987.

Cross-Reference
Gastrointestinal Radiology: THE REQUISITES, ed 2, p 41.

Comment
The patient with severe esophageal disease may require surgical bypass when he or she is no longer capable of using the native esophagus. Some surgeons use a length of colon and anastomose it from the upper thoracic or cervical esophagus to the stomach, thus bypassing the diseased esophagus. The remaining esophagus may be surgically isolated but not removed because of potential damage to nerves, lymphatics, and collateral blood flow. This procedure is most commonly performed in patients with benign diseases, such as caustic or peptic strictures, or severe motor disorders. Occasionally it is performed in patients with malignant disease, particularly if there is a good chance of survival, or if a complication, such as perforation, has occurred.

Complications are common because of the complexity of the surgery. Early complications include anastomotic leakage and possible fistula formation. Stenoses also may develop at the anastomotic sites, typically the proximal site. Aspiration of ingested contents is another problem. Later problems include stasis of swallowed material within the interposed segment and reflux of gastric contents into the colonic interposition. Malignancy has been described in these colonic interpositions, but it is rare, and any increased incidence is unlikely.

If in the course of the surgery, usually related to the pathologic process, the surgeon isolates the esophagus by surgically closing its ends, a mucocele of the esophagus may develop. This mucocele consists of mucous or proteinaceous secretions that fill the lumen of the isolated esophagus and have nowhere to drain. Usually the phenomenon is self-limited because increasing pressure within the lumen causes cessation of the mucous secretion. Rarely the mass continues to increase in size, leading to symptoms.

Notes

Diffuse Esophageal Stricture in Epidermolysis Bullosa

1. Radiation therapy to the mediastinum.

2. Epidermolysis bullosa dystrophica, pemphigoid, and rarely erythema multiforme.

3. Both Crohn's disease and eosinophilic gastroenteritis may result in stricture development.

4. Esophageal carcinoma has developed in some patients with these conditions, but the relationship is tenuous.

Reference
Tishler JM, et al: Esophageal involvement in epidermolysis bullosa dystrophica, *Am J Roentgenol* 141:1283-1286, 1983.

Cross-Reference
Gastrointestinal Radiology: THE REQUISITES, ed 2, p 24.

Comment
Diffuse esophageal stricturing can be produced by a number of conditions. The most common iatrogenic cause is radiation therapy. Ingestion of corrosive agents also produces strictures, as well as repeated episodes of inflammation. Rare skin conditions affect the esophageal mucosa, resulting in stricturing.

Epidermolysis bullosa dystrophica is a hereditary condition that can be either autosomal dominant or recessive. This condition results in minor trauma producing separation of the epidermis from the dermis, with secondary bullous formation. This disease is apparent in childhood but usually regresses in later life. Esophageal involvement develops because swallowing solid foods produces esophageal bullae and secondary mucosal sloughing and scarring, resulting in esophageal stricturing.

The term *pemphigoid* refers to two similar conditions that cause bullous changes of the skin and mucous membranes. Benign mucous membrane pemphigoid produces bullous eruptions on the mucous membranes and the esophagus. This condition affects middle-aged patients, often women. It can produce sloughing of esophageal mucosa, with subsequent stricturing. Bullous pemphigoid is a related condition that predominantly involves the skin. It occurs in elderly patients and rarely involves the esophagus. It may produce acute bullous eruptions in the esophagus but does not result in strictures. Erythema multiforme is an allergic reaction to certain medications that is quite unpredictable. In its most severe forms erythema multiforme may produce sloughing of the skin, mucous membranes, and rarely mucosa of the esophagus. As can other conditions that cause diffuse mucosal injury of the esophagus, erythema multiforme can result in stricturing.

Later development of esophageal carcinoma has been reported in patients with epidermolysis bullosa. However, these conditions are rare, and it is difficult to determine whether there is a causal relationship.

Notes

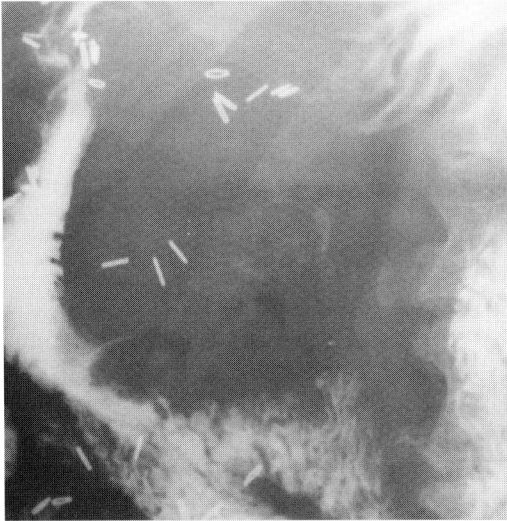

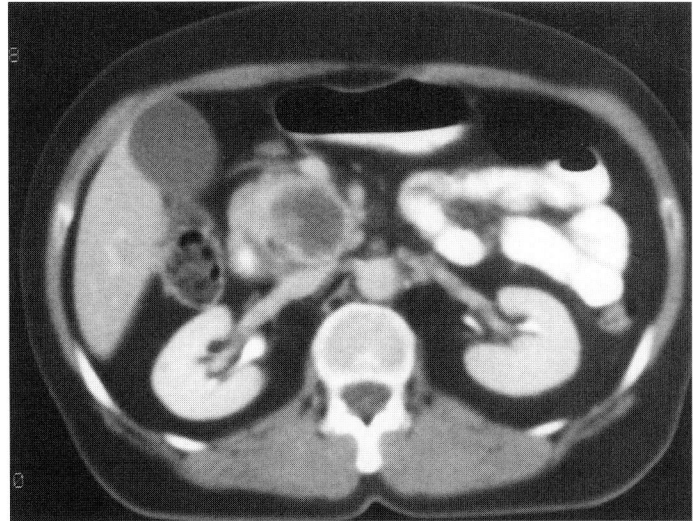

1. Does ductal adenocarcinoma of the pancreas calcify?
2. Which tumors of the pancreas calcify?
3. How often do pseudocysts calcify?
4. Which tumor produces a sunburst or stellate calcification?

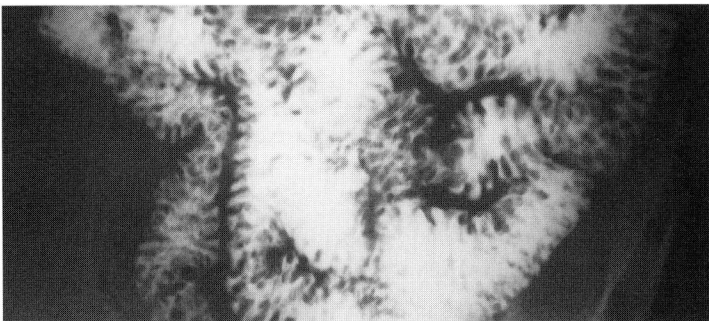

1. What process often produces regular fold thickening of the intestines?
2. What congenital problem may produce this appearance?
3. What clinical problem also may affect patients with this condition?
4. What is meant by the term *secondary lymphangiectasia?*

Calcification in a Microcystic Adenoma

1. Only rarely.

2. Cystic neoplasms, islet cell tumors, papillary neoplasms, and cystic teratomas.

3. Uncommonly (less than 10%).

4. Microcystic adenoma, or teratoma.

Reference

Friedman AC, Lichtenstein JE, Dachman AH: Cystic neoplasms of the pancreas: radiologic-pathologic correlation, *Radiology* 149:45-50, 1983.

Cross-Reference

Gastrointestinal Radiology: THE REQUISITES, ed 2, p 151.

Comment

Calcifications within the pancreas are most often attributed to chronic pancreatitis; 95% or more of calcifications in the pancreas are associated with this condition. However, both inflammatory and neoplastic masses of the pancreas can produce calcification, and sometimes these masses are the first abnormalities that are apparent radiologically. Pseudocysts calcify occasionally, but their peripheral curvilinear calcification is fairly distinctive. Calcification has been described in other tumors, however.

Microcystic adenoma is an unusual neoplasm found predominantly in women. This tumor has multiple small cysts of varying size within it. Microcystic adenoma is vascular on angiography, and a central scar or area of necrosis is often evident. This central scar tends to calcify and produce a stellate or "sunburst" type of calcification. This tumor is believed to have no malignant potential. Mucinous cystic neoplasms also calcify. The cysts in these tumors are either large and unilocular or large and multiseptate. If calcifications occur, they tend to be peripheral, simulating a pancreatic pseudocyst. Sunburst calcifications were initially attributed to mucinous cystic tumors, but this relationship is now considered rare, and many of these calcifications have been reclassified as microcystic adenomas.

Rarely, islet cell tumors may have areas of necrosis and calcification. A rare teratoma of the pancreas is another tumor that may calcify. Papillary epithelial neoplasms also have been described with calcification, although it is typically peripheral.

Notes

Lymphangiectasia

1. Edema or hemorrhage.

2. Lymphangiectasia.

3. Malabsorption and steatorrhea.

4. Lymph ducts draining the intestines become obstructed because of some underlying disease process.

Reference

Stevens RL, Jones B, Fishman EK: CT halo sign: new finding in intestinal lymphangiectasia, *J Comput Assist Tomogr* 21:1005-1011, 1997.

Cross-Reference

Gastrointestinal Radiology: THE REQUISITES, ed 2, p 111.

Comment

Edema of bowel can be present in patients with a variety of conditions. It probably occurs most commonly in patients with end-stage liver or kidney failure. Any debilitating condition that reduces the serum albumin level below 2 g also can produce edematous changes in the intestines.

Lymphangiectasia is a rarer condition, however. There are two different categories. The first is primary lymphangiectasia, which is dilation of the small lymphatic channels in the mucosa and submucosa of the bowel wall. The exact cause for the development of this condition is uncertain, but it is believed to be some type of congenital defect or weakness. As these lymph channels become dilated and engorged, particularly during the digestive process, the possibility of rupture increases. It is believed that either leakage or rupture of these dilated lymph channels leads to loss of protein and fat into the intestinal lumen. These patients lose protein into the bowel, leading to hypoproteinemia, which causes some of the edema and fold thickening that is evident on small bowel examination. Also, these patients can develop a malabsorptive condition as a result of the failure of the lymph channels to properly transport digested materials to the liver. Steatorrhea also can occur as the fat is lost back into the lumen of the bowel. Treatment consists of a low-fat diet and steroids. Radiologically these patients have thickened folds throughout the intestines but particularly proximally. Small bowel enteroclysis may demonstrate fine micronodules on the surface of the folds, measuring 1 to 2 mm in diameter. These are considered individual villi that are dilated because of the distended lymph channels.

Secondary lymphangiectasia is dilation of the lymph channels secondary to some process that may be producing obstruction of the lymph drainage from the bowel. Most typically this dilation is found in malignancies that have prominent adenopathy. Also, retroperitoneal fibrosis and fibrosis caused by radiation therapy are known causes. Rarely this process is seen in patients with Crohn's disease or Whipple's disease.

Notes

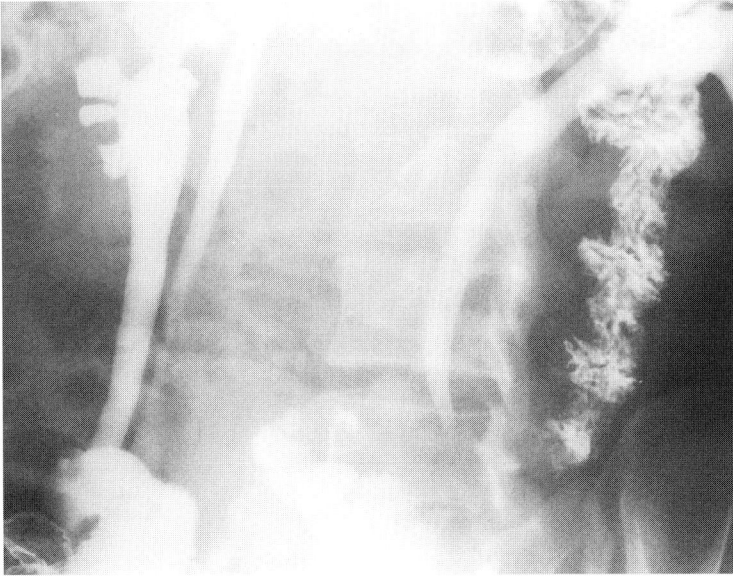

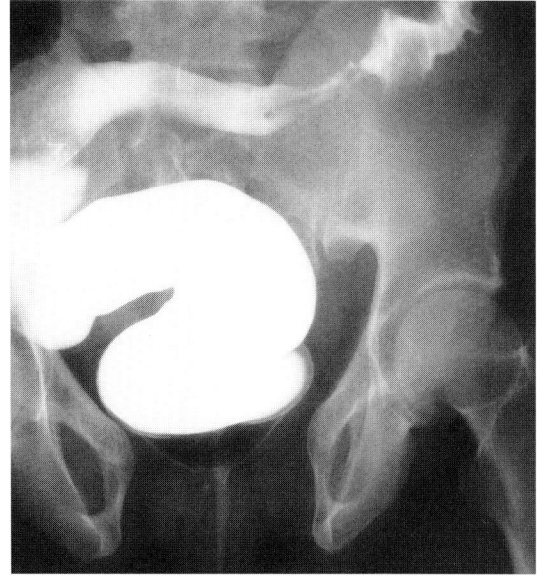

1. What stomach surgery is associated with an increased risk of carcinoma after many years?
2. What surgical procedure performed in patients with Crohn's disease is associated with a higher incidence of later malignancy?
3. What is the cause of this ureteroenteric connection?
4. What is a major complication of prolonged exposure of the gastrointestinal tract to urine?

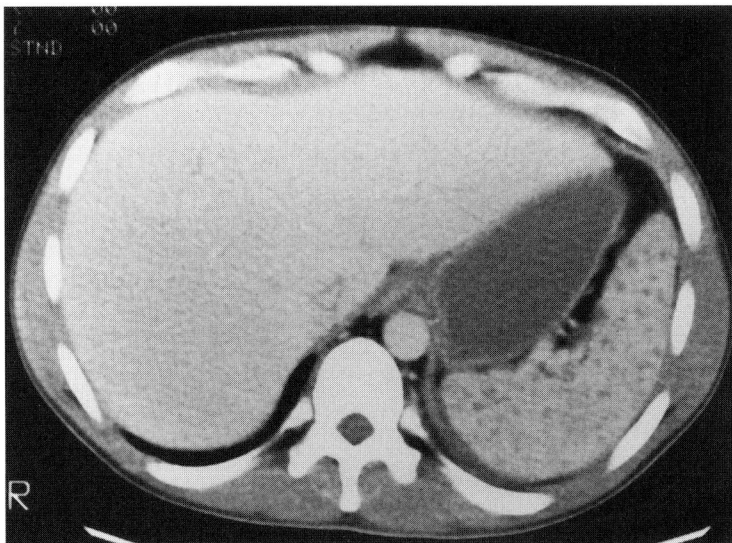

1. What underlying clinical state is often present in patients who develop this condition?
2. What common disease may mimic this condition?
3. What is the most common causative organism?
4. What other organisms also produce this appearance?

Colon Carcinoma After Ureterosigmoidostomy

1. Billroth II gastrojejunostomy.

2. Bypassing diseased loops of small bowel and not removing them.

3. Surgery.

4. Carcinoma of the intestines.

Reference

Princenthal RA, Lowman R, Zeman RK, Burrell M: Ureterosigmoidostomy: the development of tumors, diagnosis, and pitfalls, *Am J Roentgenol* 141:77-81, 1983.

Cross-Reference

Gastrointestinal Radiology: THE REQUISITES, ed 2, p 244.

Comment

It has been recognized for many years that patients undergoing gastrointestinal tract surgery for the treatment of benign disease have an increased incidence of malignancy many years after the procedure. The most well known of these procedures is the Billroth II gastrojejunostomy (for peptic ulcer disease); there is a reported increased incidence of gastric carcinoma occurring 10 or more years after this surgery. Also, patients with Crohn's disease who have had inflamed segments of bowel bypassed surgically but left in the abdomen have an increased risk of developing malignancy of the diseased segment.

Ureterosigmoidostomy is a surgical procedure that has been used for decades, and it was one of the first procedures to divert the urinary stream when the bladder could no longer function because of malignancy, congenital abnormality, or other diseases. The procedure itself has been supplanted by newer procedures for urinary diversion, but almost all of these procedures involve connecting the ureters to some portion of the intestinal tract, usually the ileum. It is now recognized that patients who had the urinary stream diverted into the colon are at a greater risk for the development of colon carcinoma. This increased risk may be a result of the effect of the urine on the colon's mucus production, other possible carcinogenic effects, and continued exposure to fecal material. Those patients with bladder exstrophy often underwent ureterosigmoidostomy, usually during childhood. Thus these patients had an entire lifespan to develop complications. Most tumors in this group develop 20 years or more after the surgical procedure. There have been only a few cases of carcinoma developing in patients who had ileal conduits performed for urinary diversion, and the neoplastic risk for this procedure is believed to be much lower.

Notes

Fungal Microabscesses

1. Immunosuppression.

2. Metastases.

3. *Candida* species.

4. *Aspergillus* and *Cryptococcus* species.

Reference

Shirkhoda A: CT findings in hepatosplenic and renal candidiasis, *J Comput Assist Tomogr* 11:795-798, 1987.

Cross-Reference

Gastrointestinal Radiology: THE REQUISITES, ed 2, p 192.

Comment

Multiple low density areas throughout the liver or spleen may be the result of metastases, which is the most common cause. However, when there are numerous tiny low density areas occurring diffusely, the possibility of microabscesses must be seriously considered. The lesions almost always occur in the setting of some type of immunosuppression (i.e., patients with acquired immunodeficiency syndrome, transplant recipients, those with leukemia, and cancer patients undergoing chemotherapy). Patients on steroid therapy comprise another subgroup to be considered. The microabscesses develop as the result of a systemic sepsis with a microorganism, usually fungal. However, many patients may have no irregular findings on blood cultures.

Candida albicans is the organism that most commonly produces this type of appearance. It is believed that the organism often resides in the immunosuppressed patient, and when the immune status of the patient reaches a certain threshold, a systemic infection occurs. Other organisms that also have been implicated include *Cryptococcus* and *Aspergillus* species. Rarely can this radiologic appearance be attributed to some type of bacterial infection. On ultrasound these abscesses have a bright central echogenic focus with a surrounding hypoechoic band and "bull's eye" lesion. Hepatic or splenic enlargement may be present. CT often reveals multiple low density areas in the liver or spleen that often do not exceed 1 cm in diameter. Sometimes there is a central area of high density. Renal involvement is common. The major differential considerations include metastases, and lymphoma may have a similar appearance.

Notes

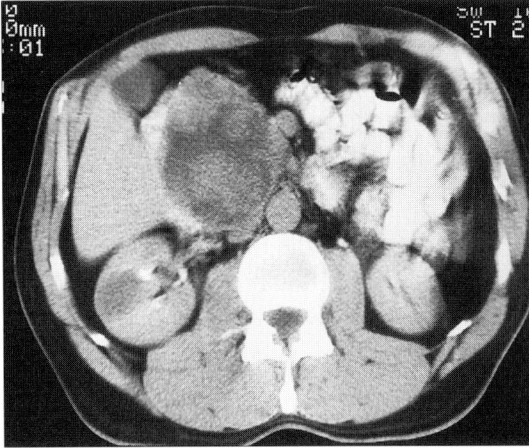

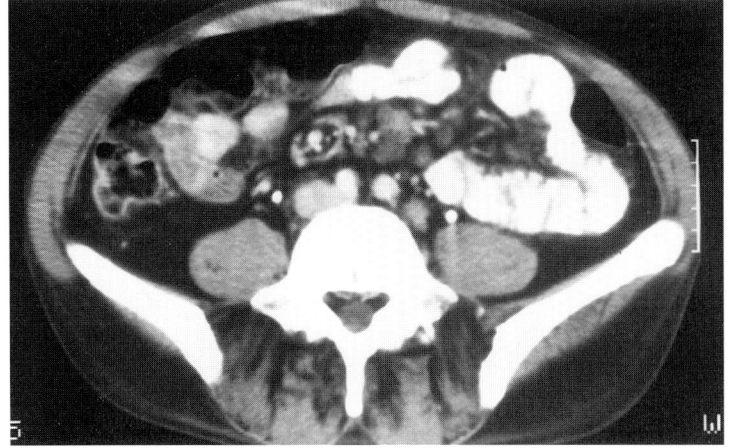

1. What necrotic or cystic masses may involve the pancreas?
2. This patient may have what underlying infection?
3. This condition also may occur after what type of surgery?
4. What neoplasm complicates the management of transplant recipients?

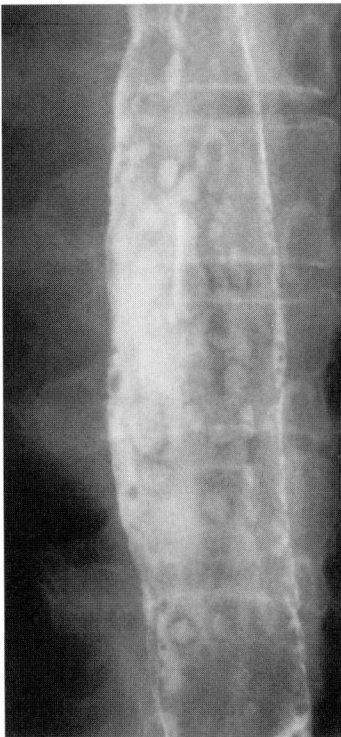

1. What conditions produce aphthous ulcers in the esophagus?
2. What two conditions produce colitis and esophagitis?
3. What is the rationale for the use of a tube esophagram?
4. Does esophageal Crohn's disease ever precede the intestinal disease?

CASE 181

Lymphoma Complicating AIDS

1. Mucinous tumors of the pancreas, necrotic adenocarcinoma, and lymphoma.

2. Human immunodeficiency virus (HIV).

3. Transplantation.

4. Lymphoma.

Reference

Redvanly RD, Silverstein JE: Intra-abdominal manifestations of AIDS, *Radiol Clin North Am* 35:1083-1098, 1997.

Cross-Reference

Gastrointestinal Radiology: THE REQUISITES, ed 2, p 311.

Comment

The CT images demonstrate a large, necrotic mass involving the region of the head of the pancreas, although there does not appear to be any associated bile duct obstruction. A soft tissue mass of the right kidney also is evident, and adenopathy is present in the peritoneum. This constellation of findings is suggestive of a multifocal neoplastic process. Neoplasms of the pancreas rarely produce adenopathy of the mesentery or result in renal masses. A renal tumor metastasizing to the pancreas is more likely. The most likely possibility is lymphoma with multiple organ involvement. Lymphoma of the pancreas is rare and almost always occurs as a manifestation of diffuse disease. Often it is a result of adenopathy in the periaortic region, with secondary invasion of the pancreatic tissue. Lymphoma does not produce vascular or biliary encasement and neither do primary pancreatic tumors.

Lymphoma involving multiple solid organs in the abdomen is uncommon but does occur in healthy patients and in those who are immunosuppressed. Patients with HIV infection are prone to the development of malignancies, particularly Kaposi's sarcoma and lymphoma. In the illustrated case the patient was known to have AIDS, and the aforementioned constellation of findings was strongly indicative of lymphoma. Another group that develops lymphoma in a rapid, diffuse fashion are transplant recipients. Lymphoma tends to occur within the first few years after transplant and is the result of the immunosuppressive drugs that are given to prevent rejection. The lymphoma is often multifocal at the time of diagnosis and may involve multiple abdominal organs.

Notes

CASE 182

Crohn's Disease of the Esophagus

1. Viral esophagitis (e.g., cytomegalovirus, herpesvirus), medication esophagitis, and Crohn's disease.

2. Crohn's disease and Behçet's disease.

3. To improve coating or distention, particularly when the patient is unable to swallow.

4. Rarely. Patients with esophageal Crohn's disease almost always have known intestinal disease.

Reference

Ghahremani GG, et al: Esophageal manifestations of Crohn's disease, *Gastrointest Radiol* 7:199-203, 1982.

Cross-Reference

Gastrointestinal Radiology: THE REQUISITES, ed 2, p 18.

Comment

An aphthous ulcer is characterized by a round or oval collection of contrast with a surrounding band of lucency. The contrast collection represents the ulcer, whereas the lucent halo is edematous tissue elevated about the ulcer crater. Typically the surrounding mucosa is normal, although in severe cases the ulceration could become diffuse. These ulcers can occur anywhere in the gastrointestinal tract. In the esophagus, viral infections, such as cytomegalovirus or herpesvirus, produce this type of ulceration. Medication ulcers produced by consumption of tetracycline or antiinflammatory agents also can have this appearance.

Two multisystem diseases cause both colitis and esophageal ulceration. The more common is Crohn's disease. The esophagus is the least common site in the gastrointestinal tract for the occurrence of Crohn's disease. Patients with Crohn's involvement of the esophagus may have not only dysphagia, but odynophagia, or painful swallowing, as well. Typically, esophageal involvement occurs well after ileocolitis. Rarely, it is the presenting complaint of Crohn's disease, or it occurs before the intestinal disease. The extent of esophageal involvement is often just a few aphthous ulcers. In severe cases there may be diffuse ulceration, sinus tracts, and even fistulas into surrounding structures. Repeated ulceration may result in stricture formation caused by fibrosis and scarring. Even postinflammatory polyposis has been reported in patients with esophageal Crohn's disease.

Behçet's disease is manifested by skin lesions and multisystem inflammation, including arthritis and colitis. Rarely, it involves the esophagus. Behçet's disease is always included in the differential diagnosis of processes that produce aphthous ulceration of the gastrointestinal tract and can produce inflammatory changes similar to those produced by Crohn's disease.

A tube esophagram is performed by passing a small (pediatric) catheter orally into the upper esophagus and injecting barium and air. It can be performed to focally study a mucosal process or stricture of the esophagus.

Notes

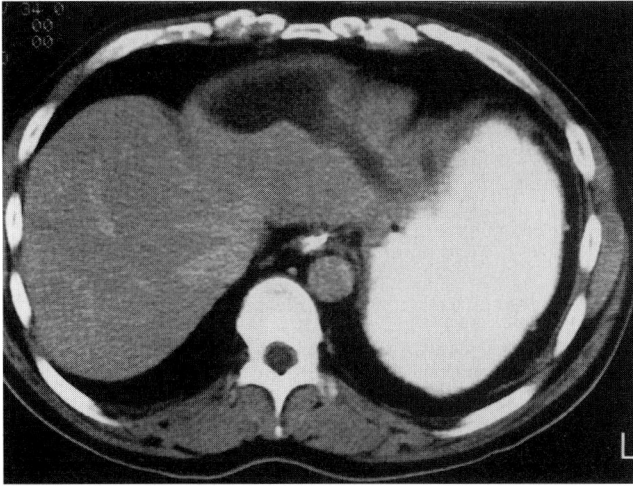

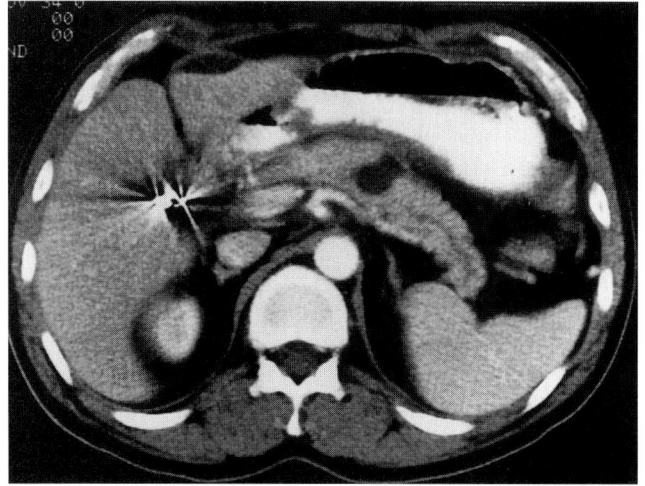

1. What is the significance of a high density pseudocyst?
2. Congenital cysts of the pancreas are related to which conditions?
3. Pathologically, what differentiates a pseudocyst from a true cyst?
4. How often do pseudocysts communicate with the pancreatic duct?

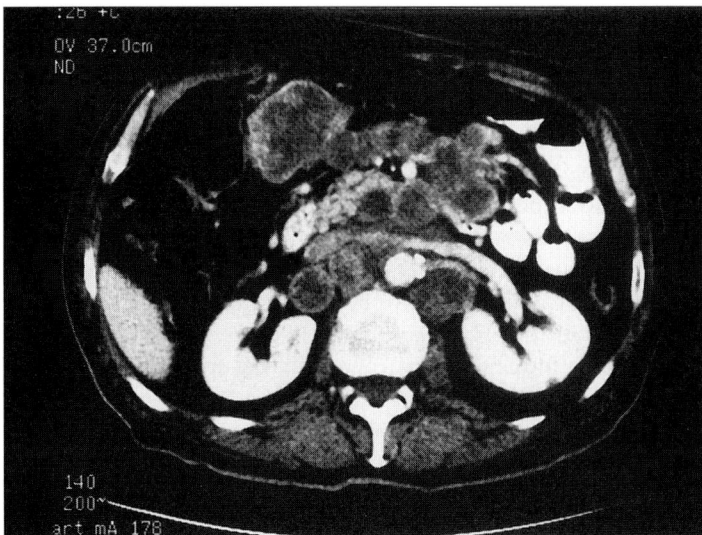

1. What infectious process may produce this change?
2. Name the neoplastic processes that may produce this change.
3. What infiltrative small bowel disease causes development of this condition?
4. With what clinical condition is this condition often associated?

Intrahepatic Pseudocyst

1. Indicates hemorrhage into the cyst.

2. Polycystic kidney disease and von Hippel-Lindau disease.

3. True cysts have an epithelial lining.

4. Uncommonly.

Reference

Ros PR, Hamrick-Turner JE, Chiechi MV, et al: Cystic masses of the pancreas, *Radiographics* 12:673-686, 1992.

Cross-Reference

Gastrointestinal Radiology: THE REQUISITES, ed 2, p 150.

Comment

There are several different types of pancreatic cysts, including true cysts, pseudocysts, and infectious (echinococcal) cysts. True cysts of the pancreas are caused by abnormal segmentation of the ducts. They have an epithelial lining that differentiates them from pseudocysts, which have a fibrous lining. True pancreatic cysts can be either solitary or multilocular in appearance and do not have an enhancing wall. Most true cysts are incidental findings. However, whenever multiple cysts of the pancreas are evident, the possibility of a congenital condition should be considered. Multiple true cysts are found in many patients with polycystic kidney disease and are present in patients with von Hippel-Lindau disease, which also is associated with a high incidence of pancreatic tumors.

Pseudocysts of the pancreas are a sequela of episodes of inflammation or pancreatitis. Fluid can be visible in or about the pancreas during acute pancreatitis. Most of this fluid is reabsorbed in the next few weeks. Fluid collections that are not reabsorbed can coalesce and organize, with a fibrous capsule surrounding them. If this process, which usually takes around 6 weeks, occurs, the growth can be termed a *pseudocyst.* Pseudocysts can have a capsule evident on CT. These pseudocysts can compress adjacent structures, producing symptoms, or can be occult. They can be found in any location within the abdomen because of the nature of their formation and even have been found in the lower chest. In this case the pseudocyst has penetrated the liver capsule. Rarely, pseudocysts resolve spontaneously as a result of drainage into the pancreatic duct or the adjacent hollow viscera. If the pseudocyst increases in density, it either has become infected or has had hemorrhage into it. Hemorrhage results in very high density pseudocysts.

Notes

Low Density Lymphadenopathy

1. Mycobacterial infection.

2. Testicular tumors and mucinous adenocarcinoma.

3. Whipple's disease.

4. Acquired immunodeficiency syndrome (AIDS).

Reference

Einstein DM, Singer AA, Chlcote WA, et al: Abdominal lymphadenopathy: spectrum of CT findings, *Radiographics* 11:457-472, 1991.

Cross-Reference

Gastrointestinal Radiology: THE REQUISITES, ed 2, p 307.

Comment

The CT image shows numerous enlarged lymph nodes in the paraaortic region and the root of the mesentery. Numerous diseases may cause this presentation. However, a distinguishing feature of this adenopathy is the low density of the nodes, particularly centrally where they are of a lower density than the periphery. This low density is present in only a few diseases and suggests certain diagnoses given enough clinical information.

Low density lymphadenopathy can present in patients with infections produced by *Mycobacterium* species. Initially, it was considered pathognomonic of *Mycobacterium avium-intracellulare* infection, which was common among AIDS patients. However, this type of adenopathy also can present in patients with *Mycobacterium tuberculosis* infections. Several tumors develop low density lymph nodes. The best known of these tumors are nonseminomatous tumors of the testes. Rarely, mucinous adenocarcinomas develop low density lymph nodes. Patients with lymphoma who are undergoing therapy may have areas of low density centrally in the adenopathy because of necrosis, but this finding is rare. Low density nodes also have been described anecdotally in epidermoid genitourinary tumors. Another disease process that results in the development of this low density adenopathy is Whipple's disease. This condition may be related to an infectious agent similar to *Mycobacterium* organisms, and it responds to antibiotics. The low density is believed to be secondary to deposition of glycogen in the lymph nodes.

Notes

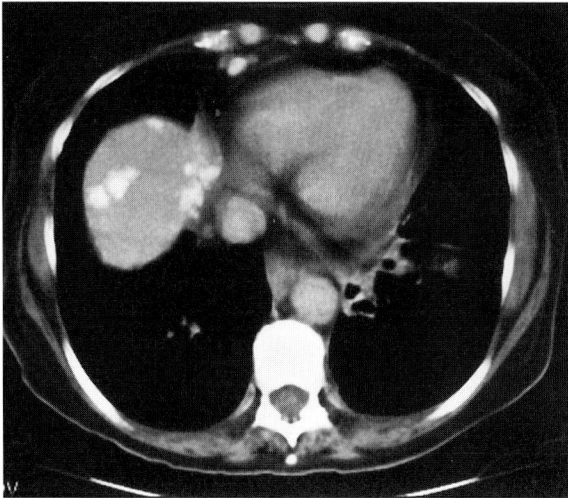

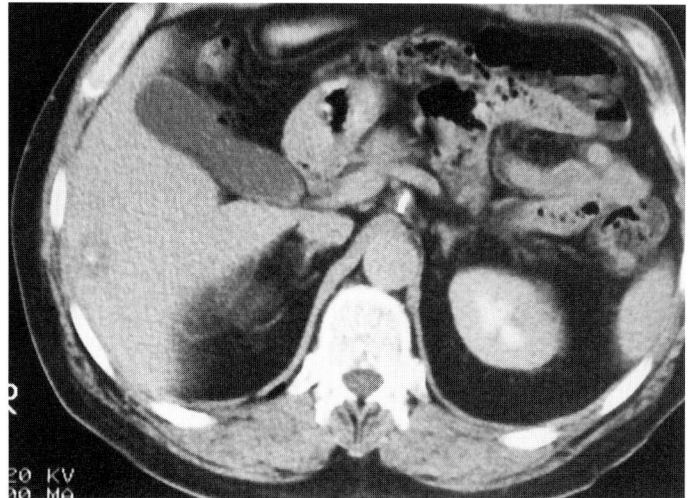

1. What is the most common cause of these liver lesions in adults?
2. What is the most common cause of these liver lesions in children?
3. What extraabdominal tumors may produce these lesions?
4. Do treated metastases ever calcify?

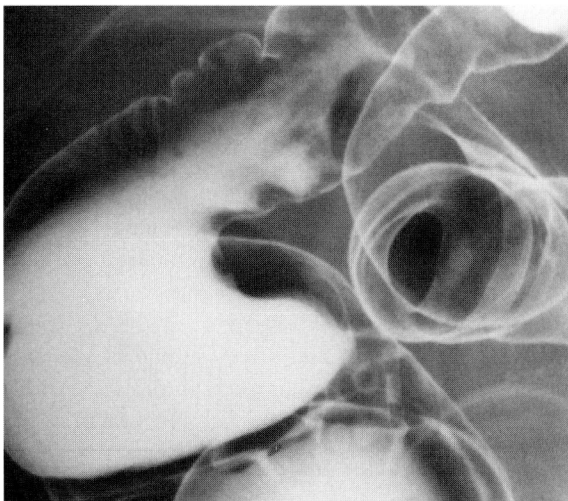

1. In a young woman, what would be the most likely diagnosis?
2. This is a good location for what type of metastases?
3. What type of abnormality is often the sequela of solitary rectal ulcer syndrome?
4. On defecography, what finding may be evident in this patient?

Calcified Liver Metastases

1. Mucinous adenocarcinoma of the colon.

2. Neuroblastoma.

3. Breast or lung carcinoma and melanoma.

4. Only rarely.

Reference

Ros PR: Malignant liver tumors. In Gore R, Levine M, Laufer I, editors: *Textbook of gastrointestinal radiology,* Philadelphia, 1994, Saunders.

Cross-Reference

Gastrointestinal Radiology: THE REQUISITES, ed 2, p 184.

Comment

The CT image demonstrates several calcified liver lesions. Primary liver tumors may calcify but typically are solitary. Infectious processes that have involved the liver, such as granulomatous infections, also may produce multiple liver calcifications. Parasitic diseases, such as echinococcal cysts, can cause calcification. However, the illustrated case shows several small lesions that are either partially or completely calcified, which is strongly suggestive of metastatic disease.

Metastases to the liver rarely calcify. In the adult population, calcification of liver metastases is typically the result of a mucinous adenocarcinoma, which produces a psammomatous type of calcification that is detectable on CT scans. Most often, mucinous adenocarcinoma is found in the colon. Other sites of mucinous carcinomas include the pancreas, stomach, and ovaries. Tumors such as osteogenic sarcoma and chondrosarcoma can produce calcification or ossification, and their metastases could have this appearance as well. In children the most likely cause is neuroblastoma; up to 25% of neuroblastoma metastases calcify. Tumors outside the abdominal cavity rarely produce calcified liver metastases, but lung tumors, breast tumors, melanoma, and testicular tumors produce these lesions on occasion. Tumors that have been treated with chemotherapy or radiation also may calcify, although admittedly this presentation is rare. Calcification has been reported in various treated tumors and in treated lymphoma of the liver.

Notes

Colitis Cystica Profunda

1. Endometriosis.

2. Peritoneal seeding into the cul-de-sac.

3. Colitis cystica profunda.

4. Internal prolapse or intussusception.

Reference

Mezwa DG, Feczko PJ, Bosanko C: Radiologic evaluation of constipation and anorectal disorders, *Radiol Clin North Am* 1375-1393, 1993.

Cross-Reference

Gastrointestinal Radiology: THE REQUISITES, ed 2, p 258.

Comment

The anterior wall of the rectum is a common location for pathologic findings. Probably the most common abnormalities in this area are diseases of the cul-de-sac, including endometriosis and numerous abdominal tumors (ovarian, gastric, pancreatic, and intestinal) that produce peritoneal seeding or drop metastases to this region. All of these processes have a similar appearance on barium enema. Primary tumors of the colon, mainly adenocarcinoma, can develop in this region.

However, the anterior wall of the rectum also is a common location for abnormalities, which occur as the sequela of anorectal defecation disorders. Patients with defecation problems, primarily constipation or chronic straining, often suffer prolapse of the rectal mucosa. The anterior wall of the rectum above the peritoneal reflection is not fixed; it is free to move. This form of prolapse or intussusception happens every time the patient attempts to defecate. This prolapse may be internal or at times even external (beyond the anal sphincter). Either way the anterior wall of the rectum becomes a vulnerable structure prone to injury. Often, ulceration occurs, leading to rectal bleeding. This condition, termed *solitary rectal ulcer syndrome,* affects all age groups but particularly younger patients.

Colitis cystica profunda is a sequela of chronic prolapse and solitary rectal ulcer syndrome. With recurrent prolapse and ulceration, there are stages of ulceration and then healing of the rectal mucosa. Over time, the regenerating mucosa may trap mucus glands underneath the mucosa. These trapped mucus glands continue to secrete mucus but do not drain because of overlying mucosa. Thus the glands become cystic structures filled with mucin, and hence the name. With time, the cysts produce one of several polypoid structures, typically along the anterior surface of the rectum because this segment is most susceptible to this trauma. This entity is difficult to diagnose in the absence of a history of long-standing defecation dysfunction. Biopsy confirms the diagnosis, and often defecography is helpful in identifying the patient's underlying defecation problems.

Notes

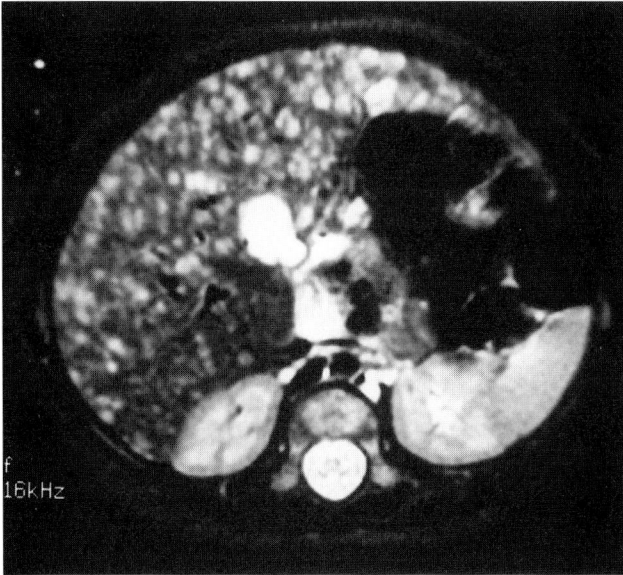

1. This lesion is in a child. What diagnostic possibilities should be considered?
2. If this were a single lesion, what abnormalities should be considered?
3. If these lesions are vascular channels, what is the diagnosis?
4. What is the long-term prognosis for the patient with this disease?

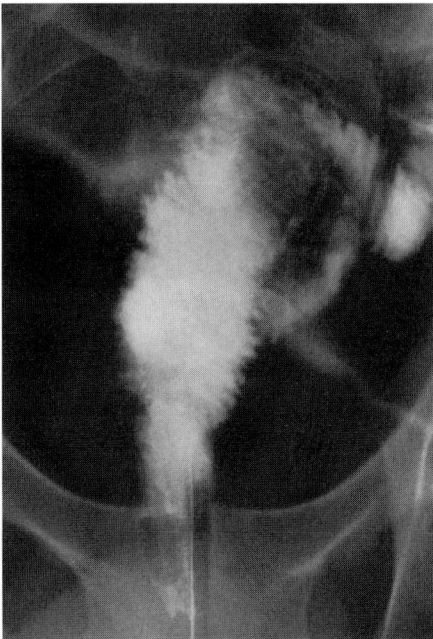

1. What surgical procedure was performed on this patient?
2. What is the most common cause for this surgery?
3. What is the most common complication of this surgery?
4. What inflammatory condition may occur?

Hemangioendothelioma of the Liver

1. Metastases from neuroblastoma, multiple hemangiomas, or cysts.

2. Cyst or hemangioma.

3. Hemangioendothelioma.

4. Tumors usually involute with age.

Reference

Dachman AH, Lichtenstein JE, Friedman AC, et al: Infantile hemangioendothelioma of the liver: a radiologic-pathologic-clinical correlation, *Am J Roentgenol* 140:1092-1096, 1983.

Cross-Reference

Gastrointestinal Radiology: THE REQUISITES, ed 2, p 183.

Comment

The MR scan of the liver demonstrates multiple high intensity lesions of the liver on this T2W image. This patient is quite young. Lesions that may have this appearance include cysts, hemangiomas, and even metastases. In the infant, metastases are the possible result of neuroblastoma. Cysts, such as those seen in infantile polycystic disease, are rare in this age group. Hemangiomas can be multiple and are a consideration. This scan demonstrates multiple hemangiomas of the liver, which in this age group is termed *infantile hemangioendothelioma.*

Infantile hemangioendothelioma is a fairly common tumor of the liver in childhood. It accounts for approximately 12% of children's liver tumors. These lesions represent proliferations of endothelial cells and form vascular channels. The vascular channels may form cavernous areas, and thus look like cavernous hemangiomas on imaging studies. There is often an association with skin angiomas.

Imaging studies demonstrate multiple vascular lesions of the liver. These lesions can be quite vascular on angiography. MRI demonstrates hyperintense lesions, which are similar to hemangiomas seen in adults. The appearance on CT scans is also similar to that of multiple hemangiomas, with the lesions showing variable degrees of enhancement after injection of intravenous contrast and puddling of contrast on delayed images.

Rarely these patients develop high output congestive heart failure because of the vascularity of the lesions. As the child grows older, the tumors tend to involute. Multiple hemangiomas may persist into adulthood, however.

Notes

Ileoanal Pouch with Leakage

1. Ileoanal pouch.

2. Chronic ulcerative colitis.

3. Small bowel obstruction.

4. Pouchitis.

Reference

Alfisher MM, Scholz FJ, Roberts PL: Radiology of ileal pouch-anal anastomosis: normal findings, examination pitfalls, and complications, *Radiographics* 17:81-98, 1997

Cross-Reference

Gastrointestinal Radiology: THE REQUISITES, ed 2, p 283.

Comment

The surgical creation of a new rectum is necessary when the entire colon, including the rectum, must be removed, usually in patients with chronic ulcerative colitis or familial adenomatous polyposis syndrome. The ileoanal pouch, or reservoir, was created so that the patient could avoid a permanent ileostomy and maintain continence with the anal sphincter mechanism. It is a complex surgical procedure that is often performed in several stages to allow the various anastomoses to heal.

The first stage of the surgery consists of the total abdominal colectomy, creation of the ileal reservoir, and the reservoir's anastomosis to the rectum. At a later stage, the small bowel is reanastomosed to the new ileoanal pouch. Sometimes this operation must be performed in three stages. The most common pouch is called a *J pouch,* referring to the folding of the ileum into a J shape with a side anastomosis to the anus. Other less common pouches are called *S* and *W pouches,* referring to how the distal ileum is folded on itself. The radiologist examines the pouch in the postoperative period to ensure the integrity of the suture lines and evaluate possible complications. This examination often is performed before the reanastomosis of the small bowel to the pouch. Barium may be used unless there is a strong suspicion of a leak, although typically leaks are well contained.

A variety of complications can occur as a result of this procedure, and they are quite common given the complexity of the operation. The most common complication is small bowel obstruction, occurring in a substantial portion of patients. This obstruction usually is caused by anastomotic strictures or adhesions in the pelvis. Another common problem is pouchitis, which is an inflammation of the pouch producing diarrhea. This complication is rarely diagnosed on the basis of radiologic studies. The most serious complication is a leak or fistula. Leaks occur at anastomoses, usually the pouch–anal anastomosis. This leak is termed *anastomotic separation.* Leaks also may occur at the staple lines of the reconstructed pouch. Often a pouch appendage, which is a blind remnant of ileum, may mimic a leak.

Notes

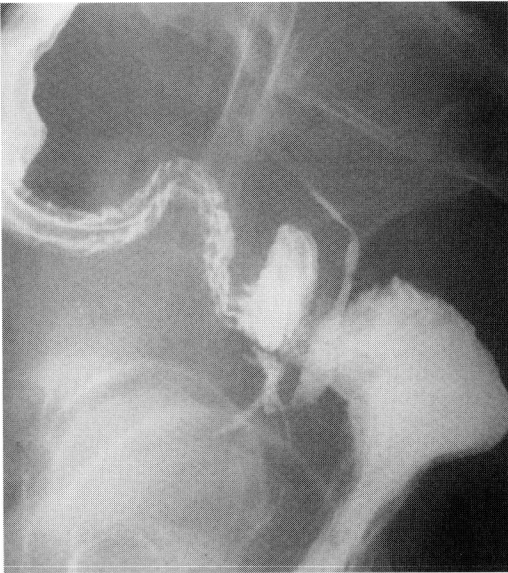

1. What is the most common cause of the abnormality shown?
2. What inflammatory process may cause this presentation?
3. What infection can cause this abnormality?
4. Besides surgery, what iatrogenic process should be considered?

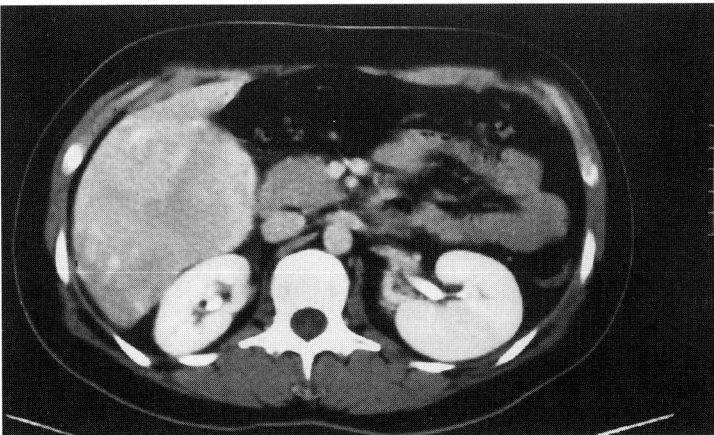

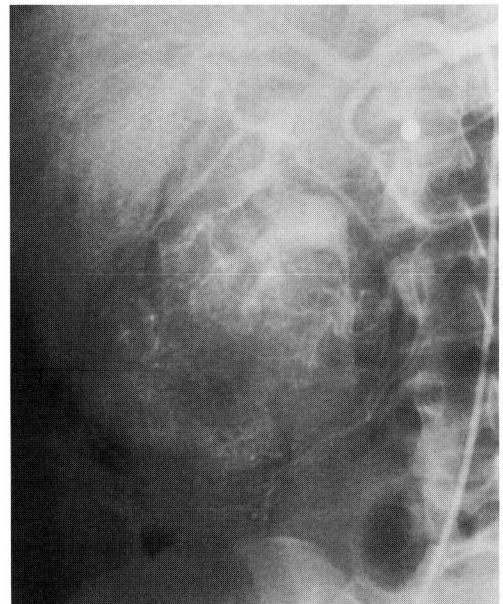

1. In which gender does this lesion predominantly occur?
2. Consumption of what drug predisposes to the development of this abnormality?
3. How does this lesion appear on a sulfur colloid liver scan?
4. Name the most common clinical presentation of this lesion.

CASE 189

Ureteroenteric Fistula

1. Surgical complication.

2. Crohn's disease or diverticulitis.

3. Tuberculosis.

4. Radiation.

Reference
Smith HJ, Berk RN, Janes JO, et al: Unusual fistulae due to colonic diverticulitis, *Gastrointest Radiol* 2:387-392, 1978.

Cross-Reference
Gastrointestinal Radiology: THE REQUISITES, ed 2, p 127.

Comment
A communication between the rectum and distal ureter is demonstrated on this barium enema. Although this type of finding is extremely rare, several disease entities may result in this abnormality. Probably the most likely scenario is that the patient has had recent pelvic surgery with resection of portions of either the rectum or ureter. Postoperative fibrosis, inflammation, or both could cause the two structures to adhere to each other, and the fistula could develop as a result of breakdown of an anastomotic line. If the patient also received radiation to the pelvis for some reason (e.g., cervical carcinoma), fistula formation could result, although there would probably have to be some prior surgery as well.

Historically, tuberculosis was the primary cause of fistula between the bowel and ureters. Inflammation of the bowel with adenopathy resulted in the development of a fistula to the retroperitoneum, producing either psoas abscesses or fistulas to structures in that region. Today, the major culprit is Crohn's disease, which mimics tuberculosis in its behavior. Diverticulitis is another cause of spontaneous fistula between the urinary tract and rectosigmoid region. Carcinoma of the colon is yet another consideration, although this condition usually produces obstruction of the ureter rather than a fistula.

Notes

CASE 190

Hepatic Adenoma

1. Women.

2. Oral contraceptives.

3. Cold defect.

4. Bleeding with right upper quadrant pain.

Reference
Ito K, Honjo K, Fujita T, et al: Liver neoplasms: diagnostic pitfalls in cross-sectional imaging, *Radiographics* 16:273-293, 1996.

Cross-Reference
Gastrointestinal Radiology: THE REQUISITES, ed 2, p 177.

Comment
Hepatic adenomas are composed of hepatocytes that are loosely arranged, have no portal tracts, and have poorly formed hepatic veins. They form bile to a slight extent. These tumors tend to be large and solitary, often exceeding 10 cm in diameter. They are also quite vascular and because of their poorly developed venous system have a propensity for spontaneous hemorrhage, which is their major clinical presentation. Usually the hemorrhage is internal within the adenoma and produces pain, but if the hemorrhage spreads into the peritoneal cavity, it could be fatal. Adenomas occur predominantly in women, usually younger women. It is believed to be an estrogen-associated tumor, and the incidence of the tumor is increased in women taking oral contraceptives. Cessation of oral contraceptive use causes the tumors to shrink. Rarely the tumor occurs spontaneously in men. Men taking anabolic steroids are at increased risk of developing a tumor that is similar to both an adenoma and a hepatocellular carcinoma. Patients with glycogen storage disease also are at greater risk of developing adenomas.

Hepatic adenomas are usually easily identifiable on cross-sectional imaging, but their differentiation from other hepatic tumors is the major concern. Ultrasound typically reveals a large hyperechoic lesion, which may have central areas of low density caused by hemorrhage or necrosis. On CT the lesion may be hypodense because of glycogen, which is often within the tumor. After contrast injection, the tumor enhances and may become isodense. At the periphery of the tumor are large vessels, which are feeding vessels for the tumor. This finding is apparent on angiography; large peripheral arteries can be seen draped around the tumor and feeding into the center of the mass. Adenomas are visible as cold defects on sulfur colloid scans; this point is important in differentiating the tumor from focal nodular hyperplasia, which appears "hot" on sulfur colloid scan. On MRI, adenomas may be hyperintense on T1W images because of the presence of glycogen and fat in the tumors.

Notes

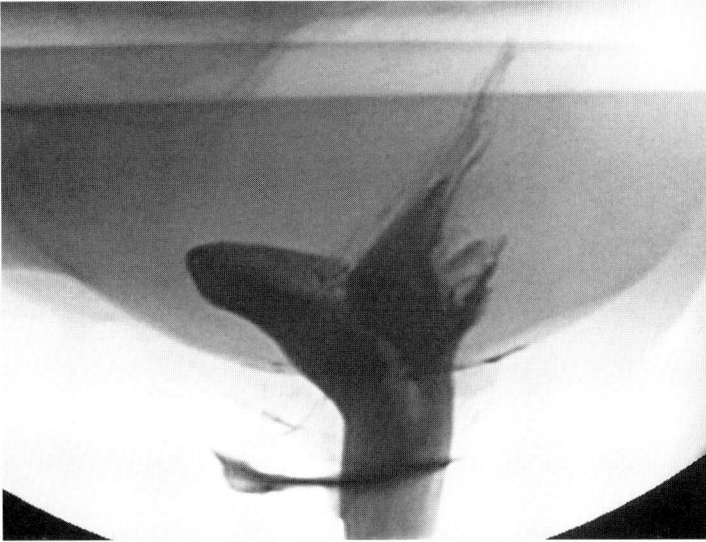

1. What abnormality is most commonly evident on defecography?
2. What must the puborectalis muscle do during defecation?
3. What abnormality visible on defecography results in solitary rectal ulcer syndrome?
4. What is considered abnormal pelvic descent?

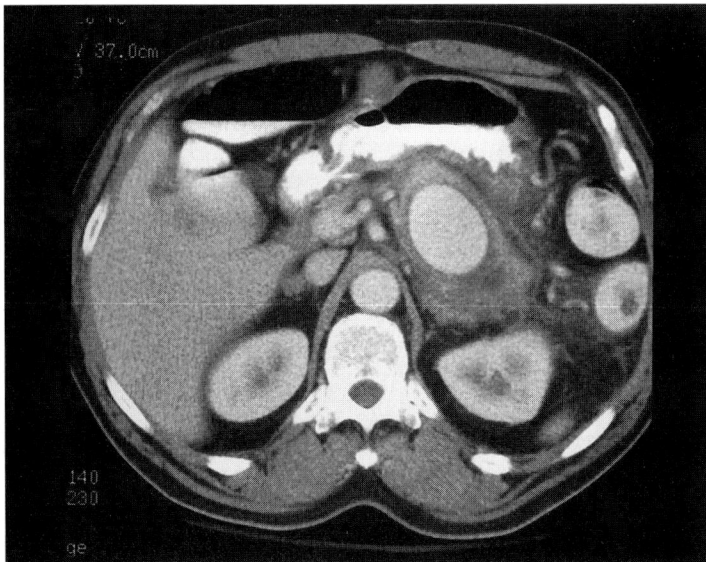

1. What is the significance of a high density pseudocyst?
2. What are vascular sequelae of pancreatitis?
3. What tumors of the pancreas tend to be hypervascular?
4. What finding is expected on Doppler sonography?

Internal Rectal Prolapse

1. Rectocele.

2. Relax.

3. Internal or external rectal prolapse.

4. Movement of the pelvic floor in excess of 3 cm during defecation.

Reference

Karasick S, Karasick D, Karasick SR: Functional disorders of the anus and rectum: findings on defecography, *Am J Roentgenol* 160:777-782, 1993.

Cross-Reference

Gastrointestinal Radiology: THE REQUISITES, ed 2, p 290.

Comment

Defecography is now used relatively often to assess the anatomic and functional changes of the rectum that occur during defecation. Abnormalities of defecation are extremely common in our society, and only recently has this diagnostic test been used to evaluate affected patients.

One of the more common conditions seen during defecation is internal rectal prolapse. During defecation, in some patients the upper portions of the rectum invaginate down the rectal lumen toward the anus. This invagination typically begins in the middle of the rectum because this area is much more mobile than the distal rectum, which is relatively fixed. Slight infolding of the mucosa may be noted in many healthy individuals, particularly during straining. However, if it is large enough, an intraluminal mass of tissue can be identified during defecography. If the intussusceptum remains within the rectum or extends only into the proximal anal canal, it is considered an internal prolapse. This condition is usually accompanied by a rectocele, which is visible anteriorly. In this case the rectal mucosa is prolapsing into the lower rectum, producing a large filling defect superiorly. Some call this presentation a *flower* or *water lily appearance of the rectum.* If the intussusceptum extends through the anal canal, it becomes an external prolapse that may have to be manually reduced by the patient. It is visible as a soft tissue mass beyond the anal canal, often with a ringlike collection of barium around it.

Other common abnormalities noted during defecography include rectoceles, which are anterior bulges of the rectum during defecation. The puborectalis muscle must relax during defecation, creating an obtuse anorectal angle that should approach 180 degrees. This muscle's failure to relax results in severe constipation. The perineum is measured by comparing the anorectal junction with the ischial tuberosities. If the anorectal junction descends 3 to 4 cm below the ischial tuberosities, it is considered a sign of a weak perineum.

Notes

Pseudoaneurysm of the Splenic Artery After Pancreatitis

1. Indicates hemorrhage into the cyst.

2. Thrombosis of vessels or pseudoaneurysms.

3. Islet cell tumors.

4. Evidence of blood flow.

Reference

Vujic I: Vascular complications of pancreatitis, *Radiol Clin North Am* 27:81-91, 1989.

Cross-Reference

Gastrointestinal Radiology: THE REQUISITES, ed 2, p 150.

Comment

The CT scan of the pancreas demonstrates a well-defined lesion of high density. This lesion is much denser than the surrounding pancreatic tissue. Given the fact that this scan was obtained after intravenous injection of contrast, the indication is that the abnormality is highly vascular. Another possibility is that this is an area of relatively severe hemorrhage, which would appear high density. Because the lesion is well defined, a pseudocyst with severe hemorrhage into it is a primary consideration in this instance. Vascular tumors, such as islet cell tumors, may be slightly denser but usually are not this dense or as smoothly defined. The other consideration in this case is a pseudoaneurysm, with the density being attributed to the contrast in the lumen of the pseudoaneurysm.

Several vascular complications are associated with pancreatitis. The most common is thrombosis of venous structures. The splenic vein is prone to thrombosis as it courses along the superior or posterior aspect of the pancreas. Thrombosis of the superior mesenteric vein and other venous structures also has been reported. Sometimes this thrombosis can extend into the portal vein. Collateral channels or varices may be evident.

Pseudoaneurysms after pancreatitis develop as a result of inflammatory weakening of the wall of an artery, which is caused by the pancreatic enzymes. This weakening results in bulging or dilation of the artery. The pseudoaneurysm persists long after the inflammatory changes of pancreatitis have subsided. Typically these pseudoaneurysms develop in the splenic artery (as illustrated in this case) or the gastroduodenal arteries. The major complication associated with pseudoaneurysms is sudden, life-threatening hemorrhage. Identification of this complication is important, and further imaging is necessary to confirm the diagnosis.

Notes

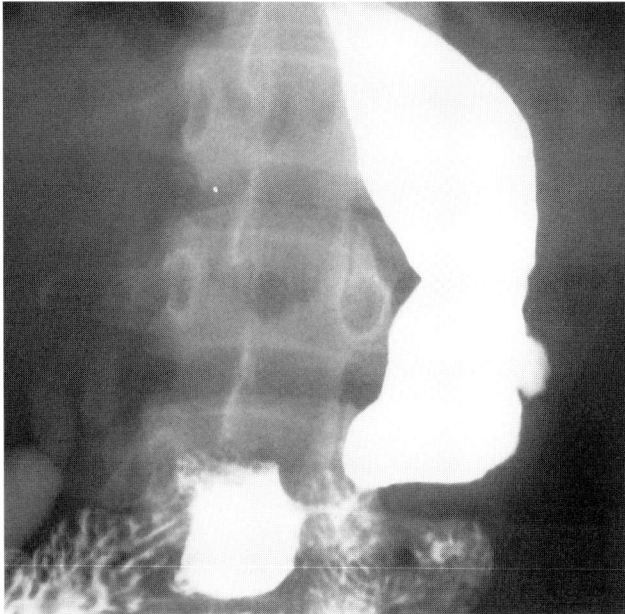

1. What most commonly causes this appearance of the stomach?
2. Metastases from which primary tumor also may cause this appearance?
3. Name some infectious processes that produce narrowing of the stomach.
4. If there is associated small bowel disease, what diagnoses should be considered?

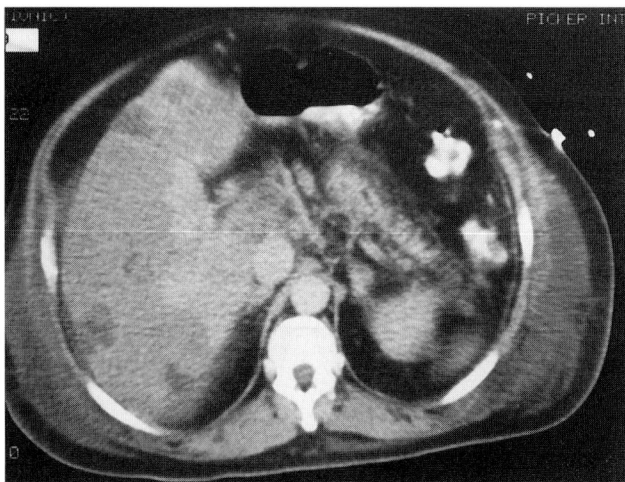

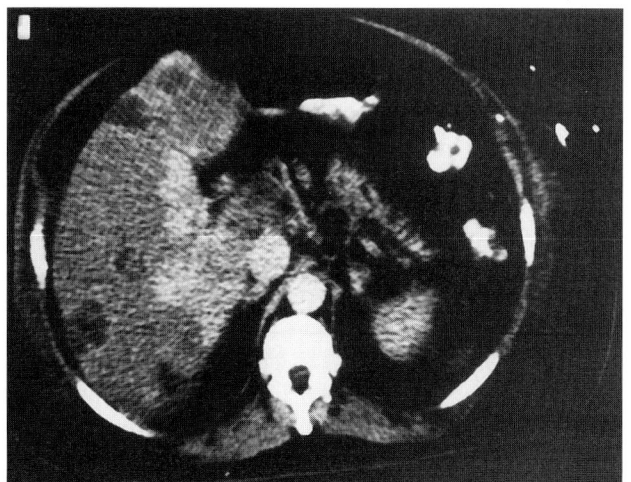

1. Besides the metastatic disease, what other condition is affecting the liver?
2. Why is the caudate lobe spared?
3. What neoplasm most commonly produces this condition?
4. Name some drugs that may cause this condition.

Syphilis of the Stomach Producing a Linitis Plastica Appearance

1. Gastric adenocarcinoma.

2. Breast cancer.

3. Syphilis and tuberculosis.

4. Crohn's disease, eosinophilic gastroenteritis, and lymphoma.

Reference

Feczko PJ, Collins DD, Mezwa DG: Metastatic disease involving the gastrointestinal tract, *Radiol Clin North Am* 31:1359-1374, 1993.

Cross-Reference

Gastrointestinal Radiology: THE REQUISITES, ed 2, p 55.

Comment

Narrowing of the stomach is commonly referred to as a *linitis plastica appearance,* although the term *leather bottle stomach* was used in the past. Numerous entities have been associated with this appearance, and a certain number of them warrant review.

Traditionally the most common cause for this appearance is scirrhous gastric adenocarcinoma. In certain instances the tumor grows by infiltrating along the wall of the stomach, stimulating a desmoplastic response in the tissues. This response produces contraction of the lumen, rigidity, and aperistalsis. The stomach assumes a tubelike appearance. Rarely, lymphoma (typically Hodgkin's disease) may cause this appearance as well. Another common malignancy that produces this change is metastatic breast carcinoma to the stomach. Particularly in poorly differentiated tumors, the hematogenous metastases diffusely infiltrate the wall of the stomach submucosally. Rarely, other tumors, such as pancreatic and other diffuse abdominal metastases (e.g., ovarian), secondarily invade the stomach and produce these changes.

Infectious processes may produce rigidity and narrowing of the stomach. Although rare today, both tertiary syphilis and chronic tuberculous infection may result in narrowing of the gastric lumen. Occasionally, other infections, such as histoplasmosis and actinomycosis, narrow the stomach. Several diseases that also involve the small bowel may produce gastric narrowing. Perhaps the best known of these conditions is Crohn's disease. Crohn's disease has a predilection for the distal stomach, producing ulceration, bowel wall thickening, and rigidity. In severe cases the disease spreads into the proximal duodenum, resulting in a continuous rigid tube, the so-called ram's horn sign. Eosinophilic gastroenteritis may produce rigidity of the gastric wall in patients with severe disease. Other entities that cause gastric narrowing are chronic ulcer disease, corrosive ingestion, radiation therapy, arterial infusion of chemotherapeutic agents, and sarcoidosis.

Notes

Budd-Chiari Syndrome

1. Budd-Chiari syndrome (BCS).

2. The hepatic veins drain differently into the inferior vena cava (IVC).

3. Hepatocellular carcinoma.

4. Oral contraceptives and chemotherapeutic agents.

Reference

Kawamoto S, Soyer PA, Fishman EK, et al: Nonneoplastic liver disease: evaluation with CT and MR imaging, *Radiographics* 18:827-848, 1998.

Cross-Reference

Gastrointestinal Radiology: THE REQUISITES, ed 2, p 165.

Comment

Budd-Chiari syndrome is produced by obstruction of the hepatic venous outflow, either in the hepatic veins or in the IVC above the diaphragm. The onset of the condition may be sudden or slow and progressive. The clinical symptoms often are related to the speed and extent of the blockage. In the severe form there is simultaneous obstruction of all the hepatic veins and often sudden onset of pain, hepatomegaly, ascites, and even hypotension. There may be a marked increase in liver function, with ensuing liver failure. In the long-standing form, pain and hepatomegaly may be minimal. Liver function tests may be only minimally abnormal, and the changes may mimic cirrhosis of the liver.

There are numerous causes of BCS. Primary BCS is believed to be caused by a membrane obstructing portions of the hepatic veins, and this disorder is commonly seen in the Far East. Secondary BCS is more typically seen in North America and Europe and can result from a variety of causes. Hepatocellular carcinoma is the most common cause, although metastatic disease, hypernephroma, and other tumors have been described. Use of numerous drugs has been implicated as well, although the best known are oral contraceptives and chemotherapeutic agents, which are given to patients with carcinoma. Diseases that predispose an individual to venous thrombosis, such as polycythemia vera, often produce BCS. Parasitic diseases of the liver can produce secondary BCS, although this presentation is typically seen in underdeveloped countries.

Diagnosis can be difficult regardless of the imaging modality used. Perhaps the best way to demonstrate BCS is by detecting thrombosis of the hepatic veins or IVC, which can be visible on ultrasound, CT, or MRI. Another feature of the disease is the relative sparing of the caudate lobe and its eventual enlargement. The caudate lobe is spared because it has a different drainage to the IVC than the rest of the liver.

Notes

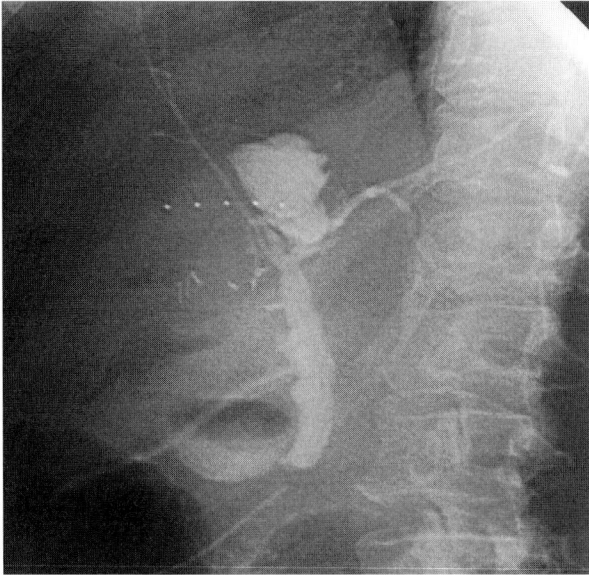

1. How often do simple hepatic cysts communicate with the biliary system?
2. Do echinococcal cysts ever communicate with the biliary tree?
3. If the patient has had recent cholecystectomy, what is the likely diagnosis?
4. What is the major complication associated with this abnormality?

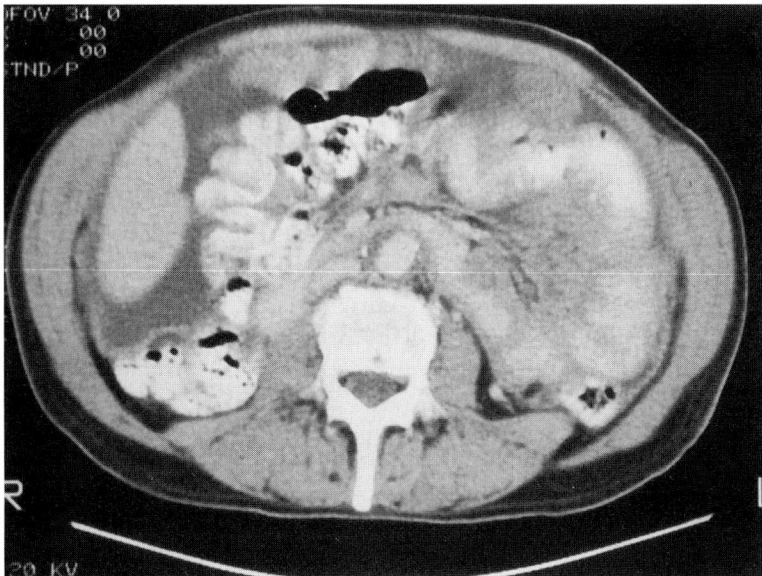

1. What is the most common cause for this appearance?
2. What pleural lesion also may affect the peritoneal cavity?
3. With what material is this lesion associated?
4. Is this condition always associated with the pulmonary disease?

CASE 195

Intrahepatic Bile Duct Perforation

1. Rarely.

2. Yes. They may rupture spontaneously.

3. Intraoperative perforation of the bile duct.

4. Infection or biloma formation.

Reference

Ghahremani GG, Crampton AR, Bernstein JR, et al: Iatrogenic biliary tract complications: radiologic features and clinical significance, *Radiographics* 11:441-456, 1991.

Cross-Reference

Gastrointestinal Radiology: THE REQUISITES, ed 2, p 214.

Comment

The cholangiogram demonstrates a small focus of contrast extending away from one of the small intrahepatic branches in the liver. Major diagnostic considerations include some type of cystic structure communicating with the biliary system. Simple hepatic cysts, although lined by biliary tract epithelium, rarely communicate with the biliary system, despite their common occurrence. Echinococcal cysts communicate with the biliary system, and one of their major complications is spontaneous rupture into the bile ducts. Necrotic tumors or metastases rarely communicate with the biliary tract.

The most likely cause for this intrahepatic leakage of contrast is an iatrogenic injury to the bile ducts. This injury most commonly occurs in the course of cholecystectomy. During cholecystectomy, the surgeon often inserts probes or catheters into the bile ducts to identify possible retained calculi or debris. Sometimes a small endoscope is inserted into the ducts. Because intrahepatic ducts often taper rapidly, some of these small intrahepatic ducts can rupture during passage of some of these instruments. If a cholangiogram is obtained in the immediate postoperative period, a small area of extravasation may be identified.

Usually these small intrahepatic duct perforations close spontaneously after 2 to 3 weeks. Problems arise if pressure in the biliary system is increased because of obstruction. In that case the size of the perforation may increase and form a small biloma. If the biliary tract also is infected, the bile may become infected and form an abscess. The radiologist must recognize this complication and accurately identify its true nature. This study usually can be followed by repeat cholangiogram after a few weeks.

Notes

CASE 196

Malignant Mesothelioma of the Peritoneum

1. Carcinomatosis of the abdomen.

2. Mesothelioma.

3. Asbestos.

4. Only approximately half the time.

Reference

Guest PJ, Reznek RHM, Selleslag D, et al: Peritoneal mesothelioma: the role of computed tomography in diagnosis and follow up, *Clin Radiol* 45:79-84, 1992.

Cross-Reference

Gastrointestinal Radiology: THE REQUISITES, ed 2, p 125.

Comment

The CT images demonstrate soft tissue density involving the mesentery and omentum of the abdomen. What cannot be appreciated is the fixation of the bowel loops, which is also present. The mesentery and omentum are primarily fat-containing structures with vessels and some fibrous tissue. When they become soft tissue density, it is usually a result of tumor infiltration and less commonly a result of edema or hemorrhage. The most common cause for this appearance is peritoneal metastases seeding throughout the mesentery and omentum. Typically these metastases are from abdominal malignancies, such as ovarian carcinoma and gastric, pancreatic and intestinal malignancies.

A rare intraabdominal malignancy that may have this appearance is malignant mesothelioma of the peritoneum. Mesothelioma usually arises from the pleura but can occur in the peritoneum. Like its pulmonary counterpart, mesothelioma is associated with asbestos exposure. Usually there is a long latent period of 30 to 40 years after exposure. This condition most commonly affects men. Peritoneal mesothelioma is much less common than pleural mesothelioma. Also, peritoneal mesothelioma may occur without any pulmonary abnormalities in up to half of the patients, making the diagnosis difficult. The presence of calcified pleural plaques suggests the diagnosis, however. Mesothelioma usually causes little ascites, which is a major differential consideration because ascites is often present in peritoneal metastases. Lymphoma is another differential consideration.

Notes

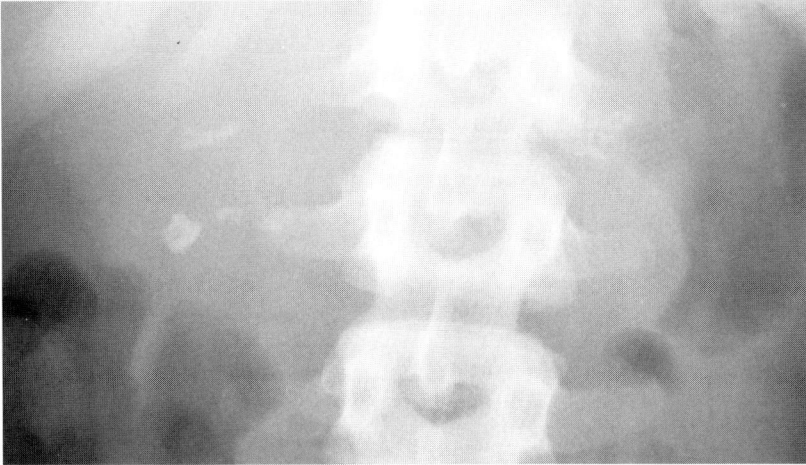

1. In this teenager, where are the calcifications located?
2. Where are the calcifications located in patients with chronic pancreatitis?
3. Name some causes of pancreatitis in children.
4. What is a major complication of hereditary pancreatitis?

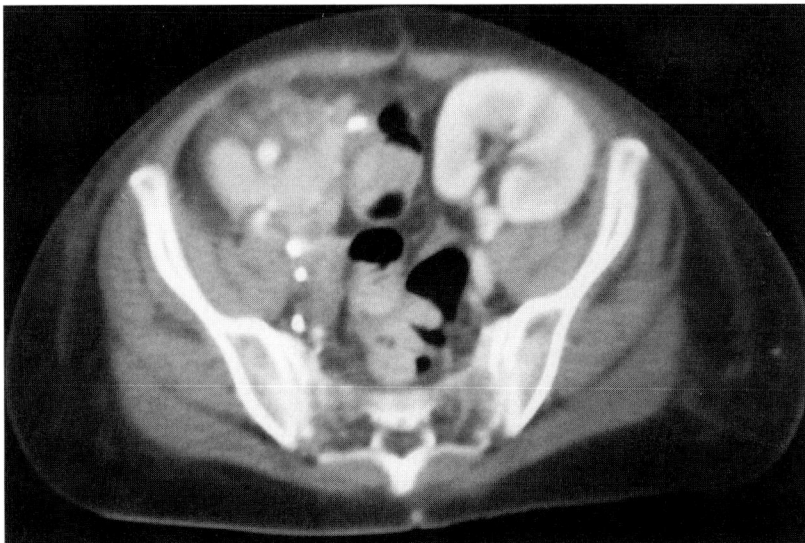

1. In pancreatic transplants, where does the pancreatic duct most commonly drain?
2. What nuclear scan is used to evaluate graft perfusion?
3. Name several causes of peripancreatic fluid collections.
4. What changes indicate graft rejection?

Hereditary Pancreatitis

1. Pancreas.

2. Pancreatic ducts.

3. Trauma, mumps, medications, cystic fibrosis, gallstones, and genetics.

4. Malignancy.

Reference

Spencer JA: Hereditary pancreatitis: early ultrasound appearances, *Pediatr Radiol* 20:293-295, 1990.

Cross-Reference

Gastrointestinal Radiology: THE REQUISITES, ed 2, p 155.

Comment

The appearance of rounded calcifications in the pancreas is usually indicative of chronic pancreatitis. The calcification of chronic pancreatitis occurs within the ducts. However, pancreatitis is an uncommon event in the pediatric age group, and chronic pancreatitis is even less common. Pancreatitis in younger patients is most often the result of trauma. In the past it was caused by viral infections, such as mumps, but this etiology is much less common today. Also, cystic fibrosis is always a consideration. Numerous drugs have been known to cause this condition, as have infections, but these causes are rare. The presence of the ductal stones suggests recurrent bouts of pancreatitis.

Hereditary pancreatitis is a familial condition transmitted by an autosomal dominant gene. It produces recurrent bouts of pancreatitis during early childhood, usually by the age of 10, and affects boys and girls equally. It causes pancreatitis throughout the lifespan of the affected patient. A diagnostic hallmark of this disease is the large ductal calcifications that develop with repeated episodes of pancreatitis. Most ductal calcifications of chronic pancreatitis are small, almost punctate. In hereditary pancreatitis the ductal calcifications are large and distinct and may even be laminated. Whenever large pancreatic ductal calcifications are encountered, hereditary pancreatitis is a consideration.

Patients with this condition have long-term complications of pancreatic insufficiency. These complications include diabetes mellitus and malabsorption resulting from diminished exocrine function. Another complication is adenocarcinoma of the pancreas, which occurs in 5% to 10% of patients and may be a sequela of the recurrent inflammation.

Notes

Pancreas Transplantation

1. Bladder.

2. Tc-DTPA.

3. Urine leak, pancreatic secretions, hemorrhage, and abscess.

4. Increasing size and edema.

Reference

Yuh WTC, Wiese JA, Abu-Yousef MM, et al: Pancreatic transplant imaging, *Radiology* 167:679-683, 1988.

Cross-Reference

Gastrointestinal Radiology: THE REQUISITES, ed 2, p 158.

Comment

The use of pancreatic transplants to minimize the complications of diabetes mellitus or loss of pancreatic function is increasing in popularity. However, the procedure is fraught with serious complications, and there is a high rate of graft failure. The surgical technique is variable but basically consists of transplanting either part or all of the pancreas into the pelvis. The blood supply comes from the iliac vessels. Exocrine pancreatic secretions are managed by diversion into the bladder or the intestines via an anastomosis.

The major immediate complications are thrombosis of the graft vessels, acute pancreatitis, sudden rejection, hemorrhage, or leakage from an anastomosis. Nuclear scintigraphy or sometimes angiography is used to evaluate the perfusion of the graft and patency of the supplying vessels. Ultrasound is of great use in that it allows evaluation of graft vascularity, with the use of Doppler, and identification of perigraft complications and fluid collections.

Later complications of pancreatic transplantation include chronic rejection, pancreatitis, or leakage at an anastomosis. Pancreatitis may be the result of an opportunistic infection, such as cytomegalovirus, in a patient who has had a transplanted pancreas for some time. If there is rejection of the graft, it often swells with edema. This increasing size and edema can be apparent on various imaging studies, including ultrasound, CT, and even MRI. Late peripancreatic fluid collections often are caused by breakdown of an anastomosis and may consist of pancreatic secretions or urine. CT or ultrasound is commonly used to evaluate these late complications, but use of MRI is increasing because it tends to be more specific.

Notes

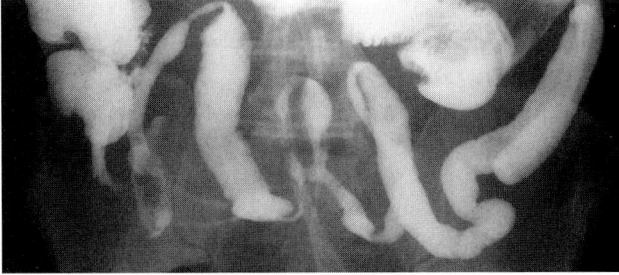

1. What chronic malabsorptive state may produce these changes?
2. What may occur during the acute phase of bone marrow transplantation?
3. When does graft-versus-host disease occur?
4. What organs are involved by graft-versus-host disease?

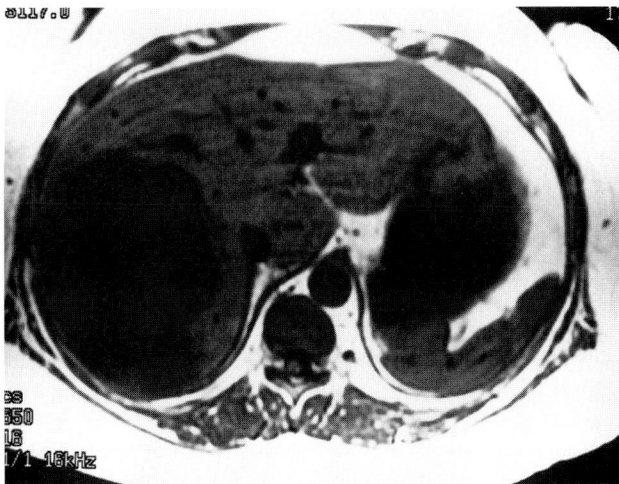

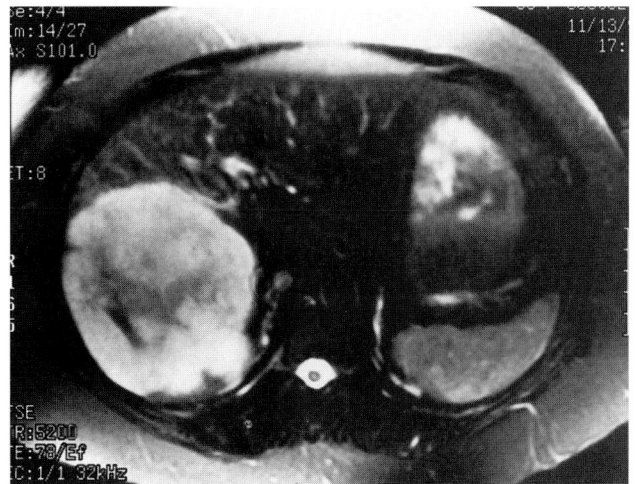

1. Name some diagnostic possibilities.
2. How does a hemangioma appear on a T2W image?
3. How does focal nodular hyperplasia appear on a T1W image?
4. How does the central scar of focal nodular hyperplasia appear on a T2W image?

Graft-Versus-Host Disease in a Bone Marrow Transplant Recipient

1. Sprue (the moulage pattern).

2. Enteritis with diarrhea and pain secondary to radiation or chemotherapy.

3. Typically within 100 days of the bone marrow transplant.

4. Gastrointestinal tract, skin, liver, and lungs.

Reference
Donnelly LF, Morris CL: Acute graft-versus-host disease in children: abdominal CT findings, *Radiology* 199:265-270, 1996.

Cross-Reference
Gastrointestinal Radiology: THE REQUISITES, ed 2, p 114.

Comment
Transplant recipients face a variety of gastrointestinal complications, which are typically related to the immunosuppressive drugs taken to prevent rejection. Peptic ulcer disease, bowel perforation, and opportunistic infections are common. Pancreatitis and hepatitis also occur more frequently in these patients.

In patients who undergo bone marrow transplants for various diseases, another set of complications can occur, in addition to those already mentioned. In the initial induction phase of therapy, during which the native bone marrow is destroyed, the patient receives high-dose radiation or chemotherapy. During this phase, acute enteritis with diarrhea, pain, and bleeding may develop because of the loss of mucosal cells lining the bowel. In the latter stages the transplanted marrow (graft) may mount an immune response against the body (host), producing the so-called graft-versus-host (GVH) disease. This rejection typically occurs within the first few months of bone marrow transplant, although later development is possible.

The major organs involved in GVH disease include the skin, gastrointestinal tract, lungs, and liver. Patients develop a diffuse rash, protein-losing diarrhea, and jaundice. Abnormalities encountered in the small bowel include fold thickening, which may progress to complete effacement of the folds; luminal narrowing; and separation of the bowel loops. Similar changes also may occur in the colon, resembling chronic ulcerative colitis. Pneumatosis of the bowel also has been reported. Gastric abnormalities include dilation and delayed gastric emptying. An unusual radiologic abnormality is prolonged barium coating of the mucosa. CT findings include bowel wall thickening, the "halo" sign caused by bowel wall edema, pericolic inflammation, and mesenteric thickening.

Notes

Giant Cavernous Hemangioma of the Liver

1. Focal nodular hyperplasia (FNH), fibrolamellar hepatoma, and giant cavernous hemangioma.

2. Hyperintense

3. Isointense.

4. Hyperintense.

Reference
Horton KM, Bluemke DA, Hruban RH, et al: CT and MR imaging of benign hepatic and biliary tumors, *Radiographics* 19:431-451, 1999.

Cross-Reference
Gastrointestinal Radiology: THE REQUISITES, ed 2, p 170.

Comment
The differentiation of benign liver tumors can be difficult at times, and this case illustrates the dilemma. There is a large well-defined, encapsulated tumor with a central irregular area or scar. The central scars occur commonly in FNH of the liver but also are present in fibrolamellar hepatoma and giant cavernous hemangioma. Hepatocellular adenomas and even carcinomas may have central irregular areas of hemorrhage or necrosis that could possibly resemble this appearance. Rarely do metastases have this appearance.

Magnetic resonance imaging is commonly used to differentiate the various liver tumors. In this instance the lesion has markedly increased intensity on the T2W image, which is characteristic of a hemangioma. The intensity on the T1W image might be the result of a hemangioma, but adenoma must be considered as well. FNH tends to be isointense with the liver parenchyma on T2W images and certainly is not associated with such a great difference in intensity between the tumor and the normal liver tissue. Also, the central scar of FNH becomes hyperintense on T2W images. The central scar in the other tumors can be of variable intensity, either hypointense or hyperintense. Adenoma of the liver may be difficult to differentiate on MRI because it also can be quite hyperintense on T2W images and of variable intensity on T1W images.

Notes